GASTROESOPHAGEAL REFLUX DISEASE AND AIRWAY DISEASE

LUNG BIOLOGY IN HEALTH AND DISEASE

Executive Editor

Claude Lenfant
Director, National Heart, Lung and Blood Institute
National Institutes of Health
Bethesda, Maryland

1. Immunologic and Infectious Reactions in the Lung, *edited by Charles H. Kirkpatrick and Herbert Y. Reynolds*
2. The Biochemical Basis of Pulmonary Function, *edited by Ronald G. Crystal*
3. Bioengineering Aspects of the Lung, *edited by John B. West*
4. Metabolic Functions of the Lung, *edited by Y. S. Bakhle and John R. Vane*
5. Respiratory Defense Mechanisms (in two parts), *edited by Joseph D. Brain, Donald F. Proctor, and Lynne M. Reid*
6. Development of the Lung, *edited by W. Alan Hodson*
7. Lung Water and Solute Exchange, *edited by Norman C. Staub*
8. Extrapulmonary Manifestations of Respiratory Disease, *edited by Eugene Debs Robin*
9. Chronic Obstructive Pulmonary Disease, *edited by Thomas L. Petty*
10. Pathogenesis and Therapy of Lung Cancer, *edited by Curtis C. Harris*
11. Genetic Determinants of Pulmonary Disease, *edited by Stephen D. Litwin*
12. The Lung in the Transition Between Health and Disease, *edited by Peter T. Macklem and Solbert Permutt*
13. Evolution of Respiratory Processes: A Comparative Approach, *edited by Stephen C. Wood and Claude Lenfant*
14. Pulmonary Vascular Diseases, *edited by Kenneth M. Moser*
15. Physiology and Pharmacology of the Airways, *edited by Jay A. Nadel*
16. Diagnostic Techniques in Pulmonary Disease (in two parts), *edited by Marvin A. Sackner*
17. Regulation of Breathing (in two parts), *edited by Thomas F. Hornbein*
18. Occupational Lung Diseases: Research Approaches and Methods, *edited by Hans Weill and Margaret Turner-Warwick*
19. Immunopharmacology of the Lung, *edited by Harold H. Newball*
20. Sarcoidosis and Other Granulomatous Diseases of the Lung, *edited by Barry L. Fanburg*

21. Sleep and Breathing, *edited by Nicholas A. Saunders and Colin E. Sullivan*
22. *Pneumocystis carinii* Pneumonia: Pathogenesis, Diagnosis, and Treatment, *edited by Lowell S. Young*
23. Pulmonary Nuclear Medicine: Techniques in Diagnosis of Lung Disease, *edited by Harold L. Atkins*
24. Acute Respiratory Failure, *edited by Warren M. Zapol and Konrad J. Falke*
25. Gas Mixing and Distribution in the Lung, *edited by Ludwig A. Engel and Manuel Paiva*
26. High-Frequency Ventilation in Intensive Care and During Surgery, *edited by Graziano Carlon and William S. Howland*
27. Pulmonary Development: Transition from Intrauterine to Extrauterine Life, *edited by George H. Nelson*
28. Chronic Obstructive Pulmonary Disease: Second Edition, Revised and Expanded, *edited by Thomas L. Petty*
29. The Thorax (in two parts), *edited by Charis Roussos and Peter T. Macklem*
30. The Pleura in Health and Disease, *edited by Jacques Chrétien, Jean Bignon, and Albert Hirsch*
31. Drug Therapy for Asthma: Research and Clinical Practice, *edited by John W. Jenne and Shirley Murphy*
32. Pulmonary Endothelium in Health and Disease, *edited by Una S. Ryan*
33. The Airways: Neural Control in Health and Disease, *edited by Michael A. Kaliner and Peter J. Barnes*
34. Pathophysiology and Treatment of Inhalation Injuries, *edited by Jacob Loke*
35. Respiratory Function of the Upper Airway, *edited by Oommen P. Mathew and Giuseppe Sant'Ambrogio*
36. Chronic Obstructive Pulmonary Disease: A Behavioral Perspective, *edited by A. John McSweeny and Igor Grant*
37. Biology of Lung Cancer: Diagnosis and Treatment, *edited by Steven T. Rosen, James L. Mulshine, Frank Cuttitta, and Paul G. Abrams*
38. Pulmonary Vascular Physiology and Pathophysiology, *edited by E. Kenneth Weir and John T. Reeves*
39. Comparative Pulmonary Physiology: Current Concepts, *edited by Stephen C. Wood*
40. Respiratory Physiology: an Analytical Approach, *edited by H. K. Chang and Manuel Paiva*
41. Lung Cell Biology, *edited by Donald Massaro*
42. Heart–Lung Interactions in Health and Disease, *edited by Steven M. Scharf and Sharon S. Cassidy*
43. Clinical Epidemiology of Chronic Obstructive Pulmonary Disease, *edited by Michael J. Hensley and Nicholas A. Saunders*
44. Surgical Pathology of Lung Neoplasms, *edited by Alberto M. Marchevsky*
45. The Lung in Rheumatic Diseases, *edited by Grant W. Cannon and Guy A. Zimmerman*

46. Diagnostic Imaging of the Lung, *edited by Charles E. Putman*
47. Models of Lung Disease: Microscopy and Structural Methods, *edited by Joan Gil*
48. Electron Microscopy of the Lung, *edited by Dean E. Schraufnagel*
49. Asthma: Its Pathology and Treatment, *edited by Michael A. Kaliner, Peter J. Barnes, and Carl G. A. Persson*
50. Acute Respiratory Failure: Second Edition, *edited by Warren M. Zapol and Francois Lemaire*
51. Lung Disease in the Tropics, *edited by Om P. Sharma*
52. Exercise: Pulmonary Physiology and Pathophysiology, *edited by Brian J. Whipp and Karlman Wasserman*
53. Developmental Neurobiology of Breathing, *edited by Gabriel G. Haddad and Jay P. Farber*
54. Mediators of Pulmonary Inflammation, *edited by Michael A. Bray and Wayne H. Anderson*
55. The Airway Epithelium, *edited by Stephen G. Farmer and Douglas Hay*
56. Physiological Adaptations in Vertebrates: Respiration, Circulation, and Metabolism, *edited by Stephen C. Wood, Roy E. Weber, Alan R. Hargens, and Ronald W. Millard*
57. The Bronchial Circulation, *edited by John Butler*
58. Lung Cancer Differentiation: Implications for Diagnosis and Treatment, *edited by Samuel D. Bernal and Paul J. Hesketh*
59. Pulmonary Complications of Systemic Disease, *edited by John F. Murray*
60. Lung Vascular Injury: Molecular and Cellular Response, *edited by Arnold Johnson and Thomas J. Ferro*
61. Cytokines of the Lung, *edited by Jason Kelley*
62. The Mast Cell in Health and Disease, *edited by Michael A. Kaliner and Dean D. Metcalfe*
63. Pulmonary Disease in the Elderly Patient, *edited by Donald A. Mahler*
64. Cystic Fibrosis, *edited by Pamela B. Davis*
65. Signal Transduction in Lung Cells, *edited by Jerome S. Brody, David M. Center, and Vsevolod A. Tkachuk*
66. Tuberculosis: A Comprehensive International Approach, *edited by Lee B. Reichman and Earl S. Hershfield*
67. Pharmacology of the Respiratory Tract: Experimental and Clinical Research, *edited by K. Fan Chung and Peter J. Barnes*
68. Prevention of Respiratory Diseases, *edited by Albert Hirsch, Marcel Goldberg, Jean-Pierre Martin, and Roland Masse*
69. *Pneumocystis carinii* Pneumonia: Second Edition, Revised and Expanded, *edited by Peter D. Walzer*
70. Fluid and Solute Transport in the Airspaces of the Lungs, *edited by Richard M. Effros and H. K. Chang*
71. Sleep and Breathing: Second Edition, Revised and Expanded, *edited by Nicholas A. Saunders and Colin E. Sullivan*
72. Airway Secretion: Physiological Bases for the Control of Mucous Hypersecretion, *edited by Tamotsu Takishima and Sanae Shimura*

73. Sarcoidosis and Other Granulomatous Disorders, *edited by D. Geraint James*
74. Epidemiology of Lung Cancer, *edited by Jonathan M. Samet*
75. Pulmonary Embolism, *edited by Mario Morpurgo*
76. Sports and Exercise Medicine, *edited by Stephen C. Wood and Robert C. Roach*
77. Endotoxin and the Lungs, *edited by Kenneth L. Brigham*
78. The Mesothelial Cell and Mesothelioma, *edited by Marie-Claude Jaurand and Jean Bignon*
79. Regulation of Breathing: Second Edition, Revised and Expanded, *edited by Jerome A. Dempsey and Allan I. Pack*
80. Pulmonary Fibrosis, *edited by Sem Hin Phan and Roger S. Thrall*
81. Long-Term Oxygen Therapy: Scientific Basis and Clinical Application, *edited by Walter J. O'Donohue, Jr.*
82. Ventral Brainstem Mechanisms and Control of Respiration and Blood Pressure, *edited by C. Ovid Trouth, Richard M. Millis, Heidrun F. Kiwull-Schöne, and Marianne E. Schläfke*
83. A History of Breathing Physiology, *edited by Donald F. Proctor*
84. Surfactant Therapy for Lung Disease, *edited by Bengt Robertson and H. William Taeusch*
85. The Thorax: Second Edition, Revised and Expanded (in three parts), *edited by Charis Roussos*
86. Severe Asthma: Pathogenesis and Clinical Management, *edited by Stanley J. Szefler and Donald Y. M. Leung*
87. *Mycobacterium avium*–Complex Infection: Progress in Research and Treatment, *edited by Joyce A. Korvick and Constance A. Benson*
88. Alpha 1–Antitrypsin Deficiency: Biology • Pathogenesis • Clinical Manifestations • Therapy, *edited by Ronald G. Crystal*
89. Adhesion Molecules and the Lung, *edited by Peter A. Ward and Joseph C. Fantone*
90. Respiratory Sensation, *edited by Lewis Adams and Abraham Guz*
91. Pulmonary Rehabilitation, *edited by Alfred P. Fishman*
92. Acute Respiratory Failure in Chronic Obstructive Pulmonary Disease, *edited by Jean-Philippe Derenne, William A. Whitelaw, and Thomas Similowski*
93. Environmental Impact on the Airways: From Injury to Repair, *edited by Jacques Chrétien and Daniel Dusser*
94. Inhalation Aerosols: Physical and Biological Basis for Therapy, *edited by Anthony J. Hickey*
95. Tissue Oxygen Deprivation: From Molecular to Integrated Function, *edited by Gabriel G. Haddad and George Lister*
96. The Genetics of Asthma, *edited by Stephen B. Liggett and Deborah A. Meyers*
97. Inhaled Glucocorticoids in Asthma: Mechanisms and Clinical Actions, *edited by Robert P. Schleimer, William W. Busse, and Paul M. O'Byrne*
98. Nitric Oxide and the Lung, *edited by Warren M. Zapol and Kenneth D. Bloch*

99. Primary Pulmonary Hypertension, *edited by Lewis J. Rubin and Stuart Rich*
100. Lung Growth and Development, *edited by John A. McDonald*
101. Parasitic Lung Diseases, *edited by Adel A. F. Mahmoud*
102. Lung Macrophages and Dendritic Cells in Health and Disease, *edited by Mary F. Lipscomb and Stephen W. Russell*
103. Pulmonary and Cardiac Imaging, *edited by Caroline Chiles and Charles E. Putman*
104. Gene Therapy for Diseases of the Lung, *edited by Kenneth L. Brigham*
105. Oxygen, Gene Expression, and Cellular Function, *edited by Linda Biadasz Clerch and Donald J. Massaro*
106. $Beta_2$-Agonists in Asthma Treatment, *edited by Romain Pauwels and Paul M. O'Byrne*
107. Inhalation Delivery of Therapeutic Peptides and Proteins, *edited by Akwete Lex Adjei and Pramod K. Gupta*
108. Asthma in the Elderly, *edited by Robert A. Barbee and John W. Bloom*
109. Treatment of the Hospitalized Cystic Fibrosis Patient, *edited by David M. Orenstein and Robert C. Stern*
110. Asthma and Immunological Diseases in Pregnancy and Early Infancy, *edited by Michael Schatz, Robert S. Zeiger, and Henry N. Claman*
111. Dyspnea, *edited by Donald A. Mahler*
112. Proinflammatory and Antiinflammatory Peptides, *edited by Sami I. Said*
113. Self-Management of Asthma, *edited by Harry Kotses and Andrew Harver*
114. Eicosanoids, Aspirin, and Asthma, *edited by Andrew Szczeklik, Ryszard J. Gryglewski, and John R. Vane*
115. Fatal Asthma, *edited by Albert L. Sheffer*
116. Pulmonary Edema, *edited by Michael A. Matthay and David H. Ingbar*
117. Inflammatory Mechanisms in Asthma, *edited by Stephen T. Holgate and William W. Busse*
118. Physiological Basis of Ventilatory Support, *edited by John J. Marini and Arthur S. Slutsky*
119. Human Immunodeficiency Virus and the Lung, *edited by Mark J. Rosen and James M. Beck*
120. Five-Lipoxygenase Products in Asthma, *edited by Jeffrey M. Drazen, Sven-Erik Dahlén, and Tak H. Lee*
121. Complexity in Structure and Function of the Lung, *edited by Michael P. Hlastala and H. Thomas Robertson*
122. Biology of Lung Cancer, *edited by Madeleine A. Kane and Paul A. Bunn, Jr.*
123. Rhinitis: Mechanisms and Management, *edited by Robert M. Naclerio, Stephen R. Durham, and Niels Mygind*
124. Lung Tumors: Fundamental Biology and Clinical Management, *edited by Christian Brambilla and Elisabeth Brambilla*
125. Interleukin-5: From Molecule to Drug Target for Asthma, *edited by Colin J. Sanderson*
126. Pediatric Asthma, *edited by Shirley Murphy and H. William Kelly*

127. Viral Infections of the Respiratory Tract, *edited by Raphael Dolin and Peter F. Wright*
128. Air Pollutants and the Respiratory Tract, *edited by David L. Swift and W. Michael Foster*
129. Gastroesophageal Reflux Disease and Airway Disease, *edited by Mark R. Stein*
130. Exercise-Induced Asthma, *edited by E. R. McFadden, Jr.*

ADDITIONAL VOLUMES IN PREPARATION

LAM and Other Diseases Characterized by Smooth Muscle Proliferation, *edited by Joel Moss*

The Lung at Depth, *edited by Claes Lundgren and John N. Miller*

Diagnostic Pulmonary Pathology, *edited by Philip T. Cagle*

Immunotherapy in Asthma, *edited by Jean Bousquet and Hans Yssel*

Neurobiology of Sleep and Circadian Rhythms, *edited by Fred Turek and Phyllis Zee*

Multimodality Treatment of Lung Cancer, *edited by Arthur T. Skarin*

Cytokines in Pulmonary Infectious Disease, *edited by Steven Nelson and Thomas Martin*

Asthma's Impact on Society: the Social and Economic Burden, *edited by Kevin B. Weiss, A. Sonia Buist, and Sean D. Sullivan*

Anticholinergic Agents in the Upper and Lower Airways, *edited by Sheldon L. Spector*

Control of Breathing in Health and Disease, *edited by Murray D. Altose and Yoshikazu Kawakami*

Chronic Lung Disease of Early Infancy, *edited by Richard D. Bland and Jacqueline J. Coalson*

The opinions expressed in these volumes do not necessarily represent the views of the National Institutes of Health.

GASTROESOPHAGEAL REFLUX DISEASE AND AIRWAY DISEASE

Edited by

Mark R. Stein

*University of South Florida College of Medicine,
Tampa, Florida*

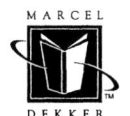

MARCEL DEKKER, INC.   NEW YORK · BASEL

ISBN: 0-8247-0230-1

This book is printed on acid-free paper.

Headquarters
Marcel Dekker, Inc.
270 Madison Avenue, New York, NY 10016
tel: 212-696-9000; fax: 212-685-4540

Eastern Hemisphere Distribution
Marcel Dekker AG
Hutgasse 4, Postfach 812, CH-4001 Basel, Switzerland
tel: 44-61-261-8482; fax: 44-61-261-8896

World Wide Web
http://www.dekker.com

The publisher offers discounts on this book when ordered in bulk quantities. For more information, write to Special Sales/Professional Marketing at the headquarters address above.

Copyright © 1999 by Marcel Dekker, Inc. All Rights Reserved.

Neither this book nor any part may be reproduced or transmitted in any form or by any means, electronic or mechanical, including photocopying, microfilming, and recording, or by any information storage and retrieval system, without permission in writing from the publisher.

Current printing (last digit):
10 9 8 7 6 5 4 3

PRINTED IN THE UNITED STATES OF AMERICA

I could never have completed this volume without the support and sacrifice of my loving wife, Phyllis. The editing assistance of my friend and colleague, Lewis Mark, M.D., and the never-ending attention to details by my office manager, Lynn Towers, were both deeply appreciated.

INTRODUCTION

Often in medicine there is the obvious—and the not-so-obvious. Such is the case with asthma, a complex disease that has many causes: the obvious ones (at least we believe we know some of them!) and the not-so-obvious ones! As pointed out by Dr. Stein in his Preface, the association between gastroesophageal reflux and lung disease has been discussed by many for centuries. Yet, it was not so long ago that a publication entitled, "Silent Gastroesophageal Reflux: An Important but Little Known Cause of Pulmonary Complications," appeared (1). Of course, one could say that this 1962 work is a bit dated. Indeed, since then we have become much more aware of the importance and prevalence of gastroesophageal reflux. This is evidenced by the following statement taken from John Murray and Jay Nadel (2):

> "Over one third of the US population have symptoms of gastroesophageal reflux and it is estimated that 10% of these individuals have respiratory symptoms that may be related to gastroesophageal reflux. This frequency of respiratory symptoms in this group is higher than expected in the general population."

Furthermore, Drs. Katz and Castell, the authors of Chapter 3 of this volume, point out that "GERD is arguably the most common disease seen in clinical practice and may present with a multitude of symptoms."

Why did it take so long to recognize the importance of the association between gastroesophageal reflux and asthma? There is no simple answer to this question but, in actuality, the question is neither important nor relevant. The fact remains that even today there is much confusion about the association between gastroesophageal reflux and asthma (and other respiratory disorders):

> "The relationship between gastroesophageal reflux and asthma is further confused by the hypothesis that respiratory disease causes gastroesophageal reflux" (2).

This volume, edited by Dr. Mark Stein, is a unique contribution to a difficult field and it is a new landmark for the series of monographs, "Lung Biology in Health and Disease." There is no doubt that physicians will find here the answers to their questions about gastroesophageal reflux and that, as a consequence, many patients will be helped.

The contributors are experts in their field, and sharing their extensive experience is a true asset to this volume.

The ultimate goal of this series of monographs is to contribute to improvements in health. The current volume exemplifies how this goal is reached. As Executive Editor, I am grateful to Dr. Stein and his contributors for the opportunity to include it in the series.

Claude Lenfant, M.D.
Bethesda, Maryland

References

1. John Hines Kennedy. Dis Chest 1962; 42:42–45.
2. John Murray and Jay Nadel. Textbook of Respiratory Medicine. Philadelphia: W.B. Saunders, 1994.

PREFACE

Clinical insights often appear to be new but may later be found to have been previously recorded and either ignored or lost. This is certainly true regarding the relationship between gastroesophageal reflux and asthma (and other airway diseases). In the Middle Ages, Maimonides noted that asthma occurred after feasting (1). In the late 1800s, Sir William Osler noted a relationship between large evening meals and worsening nocturnal asthma. He stated that "attacks may be due to direct irritation of the bronchial mucosa or . . . indirectly, too, by reflex influences from the stomach" (2). This wisdom seemed to be lost until 1934, when Bray proposed that late-evening overindulgence caused gastric distention, which led to reflex-mediated bronchoconstriction through the vagus nerve (3). References to gastroesophageal-reflux-induced airway disease began to appear with increasing frequency in the 1960s and 1970s.

Data suggesting a high incidence of hiatal hernia and gastroesophageal reflux in intrinsic asthma and in patients with idiopathic pulmonary fibrosis appeared in the 1970s (4,5). This was a stimulus for further research at several centers. In 1975, studies were initiated in Denver to explain the relationship between these two commonly occurring conditions, gastroesophageal reflux and asthma. Clinical observations that gastroesophageal reflux was worsened by theophylline led to a study demonstrating that therapeutic theophylline levels were associated with a decrease in lower esophageal sphincter pressure (6). Additional studies demonstrated aspiration of gastric contents using an isotope technique (7) and evidence for a vagally mediated reflex that permitted gastroesophageal reflux to trigger bronchospasm in both humans and a dog model (8,9).

These initial studies, together with the subsequent work of numerous investigators, have provided a scientific basis for approaching the evaluation and treatment of gastroesophageal-reflux-associated airway disease. In 1976, when a report by Mays suggested that 50% of intrinsic asthmatics had gastroesophageal reflux, many felt the study was biased and the percentage too high (4). None, at the time, would have expected that future studies could show prevalence rates of as high as 80% (see Chap. 6).

An ever-increasing body of evidence supports the importance of gastroesophageal reflux disease (GERD) as a significant factor in both upper- and lower-airway diseases. Until now, this information had not been presented in a coordinated volume enabling both primary care providers and specialists to grasp these relationships. This book is designed to fill that void, which is also present in most textbooks on asthma and respiratory diseases. It is intended to serve as an extensive review of all aspects of the subjects and to provide the reader with a better understanding of the clinical approaches to diagnosis and treatment in all age groups. It is unfortunate when patients present with severe laryngeal disease or late severe restrictive lung disease, which might have been prevented had these relationships not been missed. Hopefully, this book will provide enough useful clues to help most clinicians identify these patients earlier.

The authors have attempted to weave together broad coverage of these relationships in a format that should permit review of selected clinical topics or the entire subject. Important differences should be noted between the diagnostic approach and treatment recommendations for upper- versus lower-airway diseases.

Mark R. Stein

References

1. Maimonides M. Treatise on asthma. In: Munter S, ed. Medical Writings of Moses Maimonides. Philadelphia: Lippincott, 1963.
2. Osler WB. The Principles and Practice of Medicine, 8th ed. New York: D. Appleton, 1912.
3. Bray GW. Recent advances in the treatment of asthma and hayfever. Practitioner 1934; 34:342–348.
4. Mays EE. Intrinsic asthma in adults: association with gastroesophageal reflux. JAMA 1976; 236:2626–2628.
5. Mays EE, Dubois JJ, Hamilton GB. Pulmonary fibrosis associated with tracheobron-

chial aspiration. A study of the frequency of hiatal hernia and gastroesophageal reflux in interstitial fibrosis of obscure etiology. Chest 1976; 69:512–515.
6. Stein MR, Towner MG, Weber RW, Mansfield LE, Jacobson KW, McDonnell, JT, Nelson HS. The effect of theophylline on the lower esophageal sphincter pressure. Ann Allergy 1980; 45:238–241.
7. Reich SB, Early WC, Ravin TH, Goodman M, Spector S, Stein MR. Evaluation of gastropulmonary aspiration by a radioactive technique: concise communication. J Nucl Med 1977; 18:1079–1081.
8. Mansfield LE, Stein MR. Gastroesophageal reflux and asthma: a possible reflex mechanism. Ann Allergy 1978; 41:222–226.
9. Mansfield LE, Harneister HH, Spalding HS, Smith NJ, Glob N. The role of the vagus nerve in airway narrowing caused by intraesophageal hydrochloric acid provocation and esophageal distention. Ann Allergy 1981; 47:431–434.

CONTRIBUTORS

Brendan J. Canning, Ph.D.   Assistant Professor, Division of Clinical Immunology, Department of Medicine, The Johns Hopkins Medical Institutions, Baltimore, Maryland

Donald O. Castell, M.D.   Kimbel Professor and Chairman, Department of Medicine, Allegheny University Hospitals, Philadelphia, Pennsylvania

Steven R. DeMeester, M.D.   Assistant Professor, Departments of Surgery and Cardiothoracic Surgery, University of Southern California School of Medicine, Los Angeles, California

Tom R. DeMeester, M.D.   Professor and Chairman, Department of Surgery, University of Southern California School of Medicine, Los Angeles, California

Steven J. Filler, M.S., D.D.S.   Professor of Dentistry, Division of Hospital Dentistry, University of Alabama School of Dentistry, Birmingham, Alabama

Susan M. Harding, M.D.   Associate Professor of Medicine, Division of Pulmonary, Allergy, and Critical Care Medicine, Department of Internal Medicine, University of Alabama at Birmingham, Birmingham, Alabama

Philip O. Katz, M.D. Associate Professor and Vice Chairman, Department of Medicine, Allegheny University Hospitals, Philadelphia, Pennsylvania

Mani S. Kavuru, M.D. Director, Pulmonary Function Laboratory, Department of Pulmonary and Critical Care Medicine, The Cleveland Clinic Foundation, Cleveland, Ohio

James A. Koufman, M.D. Professor, Department of Ontolaryngology, Wake Forest University School of Medicine, Winston-Salem, North Carolina

David A. Lazarchik, D.M.D. Associate Professor of Dentistry, Division of Hospital Dentistry, University of Alabama School of Dentistry, Birmingham, Alabama

Lyndon E. Mansfield, M.D. Clinical Professor of Medicine, Texas Tech Medical School; Adjunct Professor of Biology, University of Texas; and Director, El Paso Institute of Medical Research and Development, El Paso, Texas

Stephen J. McGeady, M.D. Associate Professor of Pediatrics and Chief of Allergy and Immunology, Department of Pediatrics, Thomas Jefferson University, Philadelphia, Pennsylvania

Curtis J. Mello, M.D. Clinical Assistant Professor, Department of Medicine, Brown University School of Medicine, Providence, Rhode Island

Susan R. Orenstein, M.D. Professor of Pediatrics, Division of Pediatric Gastroenterology, University of Pittsburgh School of Medicine and Children's Hospital of Pittsburgh, Pittsburgh, Pennsylvania

Joel E. Richter, M.D. Chairman and Professor of Medicine, Department of Gastroenterology, The Cleveland Clinic Foundation, Cleveland, Ohio

Stephen J. Sontag, M.D. Department of Medicine, Veterans Affairs Hospital, Hines, and Associate Professor of Medicine, Loyola University Stritch School of Medicine, Maywood, Illinois

Mark R. Stein, M.D. Clinical Assistant Professor of Medicine, Department of Medicine, Division of Allergy, University of South Florida College of Medicine, Tampa, Florida

CONTENTS

Introduction (**Claude Lenfant**)   *v*
Preface   *vii*
Contributors   *xi*

1. Embryologic Origins of the Relationship of GERD and Airway Disease   1
Lyndon E. Mansfield

    I. Introduction   1
    II. Comparative Embryology   2
    III. Embryology of the Human Lower Respiratory Tract   5
    IV. The Esophagus and Stomach   13
    V. Congenital Abnormalities   15
    VI. Summary   17
    References   17

2. **Inflammation in Asthma: The Role of Nerves and the Potential Influence of Gastroesophageal Reflux Disease** 19
   Brendan J. Canning

I.	Inflammation in Asthma	20
II.	Neurogenic Inflammation	24
III.	Effects of Inflammation on Airway Afferent Nerves	31
IV.	Effect of Inflammation on Airway Autonomic Nerves	34
V.	Conclusion	39
	References	40

3. **Diagnosis of Gastroesophageal Reflux Disease** 55
   Philip O. Katz and Donald O. Castell

I.	Spectrum of Gastroesophageal Reflux Disease	55
II.	Diagnosis	57
III.	Therapeutic Trials	58
IV.	Barium Radiographs	59
V.	Endoscopy	60
VI.	Laryngoscopy	61
VII.	Esophageal Biopsy	61
VIII.	Prolonged Ambulatory pH Monitoring	62
IX.	Esophageal Manometry	65
X.	Hiatal Hernia	65
XI.	Approaching the Patient with GERD-Related Airways Disease	66
	References	67

4. **The Otolaryngologic Manifestations of GERD** 69
   James A. Koufman

I.	Introduction	69
II.	Patterns and Mechanisms of Reflux in Otolaryngology Patients	72
III.	Acid and Pepsin	74
IV.	Clinical Manifestations	75
V.	Diagnosis	80
VI.	Treatment	81
VII.	Reflux, the Internal Environment, and a New Paradigm of Airway Disease	84

	VIII.	Conclusion	85
		References	85

5. GERD: A Major Factor in Chronic Cough 89
Curtis J. Mello

	I.	Introduction	89
	II.	Pathophysiology	92
	III.	Clinical Presentation	97
	IV.	Diagnosis	98
	V.	Treatment	103
	VI.	Conclusion	106
		References	106

6. The Prevalence of GERD in Asthma 115
Stephen J. Sontag

	I.	Introduction	115
	II.	Coexistence	119
	III.	Definitions	120
	IV.	Study Design and Sampling Procedures	122
	V.	Prevalence of GERD in Adults with Asthma	123
	VI.	Prevalence of GERD in Children with Asthma	129
	VII.	Bronchodilators and GER in Asthmatics	131
	VIII.	Incidence	134
	IX.	The High Prevalence of GER and the GER/Asthma Theory	134
	X.	Summary	135
	XI.	Conclusion	135
		References	136

7. GERD, Airway Disease, and the Mechanisms of Interaction 139
Susan M. Harding

	I.	Pathophysiology of Esophageal Acid–Induced Bronchoconstriction	140
	II.	Factors That Could Promote GERD in Asthmatics	160
	III.	Lessons from Clinical Experience with Acid Suppression	170
		References	173

8. **Medical Treatment of Gastroesophageal Reflux Disease
   and Airway Disease**   179
   Mani S. Kavuru and Joel E. Richter

I.	Introduction	179
II.	Methodology Issues	180
III.	Medical Treatment	182
IV.	Surgical Therapy	196
V.	Proposed Approach to GERD-Associated Asthma	200
VI.	Future Directions	202
	References	203

9. **Surgical Treatment of Gastroesophageal Reflux Disease
   with Emphasis on Respiratory Symptoms**   209
   Steven R. DeMeester and Tom R. DeMeester

I.	Introduction	209
II.	Considerations for Surgical Therapy	210
III.	Factors to Consider When Choosing the Proper Antireflux Procedure	219
IV.	Types of Antireflux Operations	223
V.	Surgical Complications	226
VI.	Results of Surgery	229
VII.	Summary	233
	References	234

10. **GERD and Airways Disease in Children and Adolescents**   237
    Stephen J. McGeady

I.	Introduction	237
II.	Upper Airway Manifestation of GERD	238
III.	GERD and Lower Respiratory Tract	244
IV.	Diagnosis of GERD	250
V.	Treatment of GERD	254
	References	260

11. **Respiratory Complications of Reflux Disease in Infants**   269
    Susan R. Orenstein

I.	Physiology: Infants Versus Older Children and Adults	269
II.	Gastroesophageal Reflux Disease in Infants	272

III.	Vicious Cycles Between Reflux and Respiratory Disease	273
IV.	Respiratory Diseases in Infants	274
V.	Diagnosis of Reflux in Infantile Respiratory Disease	276
VI.	Therapy of Reflux in Infantile Respiratory Disease	277
VII.	Conclusion	279
	References	279

12. Oral Manifestations of GERD — 285
David A. Lazarchik and Steven J. Filler

I.	Introduction	285
II.	Oral Soft Tissue Manifestations	286
III.	Hard Tissue Manifestations	287
IV.	Relationship of Dental Erosion to Salivary Parameters	291
V.	Differential Diagnosis of Dental Erosion	292
VI.	Prevention of Oral Manifestations	297
VII.	Treatment of Oral Manifestations	298
VIII.	Conclusion	299
	References	300

13. Odds and Ends and the State of the Art — 303
Mark R. Stein

I.	GERD in the Geriatric Patient	304
II.	GERD and Airway Disease During Pregnancy	314
III.	State of the Art	314
IV.	Conclusions	318
	References	318

Author Index	*323*
Subject Index	*353*

1

Embryologic Origins of the Relationship of GERD and Airway Disease

LYNDON E. MANSFIELD

Texas Tech Medical School
University of Texas
El Paso Institute of Medical Research and Development
El Paso, Texas

I. Introduction

There are important interactions between the esophagus, stomach, and respiratory system that are a part of normal day-to-day living. These are physiologic events that involve coordination of the breathing and swallowing functions through a rich array of neural reflexes. Derangement in any of these three organs can have deleterious effects on one or the other neighboring organ's functions. The purpose of this chapter on embryology is to remind the reader that these important interactions begin early in human embryogenesis.

This review is not an extremely detailed embryologic recounting. The references offered at the chapter's end are provided for the reader who desires more in-depth information. I have tried to minimize the introduction of special argot, whenever possible.

Embryology can become very confusing, especially human embryology, as the organs move and change orientation, which then distorts the segmental arrangement and relationship of the early embryo.

Most health care providers understand the anatomic relationship of postembryonic life. Therefore, the text is arranged to focus on individual organ development, as they are in the postuterine pattern, rather than using a time-line approach

Table 1 Time Line

Gestation	Respiratory tract	Stomach/Esophagus
Week 2		Gut partially separated from yolk sac
Week 3	Laryngotracheal groove	Esophagus
Week 4	Primary laryngeal bud	Stomach dilation appears
Week 5	Division into R + L mainstem bronchi and upper lower middle divisions	
Week 6	Larynx—dilation appears in primary laryngotracheal bud	
Week 7	Larynx begins chondrification lung growth	Esophagus elongates
Month 3	Epiglottis present	Stomach rotates
Months 4–5	Ciliated cells in trachea, bronchi	Acid glands in stomach
Months 6–7	Terminal sacs appear Surfactant, alveolus monolayers	
Months 8–9	Surfactant sufficient for ex utero	

(Table 1). The reader must keep in mind that while the described organ is developing, other processes are occurring which may influence its ultimate maturation.

The most important messages derived from the embryology of the respiratory tract, esophagus, and stomach are:

1. They all have a common origin from the embryonic foregut, as shown in Figure 1.
2. They have the same pattern of innervation, predominantly through the vagus nerve.

II. Comparative Embryology

The lower respiratory tract, the stomach, and the esophagus alter during the evolutionary process in a complex process.

A. Fish

Of all the vertebrates, fish have the most unique respiratory apparatus, as respiratory gas exchange occurs in a liquid media. In fish, a series of branchial (*branchia*

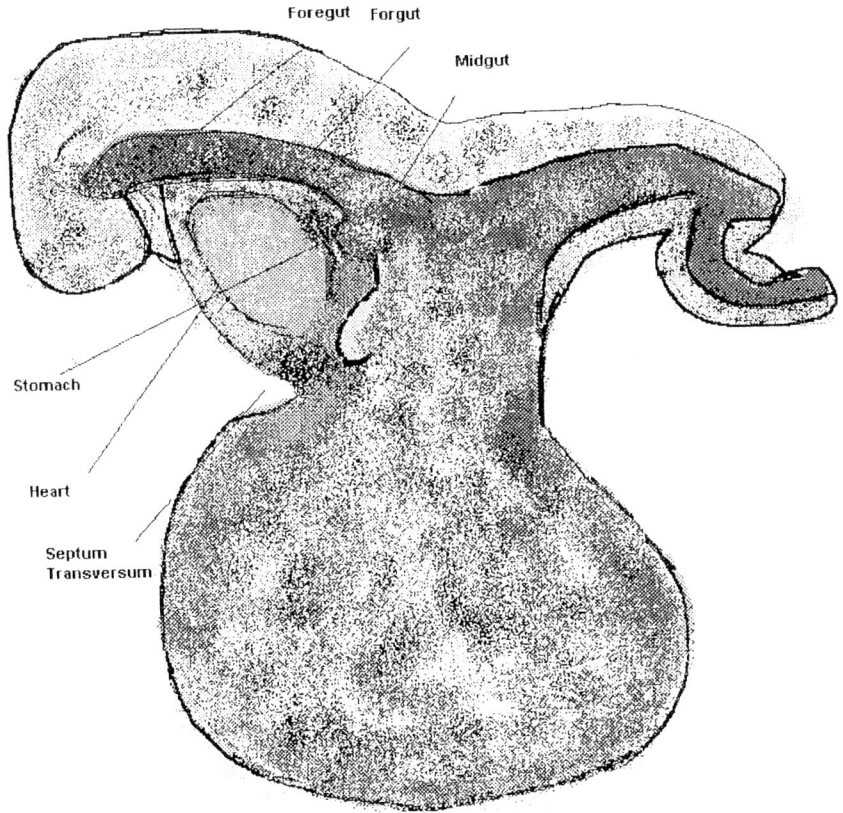

Figure 1 The human embryo at 4 weeks. The laryngotracheal groove has not yet formed a laryngotracheal bud. The future stomach is present as a small dilation at the caudal end of the foregut.

= Gr., gill) arches and clefts appear just caudal to the future head. Water is pumped over the highly vascular tissue of the branchia by specialized branchial muscles. Gas exchange occurs as water enters through the mouth is pumped over the gills, and exhausted through the gill slits.

It is clear the branchia are not the forerunner of lungs in air-breathing animals. This role belongs to an organ called the swim bladder, in which the fish store gas, usually oxygen. The swim bladder controls the buoyancy of the fish. The swim bladder is a simple highly vascularized sac, with an opening into the ventral foregut just cephalad to the esophagus. There are two tissue folds surrounded by muscle similar to that of the esophagus, which open and close the entrance to the swim bladder. These folds are analogous to the true vocal cords. The swim bladder is modified in the air-breathing lung fish.

The esophagus of the fish is a short muscular tube. Both the glottis and the esophagus are enervated by branches of the vagus nerve, which contain both the afferent and visceral motor efferent fibers. The nerve fibers converge in areas of the fish hindbrain. This basic neurologic relationship is retained throughout the evolutionary changes.

B. Amphibians

Amphibians have structures that can really be called a lung. It is a bifid organ and extends from the thoracic cavity into the abdomen. There is a distinct identifiable respiratory passageway. The gill muscles are now pharyngeal muscles, which pump air instead of water into the lungs. Body wall muscles become modified to pump the air out of the lungs. The lung is more highly vascularized and has more septation than the swim bladder. However, it is still simple compared to the lungs of the higher organisms.

C. Reptiles

Reptilian lungs show increasing septation and vascularization. The respiratory passage now consists of clearly demarcated areas of the larynx, trachea, and bronchi. The caudal lung segments still extend into the abdominal cavity. The presence of ribs and sternum allow the body wall muscles to provide a more powerful assist for inhalation and exhalation.

The pulmonary parenchyma is denser. It is more vascularized in the thoracic cavity, while the ventral and intra-abdominal lung is more sacular and markedly less vascularized. This thin-walled segment acts as a bellows or like an aspiration bulb. It collapses during exhalation and refills during inhalation.

D. Birds

Birds have a complete separation of the respiratory and bellows function of the lung. The avian lung extends into the abdomen. However, all respiratory gas exchange in birds occurs only in the chest cavity. The abdominal or caudal lung now functions solely as a sacular bellows. As the avian lungs enlarge; the length of the esophagus increases proportionately.

E. Mammals

Mammals achieve their own unique respiratory niche by completing the formation of the diaphragm. Now all of the pulmonary functions, that is, bellows and gas exchange, occur in the pleural cavity. The respiratory passage in mammals has more differentiation, with a distinctive epiglottis and second protective tissue fold, the false vocal cords.

F. Anthropoids and Humans

The bipedal upright mammals, humans and their anthropoid relatives, introduce an entirely new lung schema. In quadrupedal mammals, there are four dorsal and four ventral branches from the mainstem bronchus. In humans there are initially six divisions from the bilateral mainstem bronchi leading to the upper, middle, and lower lobes. On the left side, the heart occupies the space of the middle lobe. The left upper and middle mainstem bronchi fuse so that the bipeds have only five lobes versus the eight lobes of the other mammals.

Because of the upright stature and the change in heart position, the bipedal chest cavity is wider in the sagittal plane and narrower ventrodorsally than the chest cavity of the quadrupeds. This form is already present in the newborn, showing that this development is not based on later environmental effects.

The azygos lobe, which is large and functional in quadrupeds, disappears in the bipeds or appears as an unconnected vestigial nonfunctioning organ with its own blood supply in up to 1% of humans.

The esophageal length of humans has the greatest relative proportion compared to the size of lungs among all the animals.

The significant differences in the human relate to the adaptation of a full upright position and bipedal locomotion. Significant organ position shifts occur to accommodate the changes required by gravitational effects in the upright bipedal human. The human situation is further complicated by the fact that almost a third of the human life span is spent in a horizontal position with its own shifting effects on organs. There are effects on organ function with this daily 90 degree change in orientation. Some mechanisms may fail to operate as well in the horizontal plane.

III. Embryology of the Human Lower Respiratory Tract

A. The Epiglottis and Glottis

The epiglottis and glottis are at their most complex in humans and anthropoids. There are large sequential changes from the simple glottis of the fish, which is a simple short muscular ring around the opening into the swim bladder. The glottal muscle of the fish is similar to that found in the short piscine esophagus.

The epiglottis begins as a small prominence, the hypobranchial eminence, just behind the future tongue. By the seventh week the epiglottis is clearly separated from the tongue, which moves forward as the epiglottis moves slightly backward (Fig. 2).

During this same period, the two lateral folds appear, which connect to

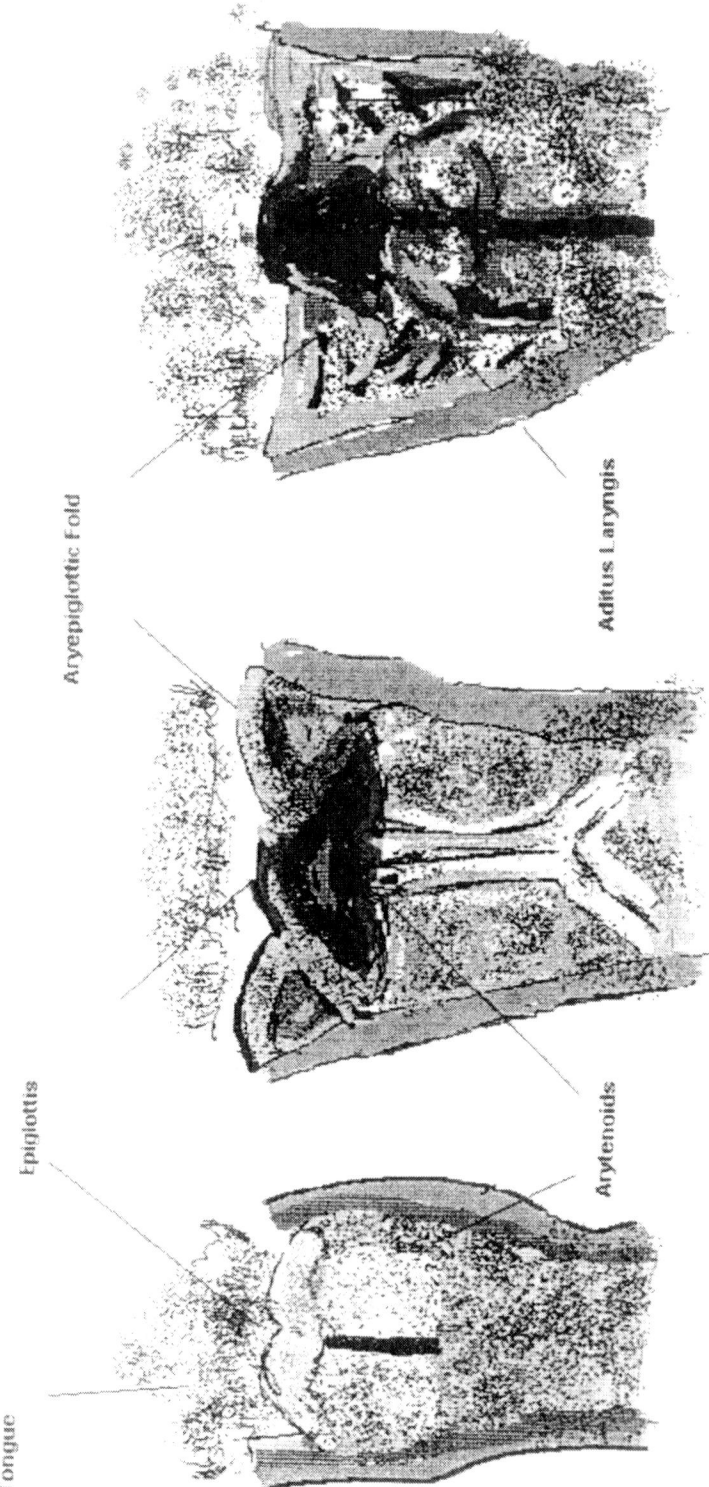

Figure 2 The complex human epiglottis and glottis develop from a simple entrance into the lower respiratory tract, with the addition of the epiglottis, the arytenoids, and the laryngeal ventricles.

base of the epiglottis. At the distant end, the arytenoid cartilages will develop after the folds are connected. The connecting folds are bent so that laryngeal closure has the characteristic "T" shape. Opening of the larynx and vocal cords occurs when the arytenoids draw backward from the epiglottis.

B. The Larynx

The anlage of the human laryngeal apparatus are the two simple movable folds that guard the orifice of the lung in the lungfish. These folds are located in the floor of the pharynx and by opening and closing regulate flow into the piscine lung.

In humans, at the fourth week of gestation, the laryngotracheal groove appears in foregut, immediately cephalad of the future esophagus. The laryngotracheal groove folds in on itself to form a bud at the ventral part of the rostral foregut. This first budding will develop into the larynx and trachea with subsequent divisions forming the bronchi and bronchioles. The primary bud elongates to become both the larynx and the trachea (Fig. 3).

The true vocal cords initially resemble the glottal folds of the fish but subsequently assume their human form and location. By the sixth or seventh week, the characteristic human superstructure to protect the vocal cords and the opening into the lower respiratory passage is present. Its components are the epiglottis, aryepiglotic folds, false vocal cords, and laryngeal ventricles.

This complex supraglottal structure is only found in mammals and not in lower animals. The false vocal cords and the laryngeal ventricles are special

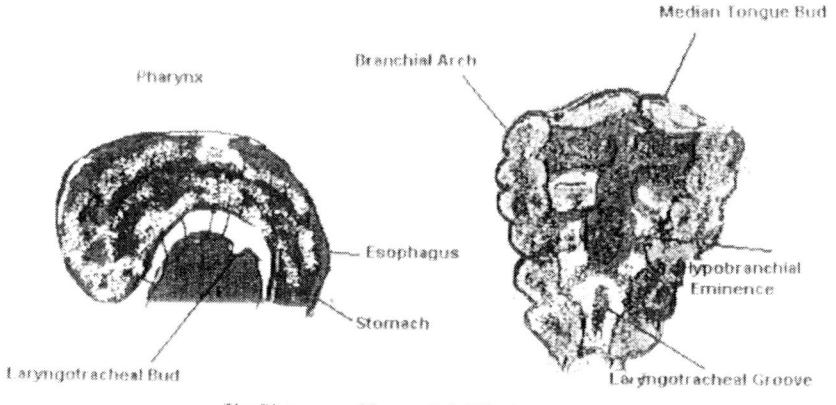

Figure 3 The epiglottis originally develops in the pharynx, and then moves back to join the laryngeal apparatus.

features of humans and anthropoids. In anthropoid apes, the ventricle may also serve a vocal function.

The thyroid cartilage is formed by the skeletal base of the fourth visceral arch. The thyroid cartilage occurs only in the mammals. The sixth visceral arch's skeletal base divides into a central portion, from which the cricoid cartilage arises, and a dorsal portion, which forms the arytenoids (Fig. 4). The muscles that support the laryngeal apparatus are from the sixth visceral segment. The nerve supply to the larynx is the inferior laryngeal nerve, a branch of the vagus.

The cricothyroid membrane and musculature is from the fourth visceral segment.

As embryogenesis proceeds, the laryngeal epithelium changes to a stratified form. Stratified epithelium in the larynx is found only in humans and anthropoids.

The laryngeal ventricles are formed in the supraglottal cavity, by an invagination above each vocal cord. The ventricular cavities are lined with a mucous membrane, in contrast to the stratified epithelium covering much of the larynx.

C. Development of the Trachea, Bronchi, and Lungs

The trachea is formed from the primary laryngotracheal bud, which elongates and also provides the laryngeal structures. The budding divisions continue into the pleuroperitoneal cavities. The endodermal buds, growing laterally, merge with the surrounding mesenchyme and become the lung with its associated bronchi and bronchioles.

From the fifth week, when the second buds enlarge to form the primary or

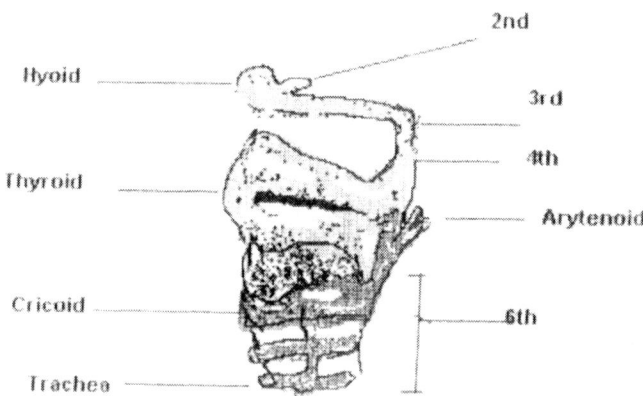

Figure 4 The cartilages forming the larynx and trachea derive from the second, third, fourth, and sixth visceral arches. In humans, the fifth arch involutes.

main stem bronchi, the budding continues until there are 16 or 17 branchings by the twenty-fourth week of gestation (Fig. 5).

The splanchnic mesenchyme provides the cartilage for the bronchi and bronchioles. This mesenchyme is also the source of pulmonary smooth muscle, connective tissue, and capillaries. A layer of visceral pleura covering the lungs is derived from the same mesenchyme. The parietal pleura is formed by the somatic mesoderm of the thoracic cavity body wall.

During these changes, lung development can be divided into four stages. The first stage is the pseudoglandular period, the second is the canalicular period, the third is the terminal sac period, and the fourth is the alveolar period.

The pseudoglandular period lasts from weeks 5 to 17. During this period the lung histology resembles an exocrine gland. By the seventeenth week, all of the major elements of the adult lung are present, except those involved with respiratory gas exchange. Successful ex utero respiration is not possible.

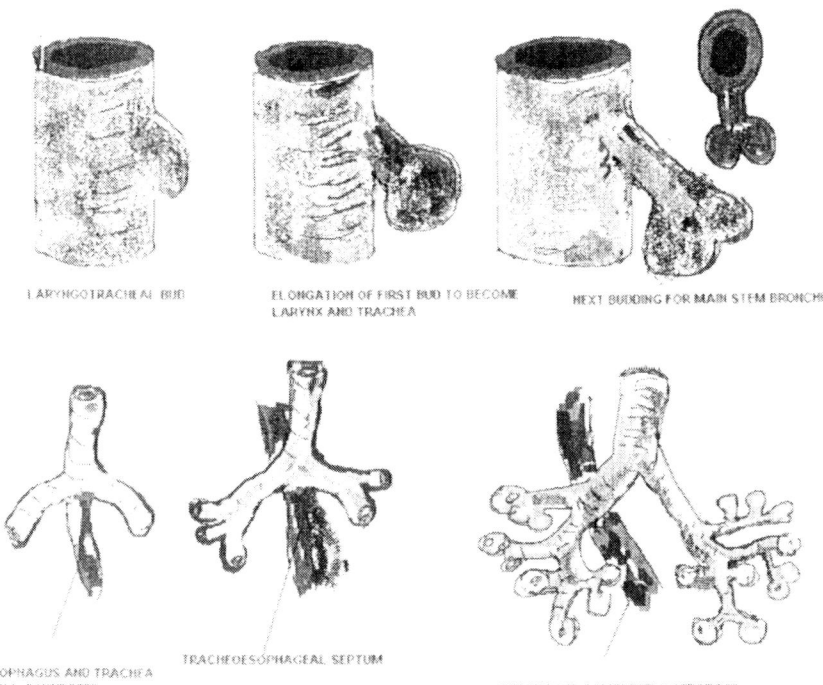

Figure 5 While the lung buds continue to subdivide, the physical separation of the esophagus is completed. The local mesenchyme provides the tissue and capillary bed of the lung.

During the canalicular period, which begins between 16 and 17 weeks and continues to week 25, there is a period of increased maturation of the lung. The lumen of the bronchi and bronchioles become larger. There is an inward migration of blood vessels. By 24 weeks each terminal bronchiole divides to form two or more respiratory bronchioles. These are thin-layered sacs in direct apposition to capillaries. At this developmental stage respiration is possible, but the fetal lung is too immature to be viable without medical intervention. There is the beginning of surfactant production by specialized alveolar pneumocytes.

During the terminal sac period, from week 24 to birth, more terminal sacs develop. The epithelium of these sacs becomes thinner until they are a simple monolayer. Increased surfactant is released from specialized endodermal epithelial known as type I alveolar pneumocytes. The capillary network continues to grow into the lung from the surrounding mesenchyme. Maturation of type II alveolar cells is critical for successful lung function in postdelivery life. Surfactant is required to facilitate the expansion of the thin terminal sacs. By the time the fetus weighs 1 kg (26–28 weeks of gestation) there are sufficient terminal sacs and alveolar surfactant to permit survival of a prematurely born infant.

The alveolar period begins during the last part of fetal development and continues to the age of 7 or 8 years. The number of alveoli increase from about 50 million at birth to 300 million with corresponding increased numbers in the tracheobronchial tree.

Respiratory reflexes exist in utero. The fetus makes tidal breathing movements before birth. During the initial breathing efforts after delivery, fluid in the lungs is cleared through three routes; through the nose and mouth from pressure on the thorax during delivery, into the lymphatics, and into pulmonary arteries, veins, and capillaries.

D. The Diaphragm

Mammals are the only animal species in which the entire lung is contained in the chest cavity completely separated from the abdominal organs. The entire lung can participate in respiratory gas exchange. No part of the lung is used for a bellows. Instead the bellows function is extrapulmonary, utilizing changes in the pleural space with the power supplied by chest wall muscles and the diaphragm.

The primary origin of the diaphragmatic muscle tissue is the cervical region near the fourth and fifth spinal segments. This is the region served by the phrenic nerve, which innervates the musculature of the diaphragm. The phrenic nerve lengthens and descends with the diaphragm as the lung continues to develop to fill the pleural cavity. The diaphragm becomes the caudad limiting factor of the thoracic cavity.

The diaphragm is formed from multiple sources (Fig. 6). The lateral parts of the diaphragm develop from the intrachondral muscles. The sternum contrib-

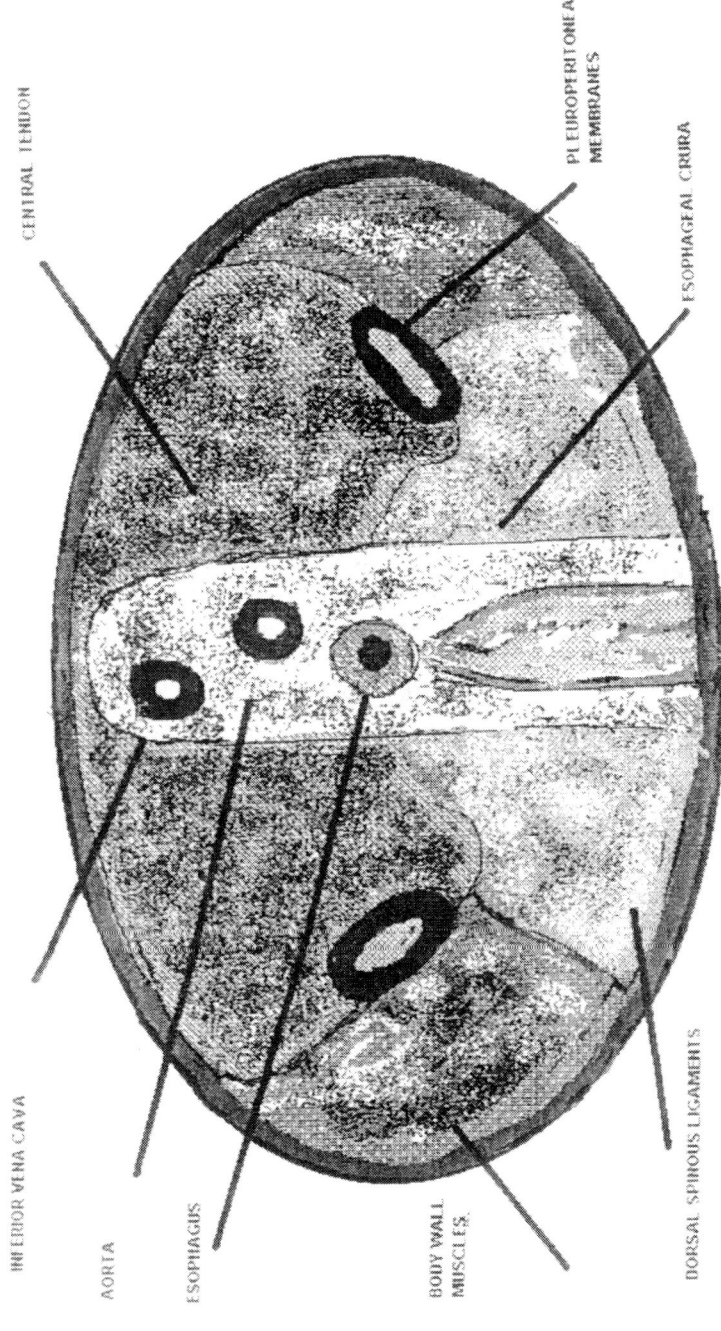

Figure 6 The diaphragm is a complex organ derived from different sources. Its primary innervation, the phrenic nerve, reflects its original position as the superior transversum behind the embryonic heart in the cervical area.

utes to the ventrolateral fibers. Ligamentous fibers arising from the spine form the dorsal part of the diaphragm. The septum transversum, which initially separated the cervical pericardial cavity, changes to become the central tendon upon which the heart comes to rest in extrauterine life.

The esophageal mesentary contributes to the formation of the diaphragm including the crura. The esophageal crura act as a part of the gastroesophageal sphincter.

Part of the septum transversum in its original location was penetrated by the aorta, esophagus, azygos vein, thoracic duct, and inferior and superior vena cava, all of which have developed in the surrounding mesenteries. In the term infant, these same organs now traverse the diaphragm. The mesentery of the foregut incorporates itself into the structures of the posterior mediastinum.

In most animals, the anterior part of the rectus abdominus reaches up from the pelvis to the first rib. In humans, the rectus divides into four sections. One part becomes the ventrolateral fibers of the diaphragm. A second division becomes the interchondral muscles of the intercostal. A third section becomes the pectoralis major, minor, and subclavus muscles. The remaining tissue becomes the abdominal rectus. The division of the rectus depends on the growth and descent of the lung into the chest.

E. Vascular System

Early in development, the lungs receive their own blood supply from the dorsal aorta. By the fifth week, connection is made to the sixth aortic arch and the pulmonary arteries (Fig. 7). The pulmonary arteries derive from the paired sixth aortic arches. The proximal part of the left arch becomes the left pulmonary artery, and the distal section involutes. The ductus arteriosus, which shunts blood away from the lung, normally involutes to become the ligamentum artriosum. The capillary networks of the lungs come from the surrounding mesenchyme.

F. Nervous System

The vagus nerve is the nerve of the foregut and its derivatives. It is formed from the fusion of the nerves of the fourth and sixth arches. The vagus carries both the visceral afferent and efferents (Fig. 8).

The larynx is enervated by the superior laryngeal nerve and the recurrent laryngeal nerves, from the fourth and sixth arch, respectively.

The sympathetic nervous system develops from neural crest cells, which migrate to form paired ganglia dorsolateral to the aorta. Ganglia are connected by neurofibers forming the sympathetic trunks. Preganglionic fibers from the spinal lateral horn sympathetic axons move into the ganglia and synapse with the ganglionic neurons to ascend or descend down the trunk. Some of the pregangli-

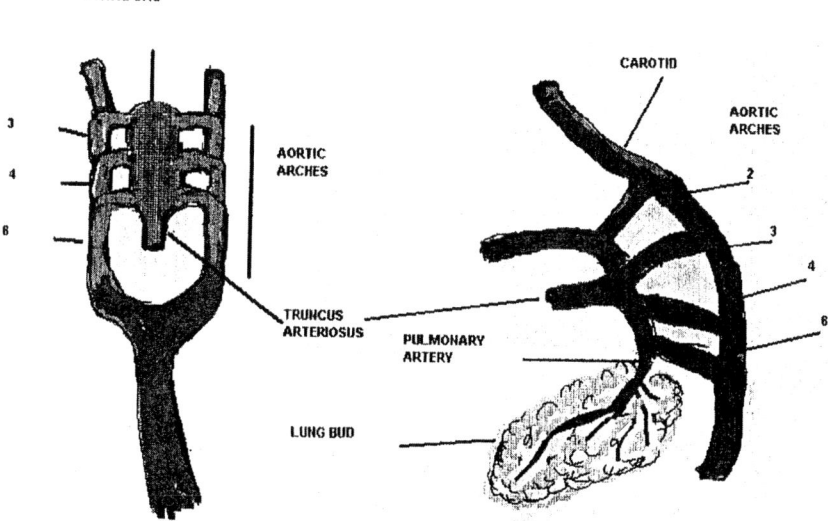

Figure 7 The dorsal aorta provides the blood supply to the future lung for a short time. By the week 4, the branches of the sixth aortic arch take over this function.

onic neurons send fibers that pass through the ganglia directly to become splanchnic nerves to the lungs.

The parasympathetic nervous system to the lung begins with fibers from brainstem nuclei. They exit the brainstem with the vagus nerve and synapse with ganglionic neurons near the lung structures. Other nerves are present, which do not use acetylcholine as the neurotransmitter but appear associated with the parasympathetic neurons. These neurons may use nitrogen oxide as their neurotransmitter and are the equivalents of the nonadrenergic noncholinergic nervous system. The pattern of innervation of the lung, esophagus, and stomach is very similar.

IV. The Esophagus and Stomach
A. The Esophagus

The esophagus develops from the portion of the foregut immediately behind the primitive pharynx and the site of the laryngotracheal bud. It is initially separated from the developing trachea by a simple groove, the laryngotracheal groove. This groove ultimately becomes a septum called the tracheoesophageal septum.

Initially the esophagus is short, but it grows rapidly as it descends into the

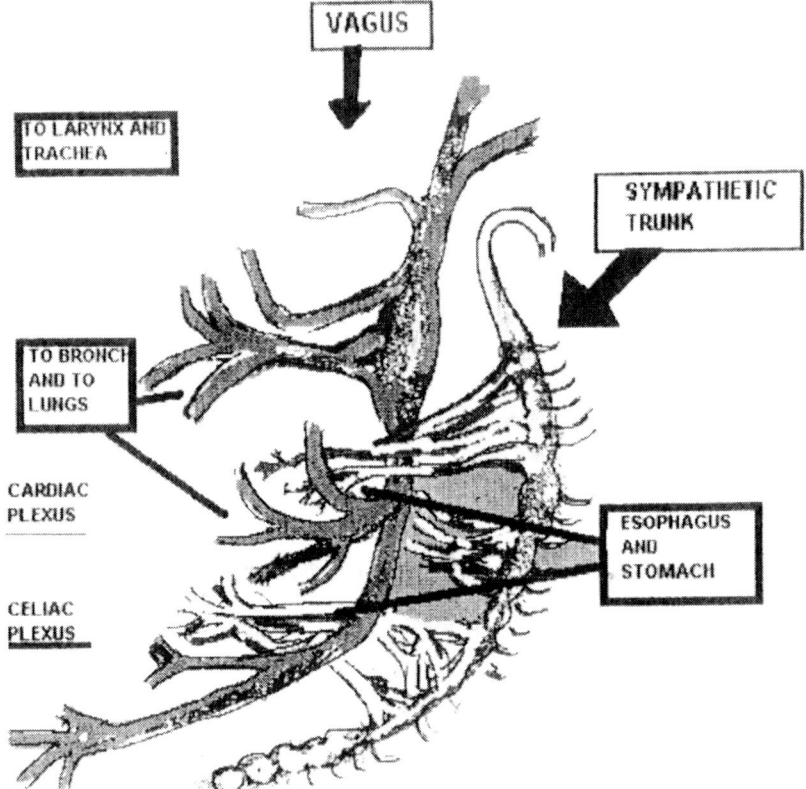

Figure 8 The respiratory tract, the esophagus, and the stomach are innervated by visceral and somatic afferents and efferents mainly via the vagus. Sympathetic fibers arise from the paravertebral ganglia of the sympathetic chain, the vagus nerve is really the combined nerve of embryonic arches 4 and 6. The nanc system is presumed to be present, but is not well studied in the embryo.

pleural cavity along with the heart and lungs. The esophagus reaches adult relative proportions compared to the lungs by the seventh week of gestation.

The epithelial glands of the esophagus are derived from the primitive endoderm. Striated muscle, which forms muscularis externa of the superior third of the esophagus, arises from the mesenchyme of the caudal branchiopharyngeal splanchnic mesenchyme.

The esophagus is enervated by branches of the vagus nerve, which were initially associated with the most caudal brancho-pharyngeal arches. In general, the innervation is similar to that of the lungs or stomach.

B. The Stomach

The distal part of the foregut is, at first, a simple tubular structure. A slight dilatation appears about the fourth week of gestation. This dilatation is oriented in the sagittal plane as it grows larger, and it then edges ventrodorsally. Since the dorsal border of the primitive stomach grows faster than its ventral border, this differential growth rate leads to the formation of the greater and lesser curvatures of the stomach. The ventrodorsal arrangement, which was apparent in the early embryo is disrupted as the embryo matures. The stomach rotates clockwise 90 degrees. The rotation moves the lesser curvature of the stomach to the right and the greater curvature to the left. The original left side of the stomach now becomes the ventral surface, and the right becomes the dorsal surface. Before rotation, the entry and exit ports of the stomach are in the same longitudinal plane. After rotating, the antrum is now to the left and inferior. The pyloric region is at the right and somewhat superior. At maturation, the stomach's long axis transverses the long axis of the body. As a result, the left vagus nerve supplies the anterior wall of the adult stomach, and the right vagus nerve supplies the posterior wall.

C. The Vascular System

The vascular supply of the stomach is by the gastro-omental arteries from the celiac division of the descending aorta.

D. The Nervous System

As mentioned above, the organs of the foregut—the esophagus, the stomach, and the respiratory tract—are innervated by visceral afferents and efferents of the vagus nerve. There are sympathetic and parasympathetic postganglionic fibers, which derive either from the tissue ganglia or the sympathetic chain. The esophagus and stomach also have a noncholinergic, nonadrenergic nervous system (see Chap. 2). The nervous array of the stomach and esophagus is the same as that found in the lungs.

V. Congenital Abnormalities

A large number of congenital abnormalities of clinical importance occur during embryogenesis of the lower respiratory tract and esophagus. A laryngeal web results from incomplete recanalization of the larynx at about the tenth week. There is partial obstruction to breathing because of the membranous web at the level of the vocal cords. The occurrence of isolated tracheal stenosis or atresia is quite rare. Most often these abnormalities are associated with tracheoesophageal fistula. An even rarer abnormality is a diverticula of the trachea, which appears as a blind bronchus. When associated with lung tissue it forms a small tracheal lobe of the lung.

The most frequent combined abnormality is the tracheoesophageal fistula. This abnormality appears in up to 1 of 2500 births. The disorder results from incomplete fusion of the tracheoesophageal folds or incomplete development of the tracheoesophageal septum. There are four recognized forms of tracheoesophageal fistula (Fig. 9):

1. The most common type involves the upper esophagus ending blindly, while the lower portion of the esophagus joins the trachea near the bifurcation.
2. In a second type, the so-called "H" type, there is a tubular connection between the esophagus and the trachea.
3. A third type has the upper esophagus connecting to the trachea with the lower portion connecting to the stomach, but ending blindly.
4. A fourth type has the upper esophagus entering into the trachea, with the lower esophagus exiting the trachea and connecting to the stomach.

Congenital diaphragmatic hernia occurs in up to one of every 3000 births. There is a posteriolateral defect of the diaphragm, which allows the abdominal contents to migrate into the pleural cavity, usually on the left side. Because of the space taken up by the abdominal organs, the ipsilateral lung is hypoplastic. Early recognition is important as the abnormality can be surgically repaired. When the defect is closed, the hypoplastic lung will usually grow and develop normally.

Eventration of the diaphram is a similar disorder which involves defective musculature that balloons into the thoracic cavity. Again the abdominal viscera moves into the chest cavity, inhibiting lung growth. Early recognition and surgical repair usually mean a good prognosis.

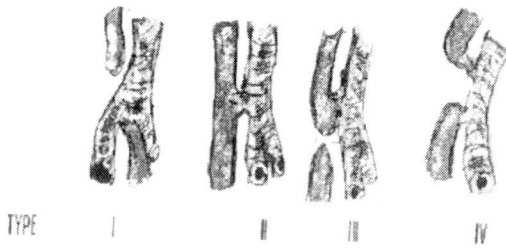

Figure 9 The type 1 anomaly, consisting of an atretic upper portion of the esophagus with connection of the lower esophagus to the trachea at the bifurcation, is the most frequent type of tracheoesophageal fistula.

VI. Summary

The lower respiratory tract, the esophagus, and the stomach begin embryonic development as part of the foregut. Because of this, they share similar nervous innervation, most significantly the visceral afferents and efferents of the vagus. These nerves will serve to provide the coordination required of the lungs and upper digestive system in extrauterine life. This intimate relationship continues in the infant and adult.

References

1. Allan FD. Essentials of Human Embryology, 2nd ed. New York: Oxford University Press, 1969.
2. Heisler JC. A Text-Book of Embryology for Students of Medicine. Philadelphia: W.B. Saunders, 1899.
3. Keith A. Human Embryology and Morphology, 5th ed. Baltimore: W. Wood & Co., 1933.
4. Langebartel DA. The Anatomical Primer: An Embryological Explanation of Human Gross Morphology. Baltimore: University Park Press, 1977.
5. Langman J. Medical Embryology, 4th ed. Baltimore: Williams & Wilkins, 1981.
6. Moore KL. Color Atlas of Clinical Embryology. Philadelphia: Saunders, 1994.
7. Moore KL. The Developing Human: Clinically Oriented Embryology, 5th ed. Philadelphia: Saunders, 1993.
8. Patten BM. Patten's Human Embryology: Elements of Clinical Development. New York: McGraw-Hill, 1976.

2

Inflammation in Asthma
The Role of Nerves and the Potential Influence of Gastroesophageal Reflux Disease

Brendan J. Canning

The Johns Hopkins Medical Institutions
Baltimore, Maryland

The National Institutes of Health of the United States described asthma as "a chronic inflammatory disorder of the airways . . . [which] causes recurrent episodes of wheezing, breathlessness, chest tightness and cough, particularly at night and/or in the early morning" (1). This description reflects a seemingly general consensus among clinicians and basic scientists alike that inflammation is not only a characteristic of the asthmatic airways and lungs, but may be the underlying pathogenesis of the disease.

Identifying inflammation as the cause, not just a feature, of asthma has led to the concept that reversing and/or preventing the inflammatory processes of asthma may be the most appropriate therapeutic strategy for treating the chronic disease. This belief is reflected in the increasing advocacy of anti-inflammatory agents such as steroids (2,3), the opposition to continuous use of short-acting beta agonists (4,5), and myriad therapeutic strategies currently in development that have been designed to disrupt the inflammatory processes associated with the airway disease (6,7).

It is indisputable that gastroesophageal reflux disease (GERD) can initiate symptoms attributed to inflammation in current definitions of asthma (8). It is also indisputable that treatment, particularly surgical treatment, of an underlying reflux disorder can completely cure asthma in some patients and in others markedly reduce their dependency on corticosteroids for control of their asthmatic condition (9–14). Does reflux, with its potential for aspiration of gastric contents into the airway spaces and lungs, initiate inflammation characteristic of asthma? Alternatively, is the identity of inflammation as the cause of asthma too rigid to adequately describe the asthmatic syndrome that may have many causes, including reflux and inflammation? These are questions that need to be addressed in future clinical research endeavors.

A potential link between reflux and asthmatic inflammation is the nervous system. The nervous system has long been recognized as a key element in inflammatory processes throughout the body (15–18), and asthma has also been attributed to a dysfunction of airway nerves (19). The chest pain (20), coughing (8,21,22), and reflex bronchoconstriction (23–26) associated with reflux provide compelling evidence that the nervous system plays a key role in the pathogenesis of GERD. In this chapter the inflammatory attributes of asthma are reviewed as are the potential roles of nerves and GERD in chronic airway disease.

I. Inflammation in Asthma

In their classic treatise on the pathology of asthma, Huber and Koessler (27) described the inflammation in asthma with its associated vascular engorgement (due to dilation of pulmonary blood vessels), mucosal edema (due to an increase in vascular permeability), and inflammatory cell infiltrates (predominantly eosinophils and mononuclear cells). Subsequent autopsy studies (28,29) and more recent studies utilizing bronchial biopsies (30) and bronchoalveolar lavage (31–33) confirmed that inflammation, particularly mucosal edema and inflammatory cell infiltration, is a consistently observed feature of asthmatic airways.

The inflammation associated with asthma that Huber and Koessler described is now known to be mediated by a variety of proinflammatory autacoids and cytokines (34). These substances act directly on target cells within the airways to induce bronchoconstriction, vasodilatation, plasma extravasation, epithelial damage, and edema. They can also act indirectly by inducing expression of inflammatory cell adhesion molecules and chemoattractants, which are necessary for the selective recruitment and migration of inflammatory cells into the airway walls and spaces. The many cells, autacoids, and cytokines that contribute to this inflammatory process are targets for asthma therapy. Table 1 lists selected proinflammatory cytokines and autacoids associated with asthma, their potential source, and their role in inflammation.

Eosinophils are the inflammatory cells most commonly associated with asthma (36). Present in lung tissues from patients who have died during an attack of asthma and in bronchial biopsies and lavages recovered from asthma sufferers, eosinophils produce a variety of mediators that might precipitate the symptoms of the disease. Consistent with the hypothesis that eosinophilia might underlie the pathogenesis of asthma, eosinophil numbers or activation indices in biopsies or lavage are correlated with disease severity in both asthmatics and animal models of asthma (31,55,56). Furthermore, therapeutic strategies aimed at preventing airway inflammation (such as corticosteroids) in asthma or specifically designed to suppress eosinophil recruitment and activation in models of asthma markedly improve disease severity, most notably, airways hyperresponsiveness, and the need for bronchodilators (32,56,57).

The association of atopy with asthma and the correlation of serum IgE with asthma severity make the mast cell, with its high-affinity receptor for IgE, a likely effector in asthma (34,40,58,59). Allergen-induced bronchospasm elicited in a clinical setting closely resembles an acute exacerbation of chronic asthma, and both conditions are effectively treated by drugs that inhibit the actions or release of mast cell–derived autacoids (38,40). Human lung mast cells may also produce proinflammatory cytokines (60). The ability of mast cell activation to precipitate an inflammatory response that is essentially indistinguishable from that associated with chronic asthma provides further evidence for the potential role of mast cells in asthma but also reveals that mast cell activation may not be a sufficient condition. Many atopic individuals will bronchoconstrict and develop a profound inflammatory response to inhaled allergen and yet have no chronic symptoms of asthma (e.g., recurrent wheezing and cough, airways hyperresponsiveness) (61). Furthermore, IgE-deficient mice still develop airways hyperresponsiveness and eosinophilia following allergen challenge (62). This suggests that factors in addition to atopy (e.g., GERD) and high-affinity IgE receptor activation may be necessary for expression of the asthmatic phenotype.

The mononuclear cells of the inflammatory cell infiltrates in asthmatic airways are comprised of both lymphocytes and macrophages (30,34,54,63). These cells produce a wide variety of cytokines that play an essential role in orchestrating the processes of lung defense and inflammation. Given their key role in the inflammatory process, the biology and pathobiology of these cells has become perhaps the most intensely investigated field of asthma research. Particular emphasis has been placed on the CD4+ T helper (Th) lymphocyte. Based on their production of cytokines associated with cellular immunity and delayed-type hypersensitivity (e.g., IFN-γ, IL-2) or humoral immunity and allergic inflammatory reactions (e.g., IL-4, IL-13, MIP-1α), murine Th cells can be subclassified into Th_1 and Th_2 subtypes, respectively (64). It has been postulated that if the Th_1/Th_2 classification of lymphocytes is applicable to humans, Th_2 lymphocytes might be critical in asthma (63). While evidence against the Th_1/Th_2 classification of T lymphocytes in humans has been presented, the hypothesis continues to be invoked as a potential explanation for the development of the asthmatic phenotype (35,65,66).

Neutrophils and basophils can also be found in asthmatic airways (30,33). Their presence in biopsies and in bronchoalveolar lavage coupled with the obser-

Table 1 Various Inflammatory Mediators Associated with the Pathogenesis of Asthma[a]: Cellular Source and Potential Effects in the Lung

Mediator	Cellular source[b]	Potential role in asthma	Ref.
Cysteinyl-leukotrienes (LTC$_4$, D$_4$, and E$_4$)	Mast cells, basophils, eosinophils	Bronchoconstriction, plasma extravasation, inflammatory cell recruitment	34,38,39
Histamine	Mast cells, basophils	Bronchoconstriction, plasma extravasation, vasodilatation	34,37,40
Major basic protein	Eosinophils	Epithelial damage, cholinergic nerve dysfunction	36,41
Tachykinins[c]	Nerves[d]	Bronchoconstriction, vasodilatation, plasma extravasation, inflammatory cell recruitment	46–50
Endothelins	Endothelium, epithelium	Bronchoconstriction, plasma extravasation	51,52
Bradykinin	Plasma kallikrein, glands	Bronchoconstriction and cough, vasodilation, plasma extravasation	53
TNF-α	Macrophages	Inflammatory cell recruitment, activation	54
IL-1	Macrophages	Inflammatory cell recruitment, activation	54

IL-4	Th lymphocytes, basophils	Inflammatory cell recruitment promotes mast cell, lymphocyte development promotes IgE and Th_2-type cytokine synthesis	34,35
IL-5	Th lymphocytes	Eosinophil, basophil maturation and survival; eosinophil, basophil recruitment and activation	7,34,55,56
IL-8	Epithelium, macrophages	Inflammatory cell recruitment and priming, airways hyperresponsiveness	6,33
RANTES	Epithelium	Inflammatory cell recruitment and priming	6,34

[a]This list is merely representative and not intended to be exhaustive. Extensive reviews on other pro-inflammatory cytokines, chemokines, and autacoids associated with the pathogenesis of asthma can be found elsewhere (6,34–37).
[b]Virtually every cell type in the lung has been implicated as a source of proinflammatory cytokines, chemokines, and autacoids. Cell sources identified above are those most often associated with a specific cytokine and/or autacoid.
[c]Substance P and neurokinin A.
[d]Eosinophils found in inflammatory cell infiltrates are potential sources of substance P (42). Interestingly, monocytes recovered from the lungs of healthy human subjects also contain both substance P messenger RNA and protein (43). This may be a potential source of the substance P found in the lavage and sputum of asthmatics (44,45).

vation that antiasthma therapies inhibit their recruitment and activation in the airways suggests that a potential role for these cells cannot be discounted (57). Indeed, both cell types—particularly the basophil, the only cell other than the mast cell to express the high-affinity IgE receptor—can produce a variety of proinflammatory cytokines (e.g., IL-4, IL-13, MIP-1α) and autacoids (e.g., cysteinyl leukotrienes, histamine) that have been implicated in the pathogenesis of asthma (67) (Table 1).

Clinical studies of the association between asthma and GERD have not always distinguished between allergic (atopic or "extrinsic") and nonallergic (nonatopic or "intrinsic") asthma (68–71). Several authors have implied, however, that asthma precipitated by GERD may be more prevalent in patients with no history of atopy (8,12,13). Interestingly, recent studies indicate that chronic airway inflammation in atopic and nonatopic asthmatics does not differ to any great extent (72–76). This suggests that whether the underlying cause of asthma is of intrinsic (e.g., GERD) or extrinsic (e.g., allergen) origin, the resulting pathology is similar. Furthermore, while direct evidence is lacking, these observations also suggest that conditions such as GERD or exercise-induced asthma may precipitate inflammation in susceptible patients.

It is unfortunate that airway inflammation has not been assessed in patients with GERD-associated asthma. Such information, particularly before and after effective reflux therapy, might profoundly influence diagnosis of the associated diseases and might also highlight the importance of considering reflux in the diagnosis of asthma. It is possible that patients with GERD-induced asthma may not possess the inflammation characteristic of allergic asthma. Indeed, some asthmatics have little or no evidence of chronic inflammation or peripheral blood eosinophilia (30,36). Alternatively, patients with GERD-associated asthma might have inflamed airways. In severe cases of reflux, patients may aspirate large volumes of gastric contents and, as a consequence, develop potentially fatal acute lung injury (77). Profound inflammation of the lungs has been noted at autopsy in patients expiring from aspiration-induced lung injury (78–80) (see also Chapter 10). In animal models the progression of this disease is dependent upon a cascade of proinflammatory cytokines (TNF-α, IL-8) which induce chemotaxis, endothelial cell adhesion (by inducing expression of endothelial cell adhesion molecules), migration, and activation of neutrophils, which mediate the potentially fatal response (Fig. 1) (78,81–83). It would be interesting to know the effect of reflux therapy on airway inflammation in asthmatic patients who are either responsive or unresponsive to effective treatment of their GERD.

II. Neurogenic Inflammation

Inflammation is a necessary defense mechanism that serves to protect the body from noxious and infectious insults. The precision of the host response to such

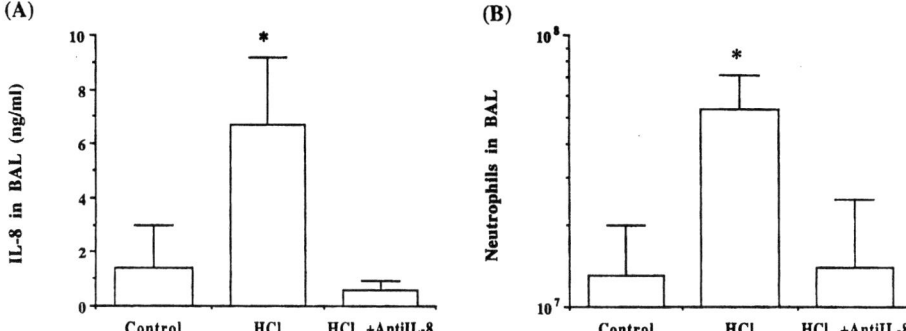

Figure 1 Effects of acid aspiration on neutrophils and IL-8 recovered by bronchoalveolar lavage (BAL) in a rabbit model of aspiration-induced acute lung injury. (A) Tracheal instillation of acid elicited marked increases in IL-8 recovered (6 hr postinstillation) by BAL. (B) Coincident with the increase in IL-8, the number of neutrophils recovered by BAL also markedly increased, an effect that was accompanied by physiological signs of severe respiratory distress, likely precipitated by acute lung injury. Administering an antibody to IL-8 subsequent to acid instillation reduced IL-8 levels in lavage and prevented neutrophil recruitment and respiratory distress. (Adapted from Ref. 82.)

insults is critical: compromised or insufficient inflammatory responses can have dire, acute consequences, while exaggerated or prolonged inflammatory responses can precipitate chronic disease. Such exaggerated inflammatory responses might precipitate chronic inflammatory diseases such as rheumatoid arthritis, inflammatory bowel disease, GERD, and asthma.

As one of the cardinal signs of the inflammatory process, pain permanently links the nervous system with the sequelae of inflammatory diseases (15–18). The pioneering studies of Bruce (15) and Lewis (16,17) early in this century suggest that neuronal activation might also be the defining event of an inflammatory response. More recent studies suggest that, like their clearly defined role in the skin of both humans and animals, peripheral nerves may also play a role in mediating and/or modulating the inflammatory processes of the viscera (18,84,85).

Dysfunction of airway nerves has long been considered an underlying cause of asthma (19,86,87). Only recently, however, has the role of nerves in asthmatic inflammation been considered. Szentivanyi (88) proposed a link between the nervous system and allergic, asthmatic inflammation, speculating that dysfunction of airway adrenergic nerves and adrenoceptors might underlie the pathogenesis of asthma. The hypothesis that autonomic nerves might modulate inflammation in asthma has been reviewed in detail elsewhere (89).

The most compelling hypothesis for a role of nerves in airway inflammation invokes a role for the axon reflex (47). First described in the skin and eye by Bruce (15) and further characterized by Lewis (16,17) and others (90), axon reflexes involve peripheral stimulation of sensory nerves and subsequent local release of proinflammatory neurotransmitters that mediate vasodilatation, plasma extravasation through leaky vessels, inflammatory cell recruitment, and, coincident with sensory nerve activation, the sensation of pain and prolonged hyperalgesia (Fig. 2). The peripheral effects of these sensory nerves are most likely due to the release of the tachykinins substance P and neurokinin A (18,84,91). These proinflammatory neuropeptides are localized to the central and peripheral nerve terminals of a specific subset of unmyelinated sensory and visceral afferent nerves. The peripheral terminals of these afferent nerves are exquisitely sensitive to a variety of chemical and mechanical stimuli. If stimulated with sufficient intensity, these nerve endings will generate bursts of action potentials coincident with local tachykinin release. Subsequent to conduction of the action potentials to the central nervous system (CNS) and release of tachykinins and other transmitters in the CNS, these nerves initiate a variety of defensive reflexes.

The lung and virtually all visceral organs (including the esophagus) in humans and animals are innervated by tachykinin-containing afferent nerves (84,92–95). Placing them in proximity to the luminal targets of inhaled and/or aspirated irritants, such fibers are readily localized to the airway epithelium (92–94). Upon stimulation, these sensory nerves orchestrate a variety of defensive reflexes that are critical for homeostasis. Failure or dysfunction of airway sensory nerves will increase susceptibility to noxious insults, infection, and consequently disease (48,96–101). One such reflex mediated by the tachykinin-containing sensory nerves is inflammation. Lundberg and Saria (102) were the first to systematically characterize the role of sensory nerves in pulmonary inflammation. Lung challenge with noxious and proinflammatory stimuli (e.g., cigarette smoke, histamine, bradykinin, and mechanical irritation) elicits marked plasma extravasation from the vasculature in the airway mucosa of rats. However, following chemical desensitization of the tachykinin-containing sensory nerves with capsaicin (an unmyelinated afferent nerve-selective neurotoxin), nearly all proinflammatory stimuli delivered to the lung were rendered ineffective at eliciting plasma extravasation. This observation is essentially identical to that described in the human skin and provides compelling evidence that tachykinin-containing sensory nerves may be key effectors of lung inflammation (16–18,47).

Neurogenic inflammation is now well characterized in the lungs of rats, mice, and guinea pigs (48,103). A wide variety of stimuli initiate plasma extravasation by activating tachykinin-containing capsaicin-sensitive nerves (Table 2). Key features of their mechanism of action highlight the role of the peripheral axon reflex. The responses are abolished or markedly inhibited by tachykinin receptor antagonists or chemical desensitization of the tachykinin-containing

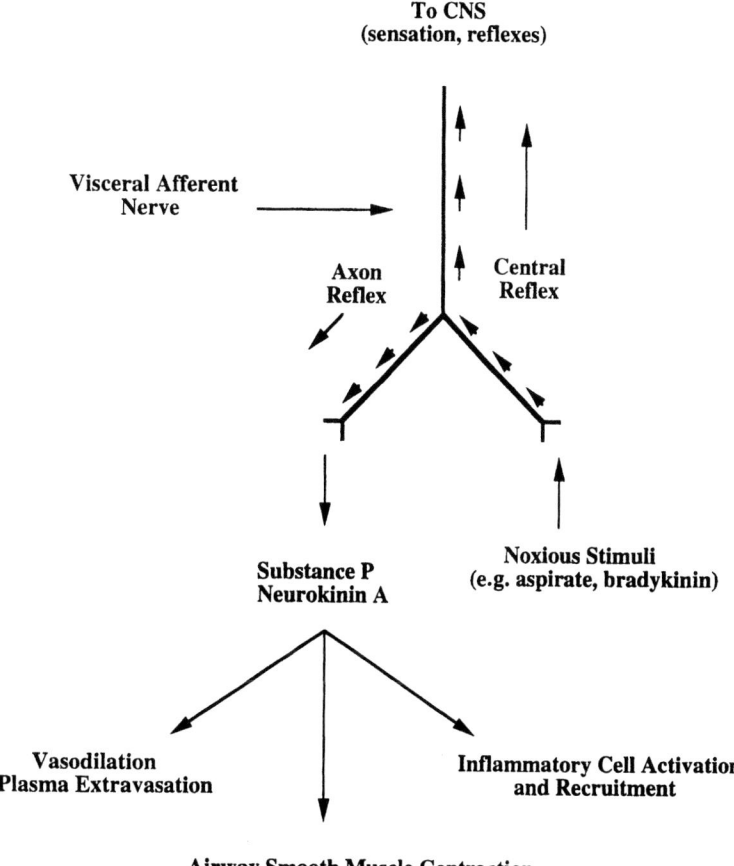

Figure 2 Schematic diagram of an afferent nerve–mediated axon reflex. Nociceptive afferent nerves are highly sensitive to a variety of mechanical and chemical stimuli. If activated with sufficient intensity, these nerves will generate action potentials resulting in peripheral release of proinflammatory neurotransmitters such as the tachykinins substance P and neurokinin A. These potent neuropeptides have multiple effects on the vasculature and cells surrounding an inflamed tissue and can either facilitate or directly mediate an inflammatory response.

nerves. They are unaffected by acute vagotomy (and thus proceed independent of central neuronal input). These neurogenic inflammatory responses are mimicked by exogenous tachykinins or electrical, antidromic stimulation of vagal afferent nerves. Other features of neurogenic inflammation described in animals highlight the potentially profound influence the axon reflex might have on the

Table 2 Stimuli Initiating Neurogenic Inflammation in the Airways[a]

Stimulus	Effect of tachykinin receptor antagonism	Ref.
Allergen	Partial inhibition	48,104
Cigarette smoke	Complete inhibition	102,105
Bradykinin	Partial inhibition	102,106
Intraesophageal acid	Complete inhibition	107
Intratracheal acid (or gastric contents)	Complete inhibition	108
Hyperpnea[b]	Complete inhibition	109
Hypertonic saline[b]	Complete inhibition	110,111

[a] All studies carried out in rats and/or guinea pigs. This list is merely representative; many other stimuli initiate neurogenic inflammation in animals (thoroughly reviewed in Ref. 48).
[b] Used as models of exercise-induced asthma.

airways. Thus, in addition to vasodilatation and plasma extravasation, activation of tachykinin-containing afferent nerves innervating the airways elicits increased excitability of airway parasympathetic ganglion neurons (112–117), mucus secretion (118), and bronchospasm (50,119).

Neurogenic inflammation in animals is also associated with inflammatory cell adhesion (in postcapillary venules, also the site of plasma leakage) and subsequent migration into airway walls (105,120,121). This effect may be indirectly mediated by the tachykinins interacting with the endothelial cells or, alternatively, may be mediated directly by the tachykinins interacting with the inflammatory cells (49,105).

Of particular relevance to GERD and its role in asthma and inflammation, airway instillation of acid or gastric contents initiates capsaicin-sensitive nerve-mediated inflammation in animals (Fig. 3) (108). In humans, inhalation of acidic solutions such as citric acid is known to elicit a variety of defensive reflexes indicative of sensory nerve stimulation and most likely due to stimulation of capsaicin-sensitive nerves (122). Interestingly, Hamamoto and colleagues (107) have presented evidence that aspiration of refluxate is not a necessary condition for induction of neurogenic inflammation in guinea pigs (Fig. 4). Upon observing that intraesophageal acid elicits neurogenic inflammation in the airways, this group speculated that either an axon reflex may exist between the esophagus and the trachea or a vascular connection between the two organs may carry inflammatory substances from the esophagus to the lung. While both vascular and neuronal projections between these two organs have been described in the guinea pig

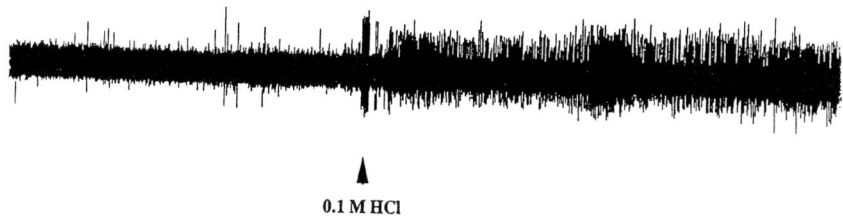

Figure 3 Effects of tracheal mucosal application of 0.1 M HCl on the activity of a capsaicin-sensitive vagal afferent nerve fiber in the guinea pig. Neuronal activity was recorded extracellularly from tracheal afferent fibers as previously described (123). Brief application of 0.5 ml HCl (0.1 M) elicited a marked increase in afferent nerve fiber activity, an increase that persisted long after mucosal pH was restored to baseline.

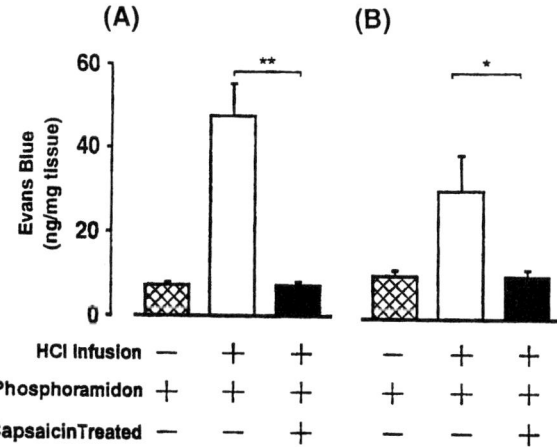

Figure 4 Effect of intraesophageal acid infusion on plasma extravasation in the guinea pig (A) trachea and (B) mainstem bronchi. Plasma extravasation was quantified by measuring the amount of serum albumin (prelabeled with Evans Blue dye) recovered in the tissues following challenge. Phosphoramidon was administered to prevent metabolism of endogenously released tachykinins. Acid was infused into the esophagus, which was sutured shut adjacent to the pharynx (thus preventing aspiration). Note that intraesophageal acid elicited marked plasma extravasation from the airways, an effect that was completely abolished by depletion of tachykinins with capsaicin. The plasma extravasation was also abolished by an NK_1 tachykinin receptor antagonist. (From Ref. 107.)

(116,124–126), the potential for such communication in humans has not been assessed.

edema, mucus ... inflammatory cell influx has been clearly demonstrated in the human upper airway (127,128). Neurogenic inflammation has also been clearly defined in the human skin (95,129). Both responses are mimicked by exogenously administered tachykinins. Does neurogenic inflammation occur in human central and peripheral airways (130)? The answer to this question is unknown, but several lines of evidence argue in favor of such a process. Thus, in humans, tachykinin receptors are present on airway smooth muscle (50,131), blood vessels (Fig. 5), glands (118), airway ganglion neurons (132), and the airway epithelium (133,134). Furthermore, both capsaicin-sensitive and tachykinin-containing nerves are present in human airways (92,135). In clinical studies, both capsaicin and tachykinins elicit bronchospasm (lower airway vascular effects of capsaicin and the tachykinins have not been assessed in a clinical setting) (135–137). In in vitro studies with human airways, both capsaicin and tachykinins induce mucus secretion and enhance excitability of airway

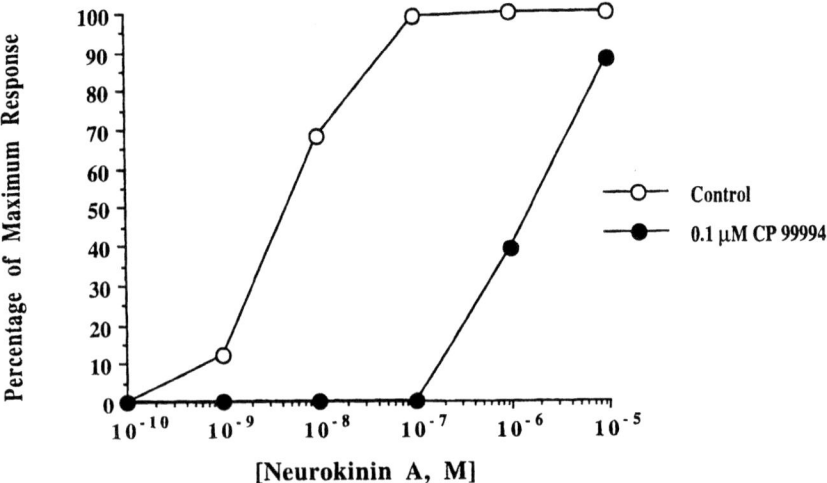

Figure 5 Neurokinin A–induced relaxations of human intrapulmonary arteries (3–5 mm outer diameter). Relaxations were endothelium-dependent and abolished by a combination of cyclooxygenase and NO synthase inhibitors (indicating they are mediated by prostanoids and nitric oxide produced by the endothelium). Similar results were obtained using substance P. Note the effect of the NK_1 selective antagonist CP 99994: tachykinin-induced relaxations of human intrapulmonary arteries were competitively antagonized by NK_1 receptor antagonists.

ganglion neurons (118,132). All of these observations suggest that axonal reflexes occur in the human airways.

Given the many proinflammatory effects mediated by tachykinins, it is possible that neurogenic inflammation might contribute to the pathogenesis of asthma. In airway biopsies taken from asthmatics, tachykinin receptor expression is greater than that seen in nonasthmatic airways, a condition that is reversed by steroid treatment (138,139). Consistent with the hypothesis that tachykinins are released during inflammatory responses, tachykinin levels are markedly increased in the lavage and sputum of asthmatics and also during acute attacks (44,45). Some investigators have even observed a marked increase in the density of tachykinin-containing nerve fibers in asthmatic airways (140), although this has not been confirmed by other investigators (141,142). Clearly then, the potential role of tachykinins and airway afferent nerves in asthma cannot be readily discounted (Table 3).

III. Effects of Inflammation on Airway Afferent Nerves

Vasodilatation and plasma extravasation resulting in the redness ("rubor"), swelling ("tumor"), and elevated temperature ("calor") of inflamed tissues along with inflammatory cell infiltration are signs of inflammation common to all tissues susceptible to inflammatory disorders (15–17,145). In the skin and in other tissues innervated by somatic nerves, other cardinal signs of inflammation are persistent pain ("dolor") and hyperalgesia and thus altered physiology ("functio laesa") in the tissues proximal to the inflamed area (85,145). It seems likely that the hyperalgesia mediated by somatic afferent nerves and the exag-

Table 3 Tachykinin Receptor–Mediated Regulation of the Airways and Lungs

End organ effects	Tachykinin receptors involved[a]	Ref.
Vasodilatation[b]	NK_1	48
Plasma extravasation	NK_1, NK_2	48
Inflammatory cell recruitment and activation	NK_1, NK_2	49,105,121
Airway smooth muscle contraction	NK_2, NK_1	50,119,131
Mucus secretion	NK_1	118
CNS-mediated reflexes[c]	NK_1, NK_2, NK_3	143,144
Modulation of parasympathetic neurotransmission	NK_3, NK_1	112–117

[a]Tachykinins mediate their effects by binding to three different neurokinin (NK) receptor subtypes. Tachykinin receptor pharmacology has been reviewed extensively elsewhere (18,46,84,91).
[b]See Figure 5.
[c]For example, sympathetic, parasympathetic reflexes, cough.

gerated autonomic reflexes mediated by afferent nerves innervating the viscera are physiologically similar phenomena.

Hyperalgesia can be precipitated by a heightened excitability of peripheral afferent nerve terminals (146,147), a heightened excitability of the secondary neurons that transform afferent input into sensation and reflex activity (148,149), or an alteration in the type or quantity of transmitters released from the central nerve terminals of the afferent nerves (150). The resulting alteration in neuronal function renders previously innocuous or moderately irritating stimuli noxious and painful, and now able to provoke inappropriate reflexes that impair maintenance of homeostasis (Fig. 6). The parallels between hyperalgesia associated with inflammation and the nonspecific airways hyperreactivity associated with asthma seem obvious.

Compelling evidence that the airway afferent nerves in asthmatics are hyperexcitable has been presented. Airways hyperreactivity renders stimuli that are without effect on lung function in normal patients (e.g., distilled water, bradykinin, adenosine, sulfur dioxide, citric acid, hypertonic saline, sodium metabisulfite) provocative. The resulting bronchospasm is generally prevented by

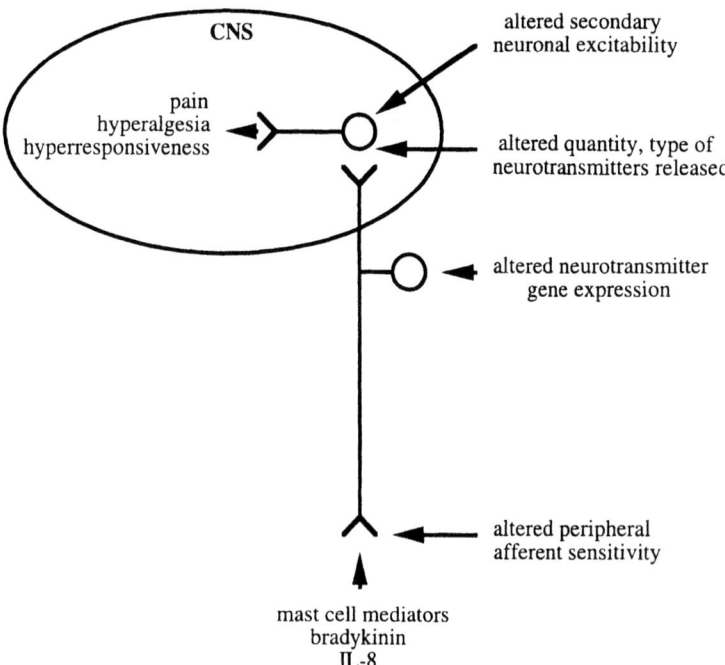

Figure 6 Schematic diagram illustrating potential mechanisms of hyperalgesia.

pretreatment with muscarinic receptor antagonists such as ipratropium bromide (151–154). This implies that each of these stimuli initiates bronchospasm by initiating a parasympathetic, cholinergic reflex. Inflammation such as that associated with allergies may induce hyperresponsiveness. In the nose, for example, the response elicited by bradykinin in seasonal allergic rhinitics is markedly enhanced in patients who are in season and symptomatic (155,156). Interestingly, a major difference in the responses of the rhinitics in season is the induction of sneezing (clearly indicating an increased neuronal excitability) and a parasympathetic reflex that is not elicited when allergy symptoms and inflammation are not present. Similar results were obtained with nasal challenge using endothelin-1 (157). These data suggest that sensitization of the afferent nerve endings induced by allergen challenge may enhance neuronal excitability. This has been directly demonstrated in the guinea pig airways and in isolated vagal afferent neurons (123,158). Furthermore, capsaicin pretreatment or tachykinin receptor antagonists reverse antigen-induced airways hyperresponsiveness in several species including nonhuman primates (159–163).

Inflammation might also alter airway afferent nerve neurotransmitter expression. Fischer and colleagues (164) observed that inhalation challenge of allergic guinea pigs with allergen induced preprotachykinin gene expression in vagal afferent neurons that normally do not produce tachykinins. Coincident with the increase in preprotachykinin gene expression, there was a three- to four-fold increase in airway nerve tachykinin content. A similar effect can be elicited by intratracheal instillation of nerve growth factor (NGF) (165). Interestingly, NGF may be produced by mast cells, and NGF levels in serum from allergic asthmatics are more than 30 times that found in healthy subjects (166).

Gastroesophageal reflux disease might induce airways hyperresponsiveness by sensitizing airway afferent nerves. Such an effect might proceed directly through the effects of refluxate contents on the afferent nerve endings or indirectly through the formation of autacoids and cytokines that might subsequently alter afferent nerve excitability. IL-8, for example, which is produced in the lung following aspiration of gastric contents (82) (Fig. 1), is known to induce hyperalgesia in animals (167). Interestingly, IL-8 also induces bronchial hyperresponsiveness in guinea pigs (168). Bradykinin is also formed at sites of plasma leakage such as that elicited by aspiration and is an extremely potent stimulant of airway afferent nerves (53). Endothelins, potent, proinflammatory peptides synthesized by epithelial and endothelial cells known to be produced during mucosal damage in the gastrointestinal tract (169), might also be produced in the airway upon aspiration (51). Endothelins have been reported to have multiple effects on airway nerves (52).

Clinical studies indicate that reflux in the absence of aspiration can also increase airways responsiveness (24,170) (see Chap. 7). It seems possible that there is a peripheral neuronal communication between the esophagus and the airways. In a study of the relaxant innervation of the guinea pig airways, for example, stimulation of capsaicin-sensitive vagal afferent nerves innervating the esophagus elicited relaxations of airway smooth muscle that were abolished by tachykinin receptor antagonists (116). A series of physiological and pharmacological analyses revealed that these relaxations were mediated by the tachykinins activating, via peripheral reflex, parasympathetic ganglion neurons that innervate the airways but have cell bodies in the esophageal myenteric plexus (which is densely innervated by tachykinin-containing nerves. Indeed, in the guinea pig, per gram of tissue, the esophagus has nearly 10 times the amount of substance P found in the airways) (116,171,172). Subsequent retrograde tracing studies confirmed that esophageal myenteric plexus neurons could be specifically labeled following injection of retrograde neuronal tracer into the airway smooth muscle (Fig. 7) (126).

Intraesophageal acid might also increase airways hyperresponsiveness through central mechanisms (Fig. 8). The central terminations of vagal afferent nerves innervating the airways, gastrointestinal tract, heart, and vasculature are distributed in several closely associated brainstem nuclei. Considerable overlap of these central terminations arising from disparate peripheral targets has been noted (175,176). Furthermore, the nuclei containing preganglionic neurons also display marked locational overlap of cell populations projecting axons to different organs (175,176). It seems likely that this lack of precise viscerotopic organization at the level of the CNS might result in alterations in preganglionic nerve activity in one organ elicited by alterations in afferent nerve activity arising from a different organ. Such a scenario might contribute to GERD-associated asthma. Indeed, it is also possible that the converse, namely, alterations in airway afferent nerve activity due to inflammation in asthma, might precipitate reflux through centrally mediated vagal reflexes. Based on such an interaction, it would be interesting to know the relative therapeutic benefit realized by anticholinergic therapy in GERD-associated asthma (153,154).

IV. Effect of Inflammation on Airway Autonomic Nerves

The airways are innervated by both sympathetic and parasympathetic nerves (136,137). A frequent error appearing in textbooks is to equate the term *parasympathetic* with both cholinergic and vagal and the term *sympathetic* with adrenergic. Using the term *vagal* to describe the parasympathetic innervation of the airways is clearly inappropriate (as are terms such as vagolytic and vagal blockade) because 70–90% of the vagal nerve fibers projecting to the airways and lungs are afferent fibers that do not specifically subserve parasympathetic reflexes (96). Likewise, the terms *cholinergic* and *adrenergic*, originally introduced by Dale (177–179) but not with the intention of replacing the terms parasympathetic and

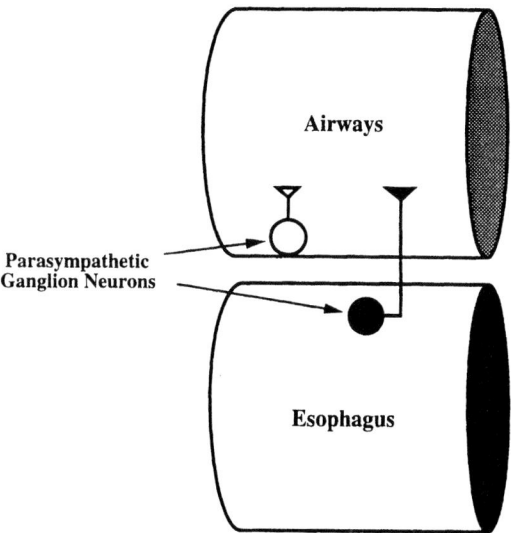

Figure 7 Schematic diagram illustrating the arrangement of the parasympathetic ganglia innervating the airways of the guinea pig. Ganglia intrinsic to the airways are labeled immunohistochemically with antisera specific for cholinergic nerves (173). Neither VIP nor NO synthase, putative mediators of noncholinergic parasympathetic nerve-mediated responses in the airway, can be localized to the ganglia intrinsic to the airway wall (125,173). Indeed, only cholinergic responses are elicited when the ganglia intrinsic to the airways are selectively stimulated (124). By contrast, noncholinergic, parasympathetic nerve–mediated responses of the airways can be elicited upon stimulating neurons intrinsic to the esophageal myenteric plexus (124). Recent retrograde tracing and immunohistochemical studies confirm that noncholinergic neurons intrinsic to the esophagus project axons to the adjacent airways (125,126,174). Similar peripheral neuronal projections between the esophagus and the airways in other species including humans have not been assessed.

sympathetic, are also inappropriate for describing the parasympathetic and sympathetic innervation of the airways. Indeed, both parasympathetic and sympathetic nerves contain many transmitters in addition to acetylcholine and noradrenaline, respectively, and it is well established that sympathetic nerves can be cholinergic (180). Accordingly, use of the terms sympathetic and parasympathetic as originally proposed by Langley (181) seems most appropriate.

The parasympathetic innervation of the airways plays a dominant role in regulating airway smooth muscle tone and mucus secretion and also regulates airway bronchial vascular tone (118,182–184). Responses mediated by parasympathetic nerve stimulation are both cholinergic and nonadrenergic, noncholiner-

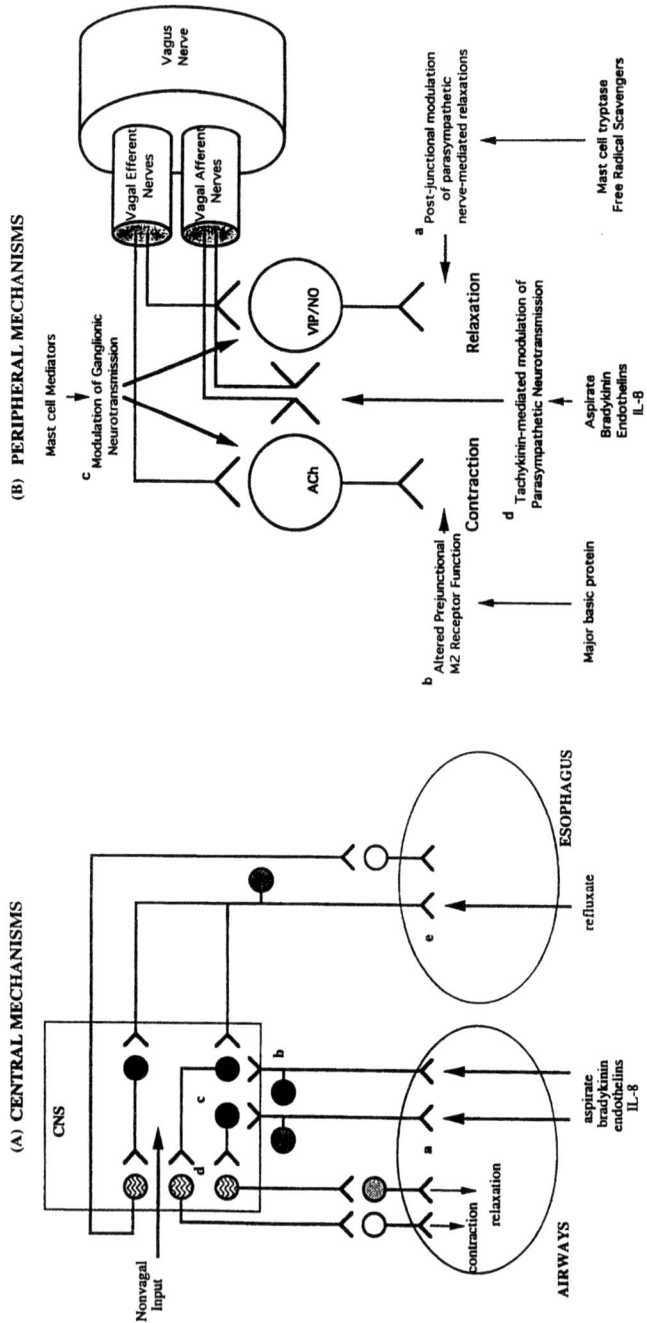

gic, or NANC in nature (118,182–184). NANC nerve–mediated responses in the airways were first described in preparations of airway smooth muscle (185–187), and their parasympathetic nature was soon described in both guinea pigs (188,189) and cats (190,191). Subsequent studies of airway glandular secretion and vascular tone revealed similar innervation of the glands and vessels of the airways in many species (118,183,184).

Immunohistochemical studies carried out in animals and humans have identified a plethora of noncholinergic neurotransmitters in the parasympathetic ganglion neurons innervating the airways, including vasoactive intestinal peptide (VIP) and related peptides (192–196), nitric oxide synthase (NOS) (195–199), calcitonin gene–related peptide (CGRP) (200), substance P (195,201), galanin (202–204), neuropeptide Y (203,205,206), and a host of other putative neurotransmitters that potentially regulate airway caliber, blood flow, and mucus secretion (206–209). Functional studies have confirmed this diversity throughout the airway tree (118,182–184). Parasympathetic, cholinergic responses have also been demonstrated throughout the airway tree (118,182–184). Recent development of an antiserum for choline acetyltransferase, the enzyme that synthesizes acetylcholine and a specific marker for cholinergic nerves, has permitted immunohistochemical studies that confirm the presence of cholinergic nerves throughout the airways (173,210).

Figure 8 Schematic diagram illustrating potential neuronal mechanisms that might precipitate airways hyperresponsiveness. (A) Central mechanisms: airway smooth muscle is innervated by parasympathetic nerves that mediate (cholinergic) contractions and (nonadrenergic, noncholinergic) relaxations. Any stimulus or disease state that increases contractile nerve activity and/or decreases relaxant nerve activity may precipitate bronchospasm and airways hyperresponsiveness. Such stimuli might increase peripheral afferent nerve terminal sensitivity (a), alter neurotransmitter gene expression in primary afferent nerves (b), alter secondary neuronal excitability (c), or alter the excitability of the preganglionic fibers regulating airway caliber (d). Alternatively, vagal afferent nerve activity arising from the esophagus (e) or nonvagal afferent nerve activity (f) arising from tissues not innervated by the vagus nerves (e.g., pharynx, nasal mucosa) might modulate the central pathways regulating airway caliber. (B) Peripheral mechanisms: inflammation might alter autonomic regulation of airway caliber by degrading and/or inactivating relaxant transmitters subsequent to release or altering airway smooth muscle responsiveness to the relaxant neurotransmitters (a) or facilitating release of acetylcholine by interacting with prejunctional receptors on the cholinergic nerve terminals (b). Inflammation might also affect synaptic neurotransmission in the ganglia by modulating the excitability of the parasympathetic ganglion neurons (c) or inducing release of neuromodulatory tachykinins from capsaicin-sensitive vagal afferent nerves that facilitate synaptic neurotransmission. See text for details and references supporting these hypotheses.

Based on the precedence of studies in other tissues (211) and the observation that both cholinergic and noncholinergic responses can be elicited by vagus nerve stimulation (188,190,191) and can be inhibited with ganglionic blockers such as hexamethonium (189–191), it has been suggested that cholinergic and noncholinergic parasympathetic neurotransmitters are co-released from a single population of postganglionic parasympathetic nerve terminals (212). This hypothesis has not, however, withstood a rigorous test in the guinea pig (124,125,173). Circumstantial and direct immunohistochemical evidence suggests that a similar situation exists in cats (213–215), ferrets (195), and humans (196,216,217). This suggests that while cholinergic and noncholinergic responses might both be mediated by parasympathetic nerves, they may be mediated by anatomically and physiologically distinct populations of nerves and, consequently, may also be regulated in a manner distinct from one another.

Surprisingly little is known about the sympathetic innervation of the airways, particularly in humans. Stimulation of adrenergic nerves has been demonstrated to elicit bronchodilatation and prevent bronchospasm in several species (191,218,219). Beta-adrenoceptor antagonists, presumably through their effects on responses mediated by adrenergic nerves and circulating catecholamines, increase bronchial hyperresponsiveness in both humans and animals (89,220,221). The observation that adrenoceptor antagonists are without effect on nerve-mediated responses in isolated human airways has led to the hypothesis that human airway smooth muscle is not innervated by sympathetic nerves (19). Nonadrenergic neurotransmitters have been localized to airway sympathetic nerves, but to date no direct evidence for a functional role of these nerves has been provided (93,222,223).

Inflammation can alter airway autonomic nerve activity in the periphery by altering the excitability of the postganglionic autonomic neurons (224), altering synaptic neurotransmission within the autonomic ganglia (225), or altering the release and/or postjunctional effects of the autonomic neurotransmitters (226) (Fig. 8). Parasympathetic nerve-mediated bronchodilation is impaired following acute allergen challenge or in chronically inflamed airways from cats (227) and rabbits (228), respectively. Similarly, mast cell tryptase markedly inhibits relaxation of human airway smooth muscle elicited by the putative NANC relaxant neurotransmitter VIP (229), and several studies have demonstrated profound inhibitory effects of inflammatory cytokines on receptor-mediated relaxations of airway smooth muscle (230). These observations may be of particular relevance to asthma because clinical studies indicate that a failure to dilate with deep inspiration, and not an excessive constriction to contractile agonists, might be the underlying cause of asthmatic airways hyperresponsiveness (231).

It has also been suggested that cholinergic neurotransmission might be adversely affected by inflammation (89). Upon release, acetylcholine mediates its effects in the airways by binding with high affinity to muscarinic M_3 receptors on the postjunctional targets of airway parasympathetic, cholinergic nerves. In addition, however, acetylcholine also activates M_2 muscarinic receptors on the prejunctional nerve terminals (232,233). When activated, the prejunctional M_2 receptors inhibit acetylcholine release, thereby serving as a brake on the cholinergic nerve terminals during periods of elevated cholinergic nerve activity. Failure of this braking system provided by the prejunctional M_2 receptors markedly potentiates the postjunctional effects of parasympathetic, cholinergic nerves (232–234). Inflammation induced by allergen (41,235), viral infection (236), or ozone exposure (237) can compromise the prejunctional M_2 receptor. Circumstantial evidence indicates that a similar dysfunction of the M_2 receptors may exist in asthmatics (89). Alternatively, inflammation such as that precipitated by allergen exposure might increase the excitability of airway parasympathetic ganglion neurons (238).

Neurogenic inflammation can also alter parasympathetic nerve excitability. Parasympathetic ganglia innervating the airways of humans (92,196), guinea pigs (117,172), ferrets (195), and rats (94) have been shown to be innervated by tachykinin-containing nerve fibers. Exogenously administered tachykinin receptor agonists potentiate responses elicited by parasympathetic nerve stimulation, and indirect evidence indicates that endogenous release of the tachykinins facilitates parasympathetic synaptic neurotransmission(112,113,115). Electrophysiological and pharmacological analyses indicate that the effects of the endogenous tachykinins are mediated by NK_3 and NK_1 receptors (114,116,172). This is another potential mechanism, namely, peripheral activation of tachykinin-containing nerves that innervate airway ganglia, whereby GERD might alter autonomic tone in the airways.

V. Conclusion

Inflammation is a hallmark feature of asthma and is likely to precipitate the symptoms and potentially life-threatening exacerbations of the chronic airway disease. Gastroesophageal reflux disease is also a cause of asthma as treatment of an underlying reflux disorder can cure or markedly improve asthma symptoms in some patients. Future clinical studies that assess airway inflammation and its association with GERD and the effects of successful GERD therapy on airway inflammation will greatly enhance our understanding of the relationship between these disorders. Finally, a potential link between airway inflammation and GERD is the nervous system. Nerves are inextricably linked to the pathogenesis of inflammatory diseases, particularly the hyperalgesia that persists long after the initial inflammatory insult. The airways are densely innervated by nerves that might precipitate inflammation and might ultimately account for the airways hyperresponsiveness that is associated with asthma and related disorders. Tachykinins, which are localized to a specific subset of afferent nerves throughout the body and in the airways of all mammalian species studied including the human, may be key mediators of neurogenic inflammation. Studies carried out in animals confirm the potential role of nerves in airway inflammation, and with the recent development of several potent and selective tachykinin receptor antagonists (46), the potential role of nerves in asthma and airway inflammation in humans may soon be addressed.

Acknowledgments

The author thanks Mr. K. F. Canning and Ms. B. Hebden for their help in the preparation of this manuscript. The author also acknowledges the assistance of Dr. B. Undem and Dr. R. Kajekar in obtaining the data presented in the figures. This work was made possible by grants from the National Institutes of Health, Bethesda, MD.

References

1. Woolcock AJ. Definitions and clinical classifications. In: Barnes PJ, Grunstein MM, Leff AR, Woolcock AJ, eds. Asthma. Philadelphia: Lippincott-Raven, 1997:27–32.
2. National Heart, Lung and Blood Institute National Asthma Education Program. Expert Panel. Guidelines for the diagnosis and management of asthma. J Allergy Clin Immunol 1991; 88:425–434.
3. International Asthma Project. International consensus report on diagnosis and management of asthma. Eur Respir J 1992; 5:601–641.
4. Page C. Asthma as a chronic inflammatory disease and the implications for future therapy. Ann Allergy 1992; 69:251–260.
5. Sears MR. Is the routine use of inhaled β-adrenergic agonists appropriate in asthma treatment? No. Am J Respir Crit Care Med 1995; 151:600–601.
6. Alam R. Chemokines in allergic inflammation. J Allergy Clin Immunol 1997; 99: 273–277.
7. Bagley CJ, Lopez AF, Vadas MA. New frontiers for IL-5. J Allergy Clin Immunol 1997; 99:725–728.
8. Harding SM, Richter JE. The role of gastroesophageal reflux in chronic cough and asthma. Chest 1997; 111:1389–1402.
9. Mansfield LE. Gastroesophageal reflux and respiratory disorders: a review. Ann Allergy 1989; 62:158–163.
10. Sontag S, O'Connell S, Greenlee H, Schnell T, Chintam R, Nemchausky B, Chejfec G, Van Drunen M, Wanner J. Is gastroesophageal reflux a factor in some asthmatics? Am J Gastroenterol 1987; 82:119–126.
11. Tardiff C, Nouvet G, Denis P, Tombelaine R, Pasquis P. Surgical treatment of gastroesophageal reflux in ten patients with severe asthma. Respiration 1989; 56: 110–115.

12. Perrin-Fayolle M, Gormand F, Braillon G, Lombard-Platet R, Vignal J, Azzar D, Forichon J, Adeleine P. Long-term results of surgical treatment for gastroesophageal reflux in asthmatic patients. Chest 1989; 96:40–45.
13. Larrain A, Carrasco E, Galleguillos F, Sepulveda R, Pope CE. Medical and surgical treatment of nonallergic asthma associated with gastroesophageal reflux. Chest 1991; 99:1330–1335.
14. Harding SM, Richter JE, Guzzo MR, Schan CA, Alexander RW, Bradley LA. Asthma and gastroesophageal reflux: acid suppressive therapy improves asthma outcome. Am J Med 1996; 100:395–405.
15. Bruce AN. Vasodilator axon reflexes. Q J Exp Physiol 1913; 6:339–354.
16. Lewis, T. The nocifensor system of nerves and its reactions. Br Med J 1937; 1: 431–435.
17. Lewis, T. The nocifensor system of nerves and its reactions. Br Med J 1937; 1: 491–497.
18. Holzer P. Local effector functions of capsaicin-sensitive nerve endings: involvement of tachykinins, CGRP and other neuropeptides. Neuroscience 1988; 24:739–768.
19. Barnes PJ. Neural control of human airways in health and disease. Am Rev Respir Dis 1986; 134:1289–1314.
20. Simpson WG. Gastroesophageal reflux disease and asthma. Arch Intern Med 1995; 155:798–803
21. Irwin RS, Zawacki JK, Curley FJ, French CL, Hoffman PJ. Chronic cough as the sole manifestation of gastroesophageal reflux. Am Rev Respir Dis 1989; 140:1294–1300.
22. Irwin RS, French CL, Curley FJ, Zawacki JK, Bennett FM. Chronic cough due to gastroesophageal reflux. Chest 1993; 104:1511–1517.
23. Mansfield L, Stein MR. Gastroesophageal reflux and asthma: a possible reflex mechanism. Ann Allergy 1978; 41:224–226.
24. Herve P, Denjean A, Jian R, Simonneau G, Duroux P. Intraesophageal perfusion of acid increases the bronchomotor response to methacholine and to isocapnic hyperventilation in asthmatic subjects. Am Rev Respir Dis 1986; 134:986–989.
25. Andersen LI, Schmidt A, Bundgaard A. Pulmonary function and acid application in the esophagus. Chest 1986; 90:358–363.
26. Wright RA, Miller SA, Corsello BF. Acid-induced esophagobronchial-cardiac reflexes in humans. Gastroenterology 1990; 99:71–73.
27. Huber HL, Koessler KK. The pathology of bronchial asthma. Arch Intern Med 1922; 30:689–760.
28. Dunnill MS. The pathology of asthma, with special reference to changes in the bronchial mucosa. J Clin Pathol 1960; 13:27–33.
29. Dunnill MS, Massarella GR, Anderson JA. A comparison of the quantitative anatomy of the bronchi in normal subjects, in status asthmaticus, in chronic bronchitis and in emphysema. Thorax 1969; 24:176–179.
30. Djukanovic R, Roche WR, Wilson JW, Beasley CRW, Twentyman OP, Howarth PH, Holgate ST. Mucosal inflammation in asthma. Am Rev Respir Dis 1990; 142: 434–457.
31. Bousquet J, Chanez P, Lacoste JY, Barneon G, Ghavanian N, Enander I, Venge

P, Ahlstedt S, Simony-Lafontaine J, Godard P, Michel F-B. Eosinophilic inflammation in asthma. N Engl J Med 1990; 323:1033–1039.
32. Robinson DS, Hamid Q, Ying S, Bentley A, Assoufi B, Durham S, Kay AB. Prednisolone treatment in asthma is associated with modulation of bronchoalveolar lavage cell IL-4, IL-5 and IFN-gamma cytokine gene expression. Am Rev Respir Dis 1993; 148:401–406.
33. Smith DL, Deshazo RD. Bronchoalveolar lavage in asthma. Am Rev Respir Dis 1993; 148:523–532.
34. Bochner BS, Undem BJ, Lichtenstein LM. Immunological aspects of allergic asthma. Ann Rev Immunol 1994; 12:295–335.
35. Corrigan CJ, Kay AB. T lymphocytes in asthma pathogenesis. In: Barnes PJ, Grunstein MM, Leff AR, Woolcock AJ, eds. Asthma. Philadelphia: Lippincott-Raven, 1997:433–452.
36. Bjornsdottir US, Quan SF, Busse WW. Eosinophils and asthma. In: Busse WW, Holgate ST, eds. Asthma and Rhinitis. Boston: Blackwell Scientific Publications, 1995: 328–346.
37. Shimizu Y, Schwartz LB. Mast cell involvement in asthma. In: Barnes PJ, Grunstein MM, Leff AR and Woolcock AJ, eds. Asthma. Philadelphia: Lippincott-Raven, 1997:353–366.
38. Holgate ST, Bradding P, Sampson AP. Leukotriene antagonists and synthesis inhibitors: new directions in asthma therapy. J Allergy Clin Immunol 1996; 98:1–13.
39. Pedersen KE, Bochner B, Undem BJ. Cysteinyl leukotriene-induced P-selectin expression via non-Cys-LT1 receptor mechanism. J Pharmacol Exp Ther 1997; 282: 655–662.
40. Holgate ST, Church MK. The mast cell. Br Med Bull 1992; 48:40–50.
41. Fryer AD, Jacoby DB. Function of pulmonary M_2 muscarinic receptors in antigen challenged guinea-pigs is restored by heparin and poly-l-glutamate. J Clin Invest 1992; 90:2292–2298.
42. Weinstock JV, Blum AM. Release of substance P by granuloma eosinophils in response to secretogogues in schistosomiasis mansoni. Cell Immunol 1990; 125: 380–385.
43. Germonpre PR, Joos GF, Bulluck GR, Pauwels RA. Expression of substance P and its receptor by human sputum macrophages. Am J Respir Crit Care Med 1997; 155:A821.
44. Nieber K, Baumgarten CR, Rathsack R, Furkert J, Oehme P, Kunkel G. Substance P and β-endorphin-like immunoreactivity in lavage fluids of subjects with and without allergic asthma. J Allergy Clin Immunol 1992; 90:646–652.
45. Tomaki M, Ichinose M, Miura M, Hirayama Y, Yamauchi H, Nakajima N, Shirato K. Elevated substance P content in induced sputum from patients with asthma and patients with chronic bronchitis. Am J Respir Crit Care Med 1995; 151:613–617.
46. Canning BJ. Potential role of tachykinins in inflammatory diseases. J Allergy Clin Immunol 1997; 99(5):579–582.
47. Barnes PJ. Asthma as an axon reflex. Lancet 1986; 1:242–245.
48. McDonald DM. Neurogenic inflammation in the airways. In: Barnes PJ, ed. Autonomic Control of the Respiratory System. Amsterdam: Harwood Academic Publishers, 1997:249–290.

49. Undem BJ, Myers AC. Neural regulation of the immune response. In: Busse WW, Holgate ST, eds. Asthma and Rhinitis, 2d ed. Boston: Blackwell Scientific Publications, in press.
50. Ellis JL, Undem BJ, Kays JS, Ghanekar SV, Barthlow HG, Buckner CK. Pharmacological examination of receptors mediating contractile responses to tachykinins in airways isolated from human, guinea pig and hamster. J Pharmacol Exp Ther 1993; 267:95–101.
51. Michael JR, Markewitz BA. Endothelins and the lung. Am Rev Respir Crit Care Med 1996; 154:555–581.
52. Hay DWP, Goldie RG. Endothelins. In: Barnes PJ, Grunstein MM, Leff AR, Woolcock AJ, eds. Asthma. Philadelphia: Lippincott-Raven, 1997:707–729.
53. Farmer SG, ed. The Kinin System. London: Academic Press, 1997.
54. Toews GB. Macrophages. In: Barnes PJ, Grunstein MM, Leff AR, Woolcock AJ, eds. Asthma. Philadelphia: Lippincott-Raven, 1997:381–398.
55. Mauser PJ, Pitman AM, Fernandez X, Foran SK, Adams III GK, Kreutner W, Egan RW, Chapman RW. Effects of an antibody to interleukin-5 in a monkey model of asthma. Am J Respir Crit Care Med 1995; 152:467–472.
56. Foster PS, Hogan SP, Ramsay AJ, Matthaei KI, Young IG. Interleukin 5 deficiency abolishes eosinophilia, airways hyperreactivity, and lung damage in a mouse asthma model. J Exp Med 1996; 183:195–201.
57. Stellato C, Schwiebert LM, Schleimer RP. Mechanisms of glucocorticoid action. In: Barnes PJ, Grunstein MM, Leff A, Woolcock AJ, eds. Asthma. Philadelphia: Lippincott-Raven Publishers, 1997:1569–1596.
58. Peat JK, Britton WJ, Salome CM, Woolcock AJ. Bronchial hyperresponsiveness in two populations of Australian schoolchildren. III. Effect of exposure to environmental allergens. Clin Exp Allergy 1987; 17:291–300.
59. Sears MR, Burrows B, Flannery EM, Herbison GP, Hewitt CJ, Holdaway MD. Relationship between airway responsiveness and serum IgE in children with asthma and in apparently normal children. N Engl J Med 1991; 325:1067–1071.
60. Church MK, Levi-Schaffer F. The human mast cell. J Allergy Clin Immunol 1997; 99:155–160.
61. Sedgwick JB, Calhoun WJ, Gleich GJ, Kita H, Abrams JS, Schwartz LB, Volovitz B, Ben-Yaakov M, Busse W. Immediate and late airway response of allergic rhinitis patients to segmental antigen challenge. Am Rev Respir Dis 1991; 144:1274–1281.
62. Mehlhop PD, Van de Rijn M, Goldberg AB, Brewer JP, Kurup VP, Martin TR, Oettgen HC. Allergen-induced bronchial hyperreactivity and eosinophilic inflammation occur in the absence of IgE in a mouse model of asthma. Proc Natl Acad Sci USA. 1997; 94:1344–1349.
63. Robinson DS, Hamid Q, Ying S, Tsicopoulos A, Barkans J, Bentley AM, Corrigan CJ, Durham SR, Kay AB. Predominant T_{H2}-like bronchoalveolar T-lymphocyte population in atopic asthma. N Engl J Med 1992; 326:298–304.
64. Mosmann TR, Coffman RL. T_{H1} and T_{H2} cells: different patterns of lymphokine secretion lead to different functional properties. Ann Rev Immunol 1989; 7:145–173.
65. Borish L, Rosenwasser L. T_{H1}/T_{H2}: doubt some more. J Allergy Clin Immunol 1997; 99:161–164.

66. Umetsu DT, DeKruyff RH. T_{H1} and T_{H2} CD4+ cells in human allergic diseases. J Allergy Clin Immunol 1997; 100:1–6.
67. Schroeder JT, MacGlashan, Jr. DW. New concepts: the basophil. J Allergy Clin Immunol 1997; 99:429–433.
68. Berquist WE, Rachelefsky GS, Kadden M, Siegel SC, Katz RM, Fonkalsrud ES, Ament ME. Gastroesophageal reflux associated with recurrent pneumonia and chronic asthma in children. Pediatrics 1981; 68:29–35.
69. Goodall RJR, Earis JE, Cooper DN, Bernstein A, Temple JG. Relationship between asthma and gastro-esophageal reflux. Thorax 1981; 36:116–121.
70. Sontag SJ, O'Connell S, Khandelwal S, Miller T, Nemchausky B, Schnell TG, Serlovsky R. Most asthmatics have reflux with or without bronchodilator therapy. Gastroenterology 1990; 99:613–620.
71. Sontag SJ, Schnell TG, Miller TQ, Khandelwal S, O'Connell S, Chejfec G, Greenlee H, Seidel UJ, Brand L. Prevalence of oesophagitis in asthmatics. Gut 1992; 33:872–876.
72. Bentley AM, Menz G, Storz C, Robinson DS, Bradley B, Jeffery PK, Durham SR, Kay AB. Identification of T-lymphocytes, macrophages, and activated eosinophils in the bronchial mucosa in intrinsic asthma—relationship to symptoms and bronchial responsiveness. Am Rev Respir Dis 1992; 146:500–506.
73. Walker C, Bode E, Boer L, Hansel TT, Blaser K, Virchow JC, Jr. Allergic and nonallergic asthmatics have distinct patterns of T-cell activation and cytokine production in peripheral blood and bronchoalveolar lavage. Am Rev Respir Dis 1992; 146:109–115.
74. Humbert M, Grant JA, Taborda-Barata L, Durham SR, Pfister R, Menz G, Barkans J, Ying S, Kay AB. High-affinity IgE receptor (FceR1)-bearing cells in bronchial biopsies from atopic and nonatopic asthma. Am J Respir Crit Care Med 1996; 153: 1931–1937.
75. Humbert M, Durham SR, Ying S, Kimmitt P, Barkans J, Assoufi B, Pfister R, Menz G, Robinson DS, Kay AB, Corrigan CJ. IL-4 and IL-5 mRNA and protein in bronchial biopsies from patients with atopic and nonatopic asthma: evidence against ''intrinsic'' asthma being a distinct immunopathologic entity. Am J Respir Crit Care Med 1996; 154:1497–1504.
76. Humbert M, Ying S, Corrigan C, Menz G, Barkans J, Pfister R, Meng Q, Damme JV, Opdenakker G, Durham SR, Kay AB. Bronchial mucosal expression of the genes encoding chemokines RANTES and MCP-3 in symptomatic atopic and nonatopic asthmatics: relationship to the eosinophil-active cytokines interleukin (IL)-5, granulocyte macrophage-colony-stimulating factor and IL-3. Am J Respir Cell Mol Biol 1997; 16:1–8.
77. Fowler III AA, Hamman RF, Good JT. Adult respiratory distress syndrome: risk with common predispositions. Ann Intern Med 1983; 98:593–597.
78. Wynne JW, Modell JH. Respiratory aspiration of stomach contents. Ann Intern Med 1977; 87:466–474.
79. Schwartz DJ, Wynne JW, Gibbs CP, Hood CI, Kuck EJ. The pulmonary consequences of aspiration of gastric contents at pH values greater than 2.5. Am Rev Respir Dis 1980; 121:119–126.
80. Goldman G, Welbourn R, Kobzik L, Valeri CR, Shepro D, Hechtman HB. Reactive

oxygen species and elastase mediate lung permeability after acid aspiration. J Appl Physiol 1992; 73:571–575.
81. Goldman G, Welbourn R, Kobzik L, Valeri CR. Shepro D, Hechtman HB. Tumor necrosis factor-α mediates acid aspiration-induced systemic organ injury. Ann Surg 1990; 212:513–520.
82. Folkesson HG, Mathay MA, Hebert CA, Broaddus VC. Acid aspiration-induced lung injury in rabbits is mediated by interleukin-8-dependent mechanisms. J Clin Invest 1995; 96:107–116.
83. Nagase T, Ohga E, Sudo E, Katayama H, Uejima Y, Matsuse T, Fukuchi Y. Intercellular adhesion molecule-1 mediates acid aspiration-induced lung injury. Am J Respir Crit Care Med 1996; 154:504–510.
84. Maggi CA, Meli A. The sensory-efferent function of capsaicin-sensitive sensory neurons. Gen Pharmacol 1988; 19:1–43.
85. Cervero F. Sensory innervation of the viscera: peripheral basis of visceral pain. Physiol Rev 1994; 74:95–138.
86. Salter HH. Asthma: Its Pathology and Treatment. New York: William Wood & Company, 1882.
87. Macklin CC. The musculature of the bronchi and lungs. Physiol Rev 1929; 9:1–60.
88. Szentivanyi A. The beta adrenergic theory of atopic abnormality in bronchial asthma. J Allergy 1968; 42:203–232.
89. Smart SJ, Casale TB. Abnormal autonomic control in respiratory disease. In: Barnes PJ, ed. Autonomic Control of the Respiratory System. Amsterdam: Harwood Academic Publishers, 1997:313–338.
90. Jancsó N, Jancsó-Gábor A, Szolcsányi J. Direct evidence for neurogenic inflammation and its prevention by denervation and by pretreatment with capsaicin. Br J Pharmacol Chemother 1967; 31:138–151.
91. Maggi CA, Patacchini R, Rovero P, Giachetti A. Tachykinin receptors and tachykinin receptor antagonists. J Auton Pharmacol 1993; 13:23–93.
92. Lundberg JM, Hökfelt T, Martling C-R, Saria A, Cuello C. Substance P-immunoreactive sensory nerves in the lower respiratory tract of various mammals including man. Cell Tiss Res 1984; 235:251–261.
93. Kummer W, Fischer A, Kurkowski R, Heym C. The sensory and sympathetic innervation of guinea-pig lung and trachea as studied by retrograde neuronal tracing and double-labeling immunohistochemistry. Neuroscience 1992; 49:715–737.
94. Baluk P, Nadel JA, McDonald DM. Substance P-immunoreactive sensory axons in the rat respiratory tract: a quantitative study of their distribution and role in neurogeneic inflammation. J Comp Neurol 1992; 319:586–598.
95. Otsuka M, Yoshioka K. Neurotransmitter functions of mammalian tachykinins. Physiol Rev 1993; 73:229–308.
96. Coleridge HM, Coleridge JCG, Schultz HD. Afferent pathways involved in reflex regulation of airway smooth muscle. Pharmacol Ther 1989; 42:1–63.
97. Hathaway T, Higenbottam T, Lowry R, Wallwork J. Pulmonary reflexes after human heart-lung transplantation. Respir Med 1991; 85 (suppl A):17–21.
98. Hobson CE, Teague WG, Tribble CG, Mills SE, Chan B, Agee J, Flanagan TL, Kron IL. Denervation of transplanted porcine lung causes airway obstruction. Ann Thorac Surg 1991; 52:1295–1299.

99. Turner CR, Stow RB, Talerico SD, Christian EP, Williams JC. Protective role for neuropeptides in acute pulmonary response to acrolein in guinea pigs. J Appl Physiol 1993; 75:2456–2465.
100. Tepper JS, Costa DL, Fitzgerald S. Role of tachykinins in ozone-induced acute lung injury in guinea pigs. Am J Physiol 1993; 75:1404–1411.
101. Bowden JJ, Baluk P, Lefevre PM, Schoeb TR, Lindsey JR, McDonald DM. Sensory denervation by neonatal capsaicin pretreatment exacerbates Mycoplasma pulmonis infection in rat airways. Am J Physiol 1996; 270:L393–L403.
102. Lundberg JM, Saria A. Capsaicin-induced desensitization of airway mucosa to cigarette smoke, mechanical and chemical irritants. Nature 1983; 302:251–253.
103. Baluk P, Thurston G, Bunnett NW, McDonald DM. Neurogenic plasma leakage in mouse airways. Am Rev Respir Crit Care Med 1997; 155:A485.
104. Bertrand C, Geppetti P, Baker J, Yamawaki I, Nadel JA. Role of neurogenic inflammation in antigen-induced vascular extravasation in guinea pig trachea. J Immunol 1993; 150:1479–1485.
105. Baluk P, Bertrand C, Geppetti P, McDonald DM, Nadel JA NK_1 receptors mediate leukocyte adhesion in neurogenic inflammation in the rat trachea. Am J Physiol 1995; 268:L263–L269.
106. Sakamoto T, Barnes PJ, Chung KF. Effect of CP-96,345, a nonpeptide NK_1 receptor antagonist, against substance P-, bradykinin- and allergen-induced airway microvascular leak and bronchoconstriction the guinea pig. Eur J Pharmacol 1993; 231: 31–38.
107. Hamamoto J, Kohrogi H, Kawano O, Iwagoe H, Fujii K, Hirata N, Ando MI. Esophageal stimulation by hydrochloric acid causes neurogenic inflammation in the airways in guinea pigs. J Appl Physiol 1997; 82:738–745.
108. Martling CR, Lundberg JM. Capsaicin-sensitive afferents contribute to acute airway edema following tracheal instillation of hydrochloric acid or gastric juice in the rat. Anesthesiology 1988; 68:350–356.
109. Garland A, Ray DW, Doerschuk CM, Alger L, Eappon S, Hernandez C, Jackson M, Solway J. Role of tachykinins in hyperpnea-induced bronchovascular hyperpermeability in guinea pigs. J Appl Physiol 1991; 70:27–35.
110. Umeno E, McDonald DM, Nadel JA. Hypertonic saline increases vascular permeability in the rat trachea by producing neurogenic inflammation. J Clin Invest 1990; 85:1905–1908.
111. Piedimonte G, Bertrand C, Geppetti P, Snider RM, Desai MC, Nadel JA. A new NK_1 receptor antagonist (CP-99,994) prevents the increase in tracheal vascular permeability produced by hypertonic saline. J Pharmacol Exp Ther 1993; 266:270–273.
112. Martling C-R, Saria A, Anderson P, Lundberg JM. Capsaicin pretreatment inhibits vagal cholinergic and non-cholinergic control of pulmonary mechanics in the guinea pig. Naunyn-Schmiedeberg's Arch Pharmacol 1984; 325:343–348.
113. Myers AC, Undem BJ. Functional interactions between capsaicin-sensitive and cholinergic nerves in the guinea pig bronchus. J Pharmacol Exp Ther 1991; 259: 104–109.
114. Myers AC, Undem BJ. Electrophysiological effects of tachykinins and capsaicin on guinea-pig bronchial parasympathetic ganglion neurones. J Physiol 1993; 470: 665–679.

115. Watson N, Maclagan J, Barnes PJ. Endogenous tachykinins facilitate transmission through parasympathetic ganglia in guinea-pig trachea. Br J Pharmacol 1993; 109: 751–759.
116. Canning BJ, Undem BJ. Evidence that antidromically stimulated vagal afferents activate inhibitory neurons innervating guinea pig trachealis. J Physiol 1994; 480: 613–625.
117. Myers AC, Undem BJ, Kummer W. Anatomical and electrophysiological comparison of the sensory innervation of bronchial and tracheal parasympathetic ganglia. J Auton Nerv Syst 1996; 61:162–168.
118. Rogers DF. Neural control of airway secretions. In: Barnes PJ, ed. Autonomic Control of the Respiratory System. Amsterdam: Harwood Academic Publishers, 1997: 201–228.
119. Ellis JL, Undem BJ. Pharmacology of non-adrenergic, non-cholinergic nerves in airway smooth muscle. Pulm Pharmacol 1994; 7:205–223.
120. McDonald DM. Neurogenic inflammation in the rat trachea. I. Changes in venules, leukocytes and epithelial cells. J Neurocytol 1988; 17:583–603.
121. Umeno E, Nadel JA, McDonald DM. Neurogenic inflammation of the rat trachea: fate of neutrophils that adhere to venules. J Appl Physiol 1990; 69:2131–2136.
122. Fox AJ, Urban L, Barnes PJ, Dray A. Effects of capsazepine against capsaicin- and proton-evoked excitation of single airway c-fibres and vagus nerve from the guinea-pig. Neuroscience 1995; 67:741–752.
123. Riccio MM, Myers AC, Undem BJ. Immunomodulation of afferent neurons in guinea-pig isolated airway. J Physiol 1996; 491:499–509.
124. Canning BJ, Undem BJ. Evidence that distinct neural pathways mediate parasympathetic contractions and relaxations of guinea-pig trachealis. J Physiol 1993; 471: 25–40.
125. Canning BJ, Undem BJ, Karakousis PC, Dey RD. Effects of organotypic culture on parasympathetic innervation of guinea pig trachealis. Am J Physiol 1996; 271: L698–L706.
126. Fischer A, Canning BJ, Undem BJ, Kummer W. Evidence for an esophageal origin of VIP- and NO synthase-IR nerves innervating the guinea pig trachealis: a retrograde neuronal tracing, immunohistochemical analysis. J Comp Neurol 1998; 394: 326–334.
127. Braunstein G, Fajac I, Lacronique J, Frossard N. Clinical and inflammatory responses to exogenous tachykinins in allergic rhinitis. Am Rev Respir Dis 1991; 144:630–635.
128. Philip G, Sanico AM, Togias A. Inflammatory cellular influx follows capsaicin nasal challenge. Am J Respir Crit Care Med 1996; 153:1222–1229.
129. Lotti T, Hautmann G, Panconesi E. Neuropeptides in skin. J Am Acad Dermatol 1995; 33:482–496.
130. Joos GF, Germonpre PR, Pauwels RA. Neurogenic inflammation in human airways: Is it important? Thorax 1995; 50:217–219.
131. Naline E, Molimard M, Regoli D, Emonds-Alt X, Bellamy J-F, Advenier C. Evidence for functional tachykinin NK_1 receptors on human isolated small bronchi. Am J Physiol. 271:L763–L767.
132. Myers AC, Hay DWP. Personal communication.

133. Carstairs JR, Barnes PJ. Autoradiographic mapping of substance P receptors in lung. Eur J Pharmacol 1986; 127:295–296.
134. Yu X-Y, Undem BJ, Spannhake EW. Protective effect of substance P on permeability of airway epithelial cells in culture. Am J Physiol 1996; 271:L889–L895.
135. Fuller RW. Pharmacology of inhaled capsaicin in humans. Respir Med 1991; 85 (suppl A):31–34.
136. Barnes PJ, Baraniuk JN, Belvisi MG. Neuropeptides in the respiratory tract. Part I. Am Rev Respir Dis 1991; 144:1187–1198.
137. Barnes PJ, Baraniuk JN, Belvisi MG. Neuropeptides in the respiratory tract. Part II. Am Rev Respir Dis 1991; 144:1391–1399.
138. Adcock IM, Peters M, Gelder C, Shirasaki H, Brown CR, Barnes PJ. Increased tachykinin receptor gene expression in asthmatic lung and its modulation by steroids. J Mol Endocrinol 1993; 11:1–7.
139. Bai TR, Zhou D, Weir T, Walker B, Hegele R, Hayashi S, McKay K, Bondy GP, Fong T. Substance P (NK_1)- and neurokinin A (NK_2)-receptor gene expression in inflammatory airway diseases. Am J Physiol 1995; 269:L309–L317.
140. Ollerenshaw SL, Jarvis D, Sullivan CE, Woolcock AJ. Substance P immunoreactive nerves in airways from asthmatics and nonasthmatics. Eur Respir J 1991; 4:673–682.
141. Howarth PH, Djukanovic R, Wilson JW, Holgate ST, Springall DR, Polak JM. Mucosal nerves in endobronchial biopsies in asthma and non-asthma. Int Arch Allergy Appl Immunol 1991; 94:330–333.
142. Lilly CM, Bai TR, Shore SA, Hall AE, Drazen JM. Neuropeptide content of lungs from asthmatics and nonasthmatic patients. Am J Respir Crit Care Med 1995; 151:548–553.
143. Daoui S, Cognon C, Emonds-Alt X, Advenier C. Effects of the specific tachykinin NK_3 receptor antagonist, SR 142801 (osanetant), on citric acid-induced cough and bronchoconstriction in guinea-pigs. Am J Respir Crit Care Med. 1997; 155:A576.
144. Bolser DC, DeGennaro FC, O'Reilly S, McLeod RL, Hey JA. Central antitussive activity of the NK_1 and NK_2 tachykinin receptor antagonists, CP-99,994 and SR 48968, in the guinea pig and cat. Br J Pharmacol 1997; 121:165–170.
145. Pain—mechanisms and management. Br Med J 1991; 47:523–675.
146. Schaible H-G, Schmidt RF. Effects of an experimental arthritis on the sensory properties of fine articular afferent units. J Neurophysiol 1985; 54:1109–1122.
147. Undem BJ, Weinreich D. Electrophysiological properties and chemosensitivity of guinea pig nodose ganglion neurons in vitro. J Auton Nerv Syst 1993;44:17–34.
148. McCarson KE, Krause JE. NK-1 and NK-3 type tachykinin receptor mRNA expression in the rat spinal cord dorsal horn is increased during adjuvant or formalin-induced nociception. J Neurosci 1994; 14:712–720.
149. Urban L, Thompson SWN, Dray A. Modulation of spinal excitability: co-operation between neurokinin and excitatory amino acid neurotransmitters. Trends Neurosci 1994; 17:432–438.
150. McCarson KE, Goldstein BD. Naloxone blocks the formalin-induced increase of substance P in the dorsal horn. Pain 1989; 38:339–345.
151. Simonsson B, Jacobs F, Nadel JA. Role of autonomic nervous system and the cough

reflex in the increased responsiveness of the airways in patients with obstructive airway disease. J Clin Invest 1968; 46:1812–1818.
152. Boushey HA, Holtzman MA, Sheller JR, Nadel JA. Bronchial hyperreactivity. Am Rev Respir Dis 1980; 121:389–413.
153. Morley J. Parasympatholytics in asthma. Pulm Pharmacol 1994; 7:159–168.
154. Gross NJ. Anticholinergic drugs. In: Barnes PJ, Grunstein MM, Leff AR, Woolcock AJ, eds. Asthma. Philadelphia: Lippincott-Raven, 1997:1555–1569.
155. Baraniuk JN, Silver PB, Kaliner MA, Barnes PJ. Perennial rhinitis subjects have altered vascular, glandular and neural responses to nasal bradykinin provocation. Int Arch Allergy Clin Immunol 1994; 103:202–208.
156. Riccio MM, Proud D. Evidence that enhanced nasal reactivity to bradykinin in patients with symptomatic allergy is mediated by neural reflexes. J Allergy Clin Immunol 1996; 97:1252–1263.
157. Riccio MM, Reynolds CR, Hay DWP, Proud D. Effects of intranasal administration of endothelin-1 to allergic and nonallergic individuals. Am Rev Respir Crit Care Med 1995; 152:1757–1764.
158. Undem BJ, Hubbard W, Weinreich D. Immunologically induced neuromodulation of guinea pig nodose ganglion neurons. J Auton Nerv Syst 1993; 44:35–44.
159. Matsuse T, Thomson RJ, Chen X-R, Salari H, Schellenberg RR. Capsaicin inhibits airway hyperresponsiveness but not lipoxygenase activity or eosinophilia after repeated aerosolized antigen in guinea pigs. Am Rev Respir Dis 1991; 144:368–372.
160. Advenier C, Daouli S, Cui Y-Y, Lagente V, Emonds-Alt X. Inhibition by the tachykinin NK_3 receptor antagonist, SR 142801, of substance P-induced microvascular leakage hypersensitivity and airway hyper-responsiveness in guinea-pigs. Am J Respir Crit Care Med 1996; 153:A163.
161. Boichot E, Germain N, Lagente V, Advenier C. Prevention by the tachykinin NK_2 receptor antagonist, SR 48968, of antigen-induced airway hyperresponsiveness in sensitized guinea pigs. Br J Pharmacol 1995; 114:259–261.
162. Turner CR, Andersen C, Patterson D, Keir R, Obach S, Lee P, Watson J. Dual antagonism of NK_1 and NK_2 receptors by CP 99994 and SR 48968 prevents airway hyperresponsiveness in primates. Am J Respir Crit Care Med 1995; 153:A160.
163. Mizuguchi M, Fujimura M, Amemiya T, Nishi K, Ohka T, Matsuda T. NK_2 receptors rather than NK_1 receptors are involved in bronchial hyperresponsiveness induced by allergic reaction in guinea pigs. Br J Pharmacol 1996; 117:443–449.
164. Fischer A, McGregor GP, Saria A, Philippin B, Kummer W. Induction of tachykinin gene and peptide expression in guinea pig nodose primary afferent neurons by allergic airway inflammation. J Clin Invest 1996; 98:2284–2291.
165. Saito H, Tsukiji J, Ikeda H, Okubo T. Nerve growth factor increases the substance P contents of the adult guinea pig airway and nodose ganglion. Am J Respir Crit Care Med 1996; 153:A163.
166. Bonini S, Lambiase A, Bonini S, Angelucci F, Magrini l, Manni L, Aloe L. Circulating nerve growth factor levels are increased in humans with allergic diseases and asthma. Proc Natl Acad Sci USA 1996; 93:10955–10960.
167. Cunha FQ, Lorenzetti BB, Poole S, Ferriera SH. Interleukin-8 as a mediator of sympathetic pain. Br J Pharmacol 1991; 104:765–767.
168. Fujimura M, Tsujiura M, Nomura M, Mizuguchi M, Matsuda T, Matsushima K.

Sensory neuropeptides are not directly involved in bronchial hyperresponsiveness induced by interleukin-8 in guinea pigs in vivo. Clin Exp Allergy 1996; 26:357–362.
169. Kurose I, Suematsu M, Miura S, Fukumura D, Serizawa H, Nagata H, Tashiro H, Imaeda H, Tashiro H, Shiozaki H, Suematsu M, Sekizuka E, Tsuchiya M. In vivo mucosal and submucosal microvascular response in the rat stomach during autonomic nervous irritation. In: Yoshikawa M, ed. New Trends in Autonomic Nervous System Research: Basic and Clinical Integration. Amsterdam: Elsevier Science Publishers, 1991:179–183.
170. Wilson NM, Chudry N, Silverman M. Role of the oesophagus in asthma induced by the ingestion of ice and acid. Thorax 1987; 42:506–510.
171. Lundberg JM, Brodin E, Saria A. Effects and distribution of vagal capsaicin-sensitive substance P neurons with special reference to the trachea and lungs. Acta Physiol Scand 1983; 119:243–252.
172. Canning BJ, Fischer A, Undem BJ. Pharmacological analysis of the tachykinin receptors mediating activation of nonadrenergic, noncholinergic relaxant nerves innervating guinea pig trachealis. J Pharmacol Exp Ther 1998; 284:370–377.
173. Canning BJ, Fischer A. Localization of cholinergic nerves in lower airways of guinea pigs using antisera to choline acetyltransferase. Am J Physiol 1997; 272: L731–L738
174. Moffatt JD. Studies on the nonadrenergic, noncholinergic innervation of airway smooth muscle. Ph.D. dissertation. University of Melbourne, Parkville, Victoria, Australia, 1997.
175. Kalia M, Mesulam MM. Brain stem projections of sensory and motor components of the vagus complex in the cat: I. The cervical vagus and nodose ganglia. J Comp Neurol 1980; 193: 435–465.
176. Kalia M, Mesulam M-M. Brain stem projections of sensory and motor components of the vagus complex in the cat: II. Laryngeal, tracheobronchial pulmonary, cardiac, and gastrointestinal branches. J Comp Neurol 1980; 193:467–508.
177. Dale HH. A survey of present knowledge of the chemical regulation of certain functions by natural constituents of the tissues. Bull Johns Hopkins Hosp 1933; 53:297–347.
178. Dale H. Pharmacology and nerve-endings. Proc R Soc Med 1935; 28:319–332.
179. Dale HH. Symposium on neurohumoral transmission. Pharmacol Rev 1954; 6:1–131.
180. Morris JL, Gibbins IL. Co-transmission and neuromodulation. In: Burnstock G, Hoyle V, eds. Autonomic Neuroeffector Mechanisms. Reading, England: Harwood Academic Publishers, 1992:33–119.
181. Langley JN. The Autonomic Nervous System. Cambridge: W. Heffer & Sons, Ltd., 1921.
182. Canning BJ, Undem BJ. Parasympathetic innervation of airway smooth muscle. In: Raeburn D, Gymbiecz M, eds. Airways Smooth Muscle: Structure Innervation and Neurotransmission. Basel: Birkhauser Verlag AG, 1994:43–77.
183. Coleridge HM, Coleridge JCG. Neural regulation of bronchial blood flow. Respir Physiol 1994; 98:1–13
184. Matran, R. Neural control of lower airway vasculature—involvement of classical transmitters and neuropeptides. Acta Physiol Scand 1991; (suppl 601):1–54.

185. Coburn RF, Tomita T. Evidence for nonadrenergic inhibitory nerves in the guinea pig trachealis muscle. Am J Physiol 1973; 224:1072–1080.
186. Coleman RA, Levy GP. A non-adrenergic inhibitory nervous pathway in guinea-pig trachea. Br J Pharmacol 1974; 52:167–174.
187. Richardson J, Beland J. Nonadrenergic inhibitory nervous system in human airways. J Appl Physiol 1976; 41:764–771.
188. Chesrown SE, Venugopalan CS, Gold WM, Drazen JM. In vivo demonstration of nonadrenergic inhibitory innervation of the guinea pig trachea. J Clin Invest 1980; 65:314–320.
189. Yip P, Palombini B, Coburn RF. Inhibitory innervation to the guinea pig trachealis muscle. J Appl Physiol 1981; 50:374–382.
190. Irvin CG, Boileau R, Tremblay J, Martin RR, Macklem PT. Bronchodilatation: noncholinergic, nonadrenergic mediation demonstrated in vivo in the cat. Science 1980; 207:791–792.
191. Diamond L, O'Donnell M. A nonadrenergic vagal inhibitory pathway to feline airways. Science 1980; 208:185–188.
192. Dey RD, Shannon WA, Said SI. Localization of VIP-immunoreactive nerves in airways and pulmonary vessels of dogs, cats, and human subjects. Cell Tissue Res 1981; 220:231–238.
193. Laitinen A, Partanen M, Hervonen A, Pelto-Huikko M, Laitinen LA. VIP-like immunoreactive nerves in human respiratory tract. Histochemistry 1985; 82:313–319.
194. Lundberg JM, Fahrenkrug J, Hökfelt T, Martling C-R, Larsson O, Tatemoto K, Änggard A. Co-existence of peptide HI (PHI) and VIP in nerves regulating blood flow and bronchial smooth muscle tone in various mammals including man. Peptides 1984; 5:593–606.
195. Dey RD, Altemus JB, Rodd A, Mayer B, Said SI, Coburn RF. Neurochemical characterization of intrinsic neurons in ferret tracheal plexus. Am J Respir Cell Mol Biol 1996; 14:207–216.
196. Fischer A, Hoffmann B. Nitric oxide synthase in neurons and nerve fibers of lower airways and in vagal sensory ganglia of man. Am J Respir Crit Care Med 1996; 154:209–216.
197. Kobzik L, Bredt DS, Lowenstein CJ, Drazen J, Gaston B, Sugarbaker D, Stamler JS. Nitric oxide synthase in human and rat lung: Immunocytochemical and histochemical localization. Am J Respir Cell Mol Biol 1993; 9:371–377.
198. Buttery LDK, Springall DR, daCosta FAM, Oliviera H, Hislop AA, Haworth SG, Polak JM. Early abundance of nerves containing NO synthase in the airways of newborn pigs and subsequent decrease with age. Neurosci Lett 1995; 201:219–222.
199. Ward JK, Barnes PJ, Springall DR, Abelli L, Tadjkarimi S, Yacoub MH, Polak JM, Belvisi MB. Distribution of human i-NANC bronchodilator and nitric oxide-immunoreactive nerves. Am J Respir Cell Mol Biol 1995; 13:175–184.
200. Keith IM, Pelto-Huikko M, Schalling M, Hökfelt T. Calcitonin gene-related peptide and its mRNA in pulmonary neuroendocrine cells and ganglia. Histochemistry 1991; 96:311–315.
201. Dey RD, Hoffpauir J, Said SI. Co-localization of vasoactive intestinal peptide- and substance P-containing nerves in cat bronchi. Neuroscience 1988; 24:275–281.

202. Cheung A, Polak JM, Bauer FE, Cadieux A, Christofides ND, Springall DR, Bloom SR. Distribution of galanin immunoreactivity in the respiratory tract of pig, guinea pig, rat and dog. Thorax 1985; 40:889–896.
203. Bowden JJ, Gibbins IL. Colocalisation of neurotransmitters in autonomic neurons supplying the respiratory tract of various species, including humans (abstr). Am Rev Respir Dis 1992; 145:A259.
204. Dey R, Zhu W. Origin of galanin nerves of cat airways and co-localization with vasoactive intestinal peptide. Cell Tiss Res 1993; 273:193–200.
205. Domeij S, Dahlqvist A, Forsgren S. Studies on colocalization of neuropeptide Y, vasoactive intestinal polypeptide, catecholamine-synthesizing enzymes and acetylcholinesterase in the larynx of the rat. Cell Tiss Res 1991; 263:495–505.
206. Krekel J, Weihe E, Nohr D, Yanaihara N, Weber E. Distribution of met-enkephalyl-arg-gly-leu in rat larynx: partial coexistence with vasoactive intestinal polypeptide, peptide histidine isoleucine and neuropeptide Y. Neurosci Lett 1990; 119:64–67.
207. Burnstock G, Allen TGJ, Hassall CJS. The electrophysiologic and neurochemical properties of paratracheal neurones in situ and in dissociated cell culture. Am Rev Respir Dis 1987; 136:S23–S26.
208. Shimosegawa T, Foda HD, Said SI. [MET]Enkephalin-arg^6-gly^7-leu^8-immunoreactive nerves in guinea-pig and rat lungs: distribution, origin, and co-existence with vasoactive intestinal polypeptide immunoreactivity. Neuroscience 1990; 36:737–750.
209. Canning BJ, Fischer A. Localization of heme oxygenase-2 (HO-2) immunoreactivity to parasympathetic ganglia of human and guinea pig airways. Am J Respir Cell Mol Biol 1998; 18:279–285.
210. Haberberger R, Schemann M, Sann H, Kummer W. Innervation pattern of guinea pig pulmonary vasculature depends on vascular diameter. J Appl Physiol 1997; 82:426–434.
211. Lundberg JM. Evidence for coexistence of vasoactive intestine polypeptide (VIP) and acetylcholine in neurones of cat exocrine glands—morphological, biochemical and functional studies. Acta Physiol Scand 1981; 496(suppl):1–57.
212. Barnes PJ. Other regulatory peptides. In: Barnes PJ, Grunstein MM, Leff AR, Woolcock AJ, eds. Asthma. Philadelphia: Lippincott-Raven, 1997:1065–1076.
213. Ichinose M, Inoue H, Miura M, Yafuso N, Nogami H, Takishima T. Possible sensory receptor of nonadrenergic inhibitory nervous system. J Appl Physiol 1987; 63:923–929.
214. Don H, Baker DG, Richardson CA. Absence of nonadrenergic noncholinergic relaxation in the cat cervical trachea. J Appl Physiol 1988; 65:2524–2530.
215. Lama A, Delpierre S, Jammes Y. The effects of electrical stimulation of myelinated and nonmyelinated vagal motor fibers on airway tone in the rabbit and the cat. Respir Physiol 1988; 74:265–274.
216. Barnes, PJ, Belvisi MG. Nitric oxide and lung disease. Thorax 1993; 48:1034–1043.
217. Fischer, A, Canning BJ, Kummer W. Correlation of vasoactive intestinal peptide and nitric oxide synthase with choline acetyltransferase in the airway innervation. Ann NY Acad Sci 1996; 805:717–722.
218. Burden DT, Parkes MW, Gardiner DG. Effect of β-adrenoceptive blocking agents

on the response to bronchoconstrictor drugs in the guinea-pig air overflow preparations. Br J Pharmacol 1971; 41:122–131.
219. Cabezas GA, Graf PD, Nadel JA. Sympathetic versus parasympathetic nervous regulation of airways in dogs. J Appl Physiol 1971; 31:651–655.
220. Drazen JM. Adrenergic influences on histamine-mediated bronchoconstriction in the guinea pig. J Appl Physiol 1978; 44:340–345.
221. Underwood DC, Mathews JK, Osborn RR, Novak LB, Bochnowitz S, Meunier L. Catecholamine and β-adrenoceptor influences on airway reactivity to antigen in guinea pigs. Int Arch Allergy Clin Immunol 1996; 109:286–294.
222. Bowden JJ, Gibbins IL. Vasoactive intestinal peptide and neuropeptide Y coexist in nonadrenergic sympathetic neurons to guinea pig trachea. J Auton Nerv Syst 1992; 38:1–20.
223. Fischer, A, Mayer B, Kummer W. Nitric oxide synthase in vagal sensory and sympathetic neurons innervating the guinea-pig trachea. J Auton Nerv Sys 1996; 56(3): 157–160.
224. Frieling T, Cooke HJ, Wood JD. Neuroimmune communication in the submucous plexus of guinea pig colon after sensitization to milk antigen. Am J Physiol 1994; 267:G1087–G1093.
225. Weinreich D, Undem BJ. Immunological regulation of synaptic transmission in isolated guinea pig autonomic ganglia. J Clin Invest 1987; 79:1529–1532.
226. Barnes PJ. Neuromodulation in airways. In: Barnes PJ, ed. Autonomic Control of the Respiratory System. Amsterdam: Harwood Academic Publishers, 1997:139–184.
227. Miura M, Ichinose M, Kimura K, Katsumata U, Takahashi T, Inoue H, Takishima T. Dysfunction of nonadrenergic noncholinergic inhibitory system after antigen inhalation in actively sensitized cat airways. Am Rev Respir Dis 1992; 145:70–74.
228. Fame TM, Colasurdo GN, Loader JE, Graves J, Larsen GL. Decrease in the airways nonadrenergic noncholinergic inhibitory system in allergen-sensitized rabbits. Ped Pulmonol 1994; 17:296–303.
229. Tam EK, Franconi GM, Nadel JA, Caughey GH. Protease inhibitors potentiate smooth muscle relaxation induced by vasoactive intestinal peptide in isolated human bronchi. Am J Respir Cell Mol Biol 1990; 2:449–452.
230. Wills-Karp M. Smooth muscle as a direct or indirect target accounting for bronchopulmonary hyperresponsiveness. Res Immunol 1997; 148:59–72.
231. Skloot, G, Permutt S, Togias A. Airway hyperresponsiveness in asthma: a problem of limited smooth muscle relaxation with inspiration. J Clin Invest 1995; 96:2393–2403.
232. Fryer AD, Maclagan J. Muscarinic inhibitory receptors in pulmonary parasympathetic nerves in the guinea-pig. Br J Pharmacol 1984; 83:973–978.
233. Matsumoto S, Nagayama T, Kanno T, Yamasaki M, Shimizu T. Evidence for the presence of function of the inhibitory M_2 receptors in the rabbit airways and lungs. J Auton Nerv Sys 1995; 53:126–136.
234. Myers AC, Undem BJ. Muscarinic receptor regulation of synaptic transmission in airway parasympathetic ganglia. Am J Physiol. 1996; 270:L630–L636.
235. Elbon CL, Jacoby DB, Fryer AD. Pretreatment with an antibody to IL-5 preserves

the function of pulmonary M_2 muscarinic receptors in antigen challenged guinea-pigs. Am J Respir Cell Mol Biol 1995;12:320–328.
236. Fryer AD, Yarkony KA, Jacoby DB. The effect of leukocyte depletion on pulmonary M_2 muscarinic receptor function in parainfluenza virus-infected guinea-pigs. Br J Pharmacol 1994; 112:588–594.
237. Gambone LM, Elbon CL, Fryer AD. Ozone-induced loss of neuronal M_2 muscarinic receptor function is prevented by cyclophosphamide. J Appl Physiol 1994; 77: 1492–1499.
238. Myers AC, Undem BJ, Weinreich D. Influence of antigen on membrane properties of guinea pig bronchial ganglion neurons. J Appl Physiol 1991; 71:970–976.

3

Diagnosis of Gastroesophageal Reflux Disease

PHILIP O. KATZ and DONALD O. CASTELL

Allegheny University Hospitals
Philadelphia, Pennsylvania

I. Spectrum of Gastroesophageal Reflux Disease

Gastroesophageal reflux disease (GERD) is a spectrum of disease that can best be defined as the symptoms and/or signs of esophageal or adjacent organ injury secondary to the reflux of gastric contents into the esophagus or beyond into the oral cavity or airways. The spectrum of symptoms are outlined in Figure 1. Injury is defined based on symptoms or organ damage resulting in esophagitis, laryngeal inflammation, or acute and/or chronic pulmonary injury.

Injury to the upper respiratory tract may be caused by direct contact of gastric contents with the mucosal surfaces of the oral cavity, trachea, or lung or by a vagal mediated reflex generated from stimulation of an afferent esophageal receptor resulting in stimulation of the airway.

GERD is arguably the most common disease seen in clinical practice and may present with a multitude of symptoms. The typical or classic symptoms are heartburn and regurgitation. Heartburn is substernal burning occurring shortly after meals or upon bending over and is relieved with antacids or other over-the-counter agents. Regurgitation is the spontaneous return of gastric contents into the esophagus or mouth. When present together, these symptoms establish a diagnosis of GERD with greater than 90% certainty. Heartburn is seen daily in 7–

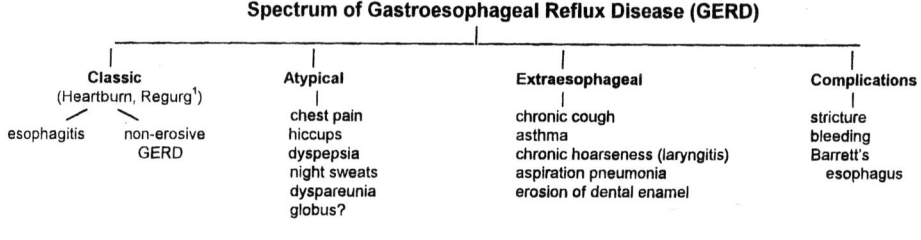

Figure 1 Spectrum of symptom presentation of gastroesophageal reflux disease.

10% of the United States population and at least monthly in about 40–50% (1–3). A similar prevalence is seen in developed countries throughout the world. Regurgitation is reported weekly by approximately 6% and at least yearly by 45% of the population in one study (2). In this same study, either heartburn or regurgitation was present in 20% of patients surveyed at least weekly and 59% at least monthly. The prevalence of heartburn appears to be inversely associated with increasing age, although the absolute differences are small.

Despite the sensitivity and specificity of these two symptoms for the diagnosis of GERD, neither the presence of heartburn and/or regurgitation nor the frequency of these symptoms are predictive of the degree of endoscopic damage to the distal esophagus. Approximately 60% of patients presenting to a physician with typical esophageal symptoms will have erosive esophagitis seen on a diagnostic endoscopic examination; approximately 40% will have a normal endoscopy and will be diagnosed as having nonerosive GERD (4).

A number of so-called atypical or extraesophageal symptoms have been associated with GERD, including unexplained substernal chest pain without evidence of coronary artery disease (noncardiac chest pain), asthma, bronchitis, chronic cough, recurrent pneumonia, hoarseness, chronic posterior laryngitis, globus sensation, otalgia, apthous ulcers, hiccups, and erosion of dental enamel. In contrast to heartburn and regurgitation, the prevalence of these atypical or extraesophageal symptoms and their frequency in the general population have not been systematically studied until recently. In a large population-based survey of Caucasians in Olmstead County, Minnesota, designed to assess the prevalence of GERD in the general population (2), unexplained chest pain was seen in 23% of the population yearly and at least weekly in 4%. The frequency of unexplained chest pain surprisingly decreased with age. Forty percent had symptoms for greater than 5 years, and 5% reported severe symptoms. Asthma was reported in approximately 9%, bronchitis in approximately 20%, and chronic hoarseness in 15% of patients who had typical GERD symptoms.

The association of these atypical symptoms with heartburn and regurgitation is controversial. In the study above one or more atypical symptoms were present in 80% of patients. Atypical symptoms were more common in patients with frequent GERD compared to patients with no GERD symptoms. The only exception was asthma. Heartburn or regurgitation was reported in more than 80% of the patients with unexplained chest pain and in 60% with globus sensation. Approximately 60% of patients with asthma, bronchitis, hoarseness, and pneumonia appeared to have typical symptoms.

Other studies of patients with atypical GERD suggest that heartburn and regurgitation are seen less frequently in these patients. Heartburn is reported to be present in 30–50% of patients with hoarseness or asthma and in about half of patients with unexplained chest pain and normal coronary arteries. Hence, the true frequency of GERD in patients with these atypical symptoms is not clear. In prospective studies using endoscopy and ambulatory pH monitoring, between 70 and 80% of asthmatics will have associated GERD (5,6). It has been estimated that 20% of patients with chronic cough will have GERD (7), while as many as 75% of patients with chronic hoarseness referred for pH monitoring will have GERD (8). Despite these high frequencies, this is not necessarily proof of a cause-and-effect relationship. Approximately 45% of patients with unexplained chest pain can be shown to have GERD (9). Esophagitis in this population is less likely, being seen in less than 10% (10). Endoscopic esophagitis is seen in 30–40% of patients with asthma (11,12).

Esophagitis may progress to severe complications including ulceration, peptic stricture, iron deficiency anemia, and Barrett's esophagus. Barrett's esophagus is most important since it is a premalignant condition found in at least 12% of patients with typical symptoms of GERD (4). The condition involves a change from normal squamous epithelial lining to a metaplastic intestinal-type epithelium with typical special stain characteristics. When Barrett's esophagus is found, periodic follow-up is needed as surveillance for malignancy (see below).

II. Diagnosis

A clinical diagnosis of GERD can be reasonably assumed if the symptoms are relieved with a therapeutic trial of antireflux therapy. The diagnosis can be based on diagnostic tests including barium radiographs, esophagoscopy, esophageal motility testing, and/or ambulatory pH monitoring. These tests allow the clinician to demonstrate that reflux occurs and to quantitate it. When used appropriately they identify end-organ effects of reflux on the esophagus and larynx. These tests can also evaluate the effects of reflux on lower esophageal sphincter (LES) pressure and esophageal acid clearance. Each study will be discussed, pointing out strengths and weaknesses, followed by general guidelines for usage (Table 1). The approach to the patient with suspected airway disease will be discussed separately (see Chap. 7).

III. Therapeutic Trials

The patient with typical heartburn and regurgitation frequently does not need diagnostic tests to support the diagnosis of GERD. A therapeutic trial of H_2 antagonists, prokinetic agents, or proton pump inhibitors for 6–8 weeks will often confirm that the symptoms are due to acid reflux. Unfortunately, heartburn is often absent in patients with extraesophageal presentations, including cough, laryngitis, and asthma. When the history for GERD is less reliable, objective diagnostic criteria become more important. Therapeutic trials may be less useful if no symptoms of GERD are present.

Clues that airway symptoms may be due to GERD include their onset after meals, onset in a recumbent position, nonseasonal onset, nonallergic onset, absence of other pulmonary pathology, and an increase or precipitation of symptoms after heavy meals or an abundance of alcohol. Patients with chronic cough, normal chest x-ray, lack of response to treatment for postnasal drip, and who are not on angiotensin-converting enzyme inhibitors are likely to have GERD (Chapter 5). Similarly, the failure of response of asthma to bronchodilator therapy should lead the clinician to consider a diagnosis of GERD-related asthma. Patients with reflux laryngitis often complain of morning hoarseness, halitosis, ex-

Table 1 Diagnostic Tests for Gastroesophageal Reflux Disease Categorized According to Specific Questions Being Asked

Is abnormal reflux present?
Barium upper gastrointestinal series
pH monitoring
Is there mucosal injury?
Barium upper gastrointestinal (air contrast) study
Endoscopy
Mucosal biopsy
Are symptoms due to reflux?
pH monitoring (with symptom index)
To obtain preoperative information:
Esophageal manometry
pH monitoring

cess phlegm, dry mouth, throat clearing, tickle in the throat, closing off of the airways or, if a singer, prolonged warm-up time. Associated chronic sore throat should be sought.

Though therapeutic trials are often used in patients with suspected GERD and airways disease, these require higher doses of antireflux therapy for longer periods of time and have not been rigorously tested. Neither cost-effectiveness nor clinical efficacy has been evaluated. Currently, it is our practice as of this writing to use twice the FDA-recommended dose of a proton pump inhibitor divided in twice-daily dosage for a minimum of 8–12 weeks as a therapeutic trial for atypical symptoms.

IV. Barium Radiographs

Barium studies are relatively inexpensive and widely available for use in diagnosis of esophageal disease. When evaluating the esophagus, a barium swallow (preferably with double contrast) should be ordered to ensure optimal evaluation. Ordering an upper GI series will often result in insufficient evaluation of esophageal function, concentrate excessively on the stomach and duodenum, and not pay careful attention to potential mucosal or motility abnormalities in the esophagus. The barium swallow is an excellent test to establish the presence of a hiatal hernia; however, up to 60% of the adult population will have a hernia (13), making this a nonspecific finding and not diagnostic of GERD. The presence of free reflux may be seen in up to 30% of normal patients and be absent in up to 60% of patients with proven GERD by pH monitoring (14), making barium an insensitive and nonspecific study to document the presence of reflux. It is often suggested that reflux above the carina or to the thoracic inlet is indicative of the potential for aspiration and is used as an aid in the diagnosis of GERD-associated airway disease. Unfortunately, no prospective or controlled studies have been done to substantiate this anecdotal information. In addition, this finding is usually reported with the patient in the supine position, causing this observation to be even less valid. There has been no association of this so-called "high" reflux on a barium study with the presence of proximal acid exposure on ambulatory pH monitoring (see below). Specific mucosal abnormalities on double contrast barium studies such as thickening of esophageal mucosal folds, erosions, or esophageal ulcers are seen in a minority of patients with GERD leaving this study relatively insensitive for this diagnosis. The diagnosis of Barrett's esophagus is rarely conclusively made by a barium swallow.

The best use of the barium study is in evaluation of suspected complications of GERD, including motility abnormalities or peptic stricture. These abnormalities are predominantly in patients presenting with solid and/or liquid dysphagia. The barium study can identify rings and webs and other obstructive lesions (including carcinoma) that may be associated with dysphagia but are rarely direct complications of GERD. A solid bolus such as a marshmallow or a barium cookie can be given to help localize the site of obstruction in a patient with solid dysphagia. In our opinion, barium swallow should be the first test in evaluation of the patient with dysphagia and should be performed in conjunction with endoscopy in this patient population. Although it may demonstrate that reflux and mucosal injury are occurring, it is rarely of value in establishing a diagnosis of GERD in patients with symptoms other than dysphagia.

Few prospective studies have been done with barium swallow in patients with GERD and airway disease, particularly asthma. In children, abnormal studies have been seen in as low as 11% (15) of patients and as high as 100% (16). In adult asthmatics, the sensitivity is usually less than 50%, though hiatal hernia is often present and demonstrable free reflux may be seen in some patients.

V. Endoscopy

Endoscopy is the single best test to document mucosal abnormalities and establish a diagnosis of erosive esophagitis or Barrett's esophagus in the patient with suspected gastroesophageal reflux disease. When patients with heartburn and regurgitation are evaluated prospectively, endoscopy reveals erosive esophagitis in 45–60% (4) of patients, with the remainder having nonerosive disease (mucosal edema, hyperemia, or a normal-appearing esophagus). Erosive esophagitis suggests a more serious form of GERD, one that is more likely to require continuous medical therapy or antireflux surgery. Therapy with a proton pump inhibitor (see Chap. 8) for relief and healing is indicated. Barrett's esophagus can be found in 10–12% (4) of reflux patients undergoing endoscopy. While there are no classic diagnostic features of Barrett's esophagus, it is most common in Caucasian males over the age of 50. Erosive esophagitis is seen with lower frequency in patients with atypical or extraesophageal symptoms. Although 50% of patients with unexplained chest pain and normal coronary arteries have GERD, the prevalence of erosive esophagitis is 10% or less (10). In GERD-associated asthma, endoscopic esophagitis has been reported in 30–40% (5,6) of adult patients. In one study by Larrain et al. (5) esophagitis was only found in 33% and was predominantly nonerosive. In a study by Sontag and colleagues from the Hines VA in Chicago (6), erosive esophagitis was seen in 39% and Barrett's esophagus in 12% of patients with asthma and GERD. It is likely that the general population is more typical of the patients described in the former study.

There are no absolute indications for endoscopy in the patient with suspected GERD. General guidelines suggest that patients with heartburn who fail to respond to a 6- to 8-week therapeutic trial of pharmacologic therapy, patients who have symptoms for more than 3–5 years, patients over the age of 50, and patients with "alarm" symptoms including dysphagia, odynophagia, weight loss, anemia, or Gl bleeding should be considered for endoscopy (17). We believe that white males with GERD should be endoscoped at least once to rule out Barrett's esophagus.

Endoscopic findings may help predict the prognosis and outcome of medical therapy. Patients with erosive esophagitis, particularly Grade 3-4, have a poor response to traditional doses of H_2 receptor antagonists and prokinetic agents and often require a proton pump inhibitor for symptom relief and healing. Patients with Grade 2 esophagitis have a variable response to H_2 blockers and prokinetics and often require proton pump inhibitors to achieve optimal symptom relief and healing. Recurrence of erosive esophagitis is seen in up to 80% of patients within 3–6 months (18); these patients usually require continuous pharmacologic therapy often with proton pump inhibitors for effective long-term relief. Because they seldom progress to more severe forms of esophagitis, patients with nonerosive esophagitis can be managed with a range of pharmacologic treatments and often respond to on-demand therapy on a long-term basis. It is our opinion that endoscopy is useful for long-term treatment planning in difficult-to-manage cases.

Because of the lower frequency of erosive esophagitis, we do not routinely perform endoscopy as our initial study in patients with suspected GERD-related chest pain, asthma, cough, or hoarseness, preferring instead to use ambulatory pH monitoring as our initial diagnostic test (see below). If extraesophageal GERD is confirmed and patients require long-term medical therapy (or antireflux surgery), we perform endoscopy to rule out Barrett's esophagus.

VI. Laryngoscopy

Laryngoscopic examination in suspected reflux-related laryngitis reveals edema and erythema of the arytenoid cartilage, posterior larynx and posterior portion of true vocal folds. Diffuse laryngitis may be seen.

VII. Esophageal Biopsy

Mucosal biopsy and cytology are of limited value in evaluation of the patient with GERD unless Barrett's esophagus or malignancy is suspected. The light microscopic signs of GERD [elongation of rete pegs and hyperplasia of the basal cell layer (19)] do not distinguish between acute and chronic disease and do not help predict the response to therapy. It is our feeling that these findings are nonspecific and do not aid in the diagnosis of GERD. Microscopic signs of acute esophagitis—polymorphonuclear leukocytes and eosinophils—are present in less than 30% of adult patients with GERD (19) and as such are insensitive diagnostic findings. Biopsy may be more useful in the pediatric population, where higher prevalence of PMNs and eosinophils has been reported (20). In today's cost-sensitive environment, we do not biopsy the esophagus in patients with GERD unless Barrett's esophagus is suspected.

If the endoscopic appearance is suggestive of Barrett's esophagus, then a systematic biopsy protocol should be followed to confirm the diagnosis and rule out dysplasia or carcinoma (21). Endoscopic surveillance with biopsies to rule out dysplasia every 1 to 2 years is currently the standard of practice for patients with Barrett's esophagus.

VIII. Prolonged Ambulatory pH Monitoring

Ambulatory pH monitoring is the best test for quantifying esophageal reflux and determining if symptoms are due to GERD. Now a widely available technology, it is usually performed by placing a 2-mm-diameter catheter transnasally into the esophagus with the distal antimony electrode placed 5 cm above the lower esophageal sphincter, which is located by esophageal manometry (Fig. 2). The probe is connected to a small microcomputer that is worn on a belt or clipped to the waist so that the patient can be monitored in an ambulatory setting. Activity

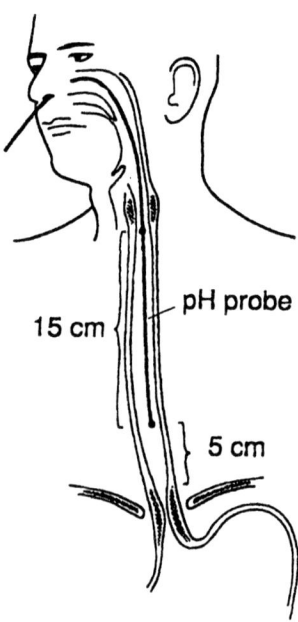

Figure 2 Placement of pH probe in relation to the lower esophageal sphincter.

can be tailored to provoke reflux in the setting in which symptoms are normally produced. For example, a patient who has nocturnal asthma after a large meal or after imbibing alcohol can be monitored with instructions to reproduce that clinical situation. A patient with chronic hoarseness who sings professionally will be reminded to sing during the study. Patients with exercise-related symptoms can be studied on a treadmill or while running or weightlifting.

Multiple electrodes can be placed simultaneously on a single catheter so that intragastric and intraesophageal pH, distal esophageal and proximal esophageal acid exposure or all three can be monitored simultaneously. This allows demonstration of acid exposure in the proximal esophagus, just below the upper esophageal sphincter (UES), predicting the potential for aspiration in patients with cough, asthma, or hoarseness, in addition to documenting abnormal distal reflux. The intragastric electrode allows monitoring of the gastric acid response to antireflux therapy. Several investigators have placed probes above the upper esophageal sphincter in the hypopharynx (22,23) in order to document reflux above the UES to be more confident of the likelihood of aspiration and/or as the cause of supraesophageal symptoms. With the currently available dual pH probe, the distance between the electrodes is fixed (Fig. 2). By placing the upper electrode above the UES, the lower electrode is no longer 5 cm above the lower esophageal sphincter (LES). This can present problems in data interpretation. Probes placed in the hypopharynx can be somewhat uncomfortable. In addition, normal values are not available and are occasionally subject to interpretation artifact. As there are normal values for distal reflux at 5 cm above the LES and for proximal reflux 20 cm above the sphincter, we believe this is a more useful standard (see Chap. 5) (24,25). Normal values vary slightly between laboratories and are included with reports from the laboratory performing the procedure. In general, the normal time (esophageal pH < 4) upright is $\leq 6\%$ and supine $\leq 1.2\%$ in the distal esophagus, and the normal time is $\leq 1.1\%$ upright and 0% supine proximally. If the problems mentioned above can be resolved, placement above the UES would be ideal.

The microcomputer (data logger) is equipped with a symptom button that allows one to record up to six symptoms during a single study. The patient is instructed to push the appropriate symptom button as well as to record the symptom on a diary card. This allows correlation of reflux events with symptoms, which is especially valuable in patients with extraesophageal symptoms such as asthma, cough, and chest pain and allows correlation between heartburn and reflux in patients who have continued symptoms on medical therapy.

Patients with typical symptoms of GERD benefit from pH monitoring to establish a diagnosis when symptoms have failed to respond to a therapeutic trial of pharmacologic therapy and endoscopy does not reveal erosive esophagitis or Barrett's esophagus. In this case, a single-channel pH probe can be placed with the distal probe 5 cm above the LES. Symptoms can then be correlated with reflux and reflux frequency assessed. Patients with known GERD who have heartburn and regurgitation not responding to medical therapy can be monitored while still on therapy with a dual channel intragastric and distal esophageal probe to assess the adequacy of gastric acid suppression and esophageal reflux frequency and to correlate symptoms with reflux events. Patients with continued esophageal acid exposure and or symptoms may require additional therapy.

Patients with asthma, cough, or other upper airway symptoms suggestive of GERD are the ideal candidates for ambulatory pH monitoring. It is our practice to perform monitoring early in the patient encounter to establish a diagnosis and symptom correlation where possible. It is also our practice to perform dual channel monitoring with one electrode 5 cm above the LES and a second probe 20 cm above in the proximal esophagus just below the UES (Fig. 2). The presence of abnormal distal esophageal acid exposure can be documented, establishing a diagnosis of GERD. More importantly, the presence of abnormal proximal reflux can be documented, suggesting the potential for aspiration and the greater probability that the extraesophageal symptom is due to GERD. If symptom correlation can be found, this will clinch the diagnosis. The presence of proximal reflux appears to predict the response to medical therapy in patients with pulmonary disease (26,27). Most importantly, a small percentage of patients will have normal distal esophageal acid exposure but demonstrable increased frequency of proximal reflux or reflux into the hypopharynx establishing a diagnosis of GERD. In one study of 10 patients with reflux laryngitis, 3 (30%) demonstrated hypopharyngeal reflux with normal distal acid exposure (22). In a larger, retrospective series, 12% of patients reviewed had only abnormal proximal reflux (26). This group would have been diagnosed incorrectly as normal had only a single-channel study been performed.

Studies in adults demonstrate abnormal amounts of acid reflux in up to 70–80% of patients with asthma whether on or off bronchodilator therapy (6). Abnormal acid exposure has been documented in both the upright and supine periods. Ambulatory monitoring is especially useful in establishing symptom correlation but results have been variable. In one study, only 50% of wheezing episodes were found to have any relationship to acid reflux (28). A final diagnosis of reflux-related asthma or cough cannot be firmly established until the symptom responds to a therapeutic intervention.

For patients with airways disease, ambulatory monitoring can be particularly valuable in assessing response to therapy, particularly in the patient who has failed to respond to a therapeutic trial. It is our practice to monitor intragastric, distal esophageal, and proximal esophageal pH in this population. Adequacy of intragastric acid suppression can be assessed, as can the presence of esophageal acid exposure and correlation between reflux events and symptoms established. Though the precise timing between a reflux event and symptoms that establish causality has not been determined, we believe that if symptoms occur within 5 minutes after a reflux episode, a strong correlation between symptoms and acid exposure can be inferred.

IX. Esophageal Manometry

Esophageal manometry is useful to establish abnormality of LES pressure or esophageal motility and to obtain preoperative information for the surgeon. Decreased lower esophageal sphincter pressure is a major determinant of gastroesophageal reflux, but a single measurement of LES pressure is rarely low in patients with GERD. In studies from our laboratory, only 4% of patients with gastroesophageal reflux disease had a low LES pressure (29). Esophageal motility abnormalities are found more frequently. The most common finding appears to be ineffective esophageal motility (amplitude of contraction in the distal esophagus less than 30 mmHg occurring with 30% or more of water swallows). In our experience, this is the most common abnormality in patients with GERD, seen in approximately 35% (29). These abnormalities appear to occur with similar frequency in patients with GERD-related asthma and cough. In general, we reserve esophageal manometry for the patient in whom antireflux surgery is being planned to establish the presence or absence of ineffective motility. Patients with asthma and other airways disease have a poor response to antireflux surgery when motility abnormalities are present compared to patients with normal motility. In addition, surgeons can be guided in their choice of antireflux surgery, usually performing a Nissen fundoplication (360 degree wrap) in patients with normal peristalsis and a Toupet procedure (240 degree wrap) in patients with peristaltic abnormalities (see Chap. 7).

X. Hiatal Hernia

Once considered of major importance in causing reflux, hiatal hernia is not predictive of reflux as a cause of the patients' symptoms. Up to 60% of patients over the age of 60 will have a hiatal hernia when barium radiographs are performed. One study suggested that only 9% of patients with a radiographically demonstrated hernia will actually have typical reflux symptoms (30).

Hernias do change the relationship of the LES and crural diaphragm. The LES is displaced above the diaphragm. The low pressure in the hernia can act as a reservoir for acid, allowing earlier reflux during LES relaxations. This may also delay esophageal clearance (31). Patients with large hernias who also have low LES pressure may be more prone to reflux (32), particularly if changes occur that increase intra-abdominal pressure.

XI. Approaching the Patient with GERD-Related Airways Disease

If a patient with suspected airways disease is seen, the following approach is suggested (Fig. 3). A thorough history, physical examination, chest x-ray, and direct laryngoscopy should be performed. If dysphagia is present, a barium swallow should be ordered to rule out esophageal obstruction or obvious motility abnormalities. When ambulatory pH monitoring is available, this is the initial diagnostic procedure of choice and should be performed (Fig. 2). An increase in the percent of time esophageal pH < 4 compared to normals in either the distal or proximal esophagus should be considered abnormal. If symptoms are present, correlation with reflux events greater than 50% (33) should be considered a positive association.

When there is a strong history of heartburn and regurgitation or other previous documentation of GERD and if pH monitoring is not available, a therapeutic trial of antireflux therapy can be attempted. A proton pump inhibitor (omeprazole 20 mg or lansoprazole 30 mg) twice daily for 8–12 weeks is indicated (34). If the patient does not improve, pH monitoring should be performed while therapy is continued. A dual-channel probe with intragastric and distal esophageal electrodes should be placed to ascertain adequate gastric acid suppression and to

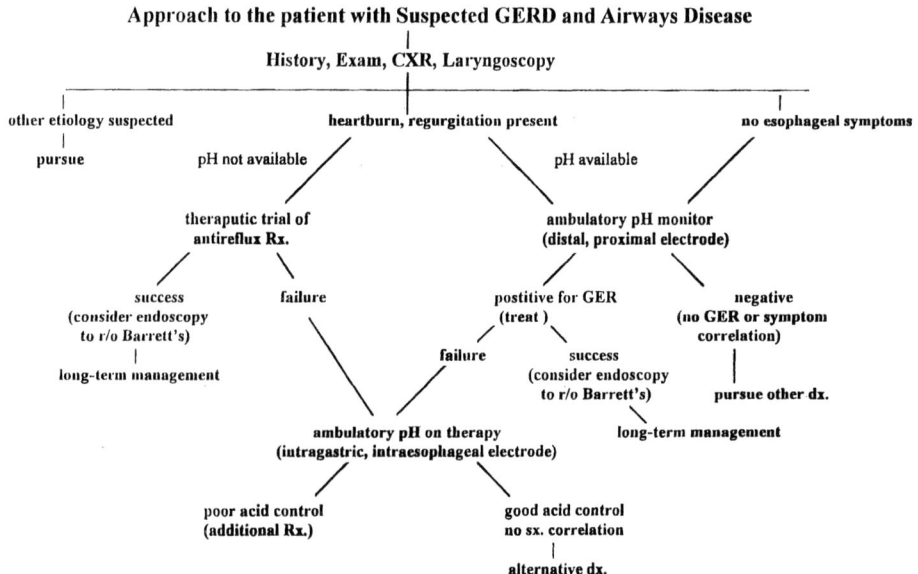

Figure 3 Suggested approach to the patient with GERD and airways disease.

assess the presence of esophageal acid exposure. Symptoms should be correlated with reflux events. If distal esophageal acid exposure is seen more than 1.2% of the time, we would consider this abnormal and would give additional medical therapy. The absence of esophageal acid exposure and adequate gastric acid suppression (pH > 4, 50% of total time) suggests adequate medical therapy, and an alternative diagnosis should be pursued. Finally, if GERD-associated airways disease is documented, we will endoscope the patient to rule out Barrett's esophagus prior to instituting long-term medical therapy or considering surgery.

References

1. A Gallup Survey on Heartburn Across America. The Gallup Organization, Inc., 1968.
2. Locke GR, Talley NJ, Fett SL, Zinsmeister AR, Melton LJ. Prevalence and clinical spectrum of gastroesophageal reflux: a population-based study in Olmstead County, Minnesota. Gastroenterology 1997; 112:5-12.
3. Nebel OT, Fornes MF, Castell DO. Symptomatic gastroesophageal reflux: incidence and precipitating factors. Dig Dis Sci 1976; 21:953-956.
4. Winters C, Spurling TJ, Chobanian SJ, et al. Barrett's esophagus: a prevalent, occult complication of gastroesophageal reflux disease. Gastroenterology 1987; 92:118-123.
5. Harding SM, Guzzo MR, Richter JE. Prevalence of GERD in asthmatics without reflux symptoms. Gastroenterology 1997; 4:A141.
6. Sontag SJ, O'Connell S, Khandelwal S, et al. Most asthmatics have gastroesophageal reflux with or without bronchodilator therapy. Gastroenterology 1990; 99:613-618.
7. Irwin RS, Corrao WM, Pratter MR. Chronic persistent cough in the adult: The spectrum and frequency of causes and successful outcome of specific therapy. Am Rev Respir Dis 1981; 123:413-422.
8. Weiner GJ, Kaufman JA, Wu WC, et al. Chronic hoarseness secondary to gastro esophageal reflux disease. Am J Gastroenterol 1989; 84:1503-1508.
9. Hewson EG, Sinclair JW, Dalton CB, et al. 24 hour esophageal pH monitoring: the most useful test for evaluating non-cardiac chest pain. Am J Med 1991; 90:576-583.
10. Cherian P, Smith LF, Bardham KD, Thorpe J, Oakley GD, Dawson D. Esophageal tests in the evaluation of non-cardiac chest pain. Dis Esophagus 1995; 8:129-133.
11. Larrain A, Carrasco E, Galleguillos F, et al. Medical and surgical treatment of non-allergic asthma associated with gastroesophageal reflux. Chest 1991; 99:1330-1336.
12. Sontag SJ, Schnell TG, Miller TQ, et al. Prevalence of oesophagitis in asthmatics. Gut 33:872-76, 1992.
13. Ott DJ, Wu WC, Gelfand DW. Reflux esophagitis revisited: prospective analysis of radiologic accuracy. Gastrointest Radiol 1981; 6:1-7.
14. Richter JE, Castell DO. Gastroesophageal reflux. Pathogenesis, diagnosis, and therapy. Ann intern Med 1982; 97:93-103.
15. Euler AR, Burne WJ, Ament ME, et al. Recurrent pulmonary disease in children: A complication of gastroesophageal reflux. J Pediatr 1984; 87:872-878.

16. Herbst JJ, Minton SD, Brooks LS. Gastroesophageal reflux causing respiratory distress and apnea in newborn infants. J Pediatr 1979; 95:763–770.
17. DeVault KR, Castell DO. Guidelines for the diagnosis and treatment of gastroesophageal reflux disease. Arch Intern Med 1995; 155:2165–2173.
18. Hetzel D, Dent J, Reed W, et al. Healing and relapse of severe peptic esophagitis after treatment with Omeprazole. Gastroenterology 1988; 95:903–912.
19. Ismail-Beigi F, Horton PF, Pope CE. Histological consequences of gastroesophageal reflux in man. Gastroenterology 1970; 58:163–174.
20. Winter CS, et al. Intraepithelial eosinophils: a new diagnostic criterion for reflux esophagitis. Gastroenterology 1982; 83:818.
21. Spechler SJ. Complications of gastroesophageal reflux disease. In: Castell DO, ed. The Esophagus. Boston: Little Brown, 1995: 533–546.
22. Katz PO, Dalton CB, Richter JE, et al. Esophageal testing in patients with noncardiac chest pain and/or dysphagia. Ann Intern Med 1987; 106:593–597.
23. Koufman JA. The otolaryngologic manifestations of gastroesophageal reflux disease: a clinical investigation of 225 patients using ambulatory pH monitoring and an experimental investigation of the role of acid and pepsin in the development of laryngeal injury. Laryngoscope 1991; 101:1–78.
24. Johnson LF, DeMeester TR. Twenty-four hour pH monitoring of the distal esophagus. Am J Gastroenterol 1974; 62:325–333.
25. Dobhan R, Castell DO. Normal and abnormal proximal esophageal acid exposure: results of ambulatory dual probe pH monitoring. Am J Gastroenterol 1993; 88:25–29.
26. Schnatz PF, Castell JA, Castell DO. Pulmonary symptoms associated with gastroesophageal reflux: use of ambulatory pH monitoring to diagnose and to direct therapy. Am J Gastroenterol 1996; 91:1715–1718.
27. Harding SM, Richter JE, et al. Asthma and gastroesophageal reflux: acid suppression therapy improves asthma outcome. Am J Med 1996; 100:395–405.
28. Sontag S, O'Connell S, Khandelwal S, et al. Does wheezing occur in association with an episode of gastroesophageal reflux? Gastroenterology 1989; 96:482–490.
29. Barrett J. Peghini P, Katz P, Castell J, Castell D. Ineffective esophageal motility (IEM): The most common abnormality in GERD (abstr). Gastroenterology 1997; 112:4.
30. Palmer ED. The hiatus hernia-esophagitis-esophageal stricture complex. Twenty year prospective study. Am J Med 1968; 44:566–572.
31. Sloan S, Kahrilas PJ. Impairment of esophageal emptying with hiatal hernia. Gastroenterology 1991; 100:596–605.
32. Sloan S, Rademaker AW, Kahrilas PJ. Determinants of gastroesophageal junction incompetence: hiatal hernia, lower esophageal sphincter, or both? Ann Intern Med 1992; 117:977–982.
33. Weiner GJ, Richter JE, Cooper JB, et al. The symptom index: a clinically important parameter of ambulatory 24 hour esophageal pH monitoring. Am J Gastroenterol 1988; 38:58–61.
34. Kuo B, Castell DO. Optimal dosing of omeprazole 40 mg daily: effects on gastric and esophageal pH and serum gastrin in healthy controls. Am J Gastroenterol 1996; 91:1532–1538.

4

The Otolaryngologic Manifestations of GERD

JAMES A. KOUFMAN

Wake Forest University School of Medicine
Winston-Salem, North Carolina

I. Introduction

It has been estimated that approximately half of otorhinolaryngology (ORL) patients with laryngeal and voice disorders have gastroesophageal reflux disease (GERD) as the primary cause or as a significant etiologic cofactor (1). This appears to be true for patients with diverse clinical manifestations (1,2); Table 1 lists the most common ORL symptoms and diseases that have been reported to be reflux-related. The mechanisms, patterns, and management of GERD in ORL patients appear to differ significantly from those of "typical" gastroenterology patients with esophagitis (1,5,20,25–29), and these differences are highlighted in this chapter.

The reported association of gastric reflux with aerodigestive tract diseases is relatively recent. In 1935, the first detailed report linking gastric reflux with esophageal disease in adults was published by Winkelstein (30); in 1950, Berenberg and Neuhauser (31) reported reflux symptoms in children; and in 1968, Cherry and Margulies (15) first reported a reflux-related laryngeal disease (contact ulcer and granuloma). Many GERD-related laryngeal diseases have only been reported in the last two decades. Summarized in Table 2 are some of the important landmarks in the history of GERD.

Table 1 Symptoms and Laryngeal Conditions Associated with GERD

A. Symptoms:
 Chronic dysphonia
 Intermittent dysphonia
 Vocal fatigue
 Voice breaks
 Chronic throat clearing
 Excessive throat mucus
 Postnasal drip
 Chronic cough
 Dysphagia
 Globus

B. Conditions associated with reflux as the cause or as a causative cofactor:
 Reflux laryngitis (2-6)
 Subglottic stenosis (2,3,7,8)
 Carcinoma of the larynx (2,6,9-13)
 Endotracheal intubation injury (2,14)
 Contact ulcers and granulomas (14-16)
 Posterior glottic stenosis (2,17)
 Unilateral or bilateral arytenoid fixation (2,14)
 Paroxysmal laryngospasm (18,19)
 Globus pharyngeus (2,20,21)
 Vocal nodules (1,2,5,22)
 Polypoid degeneration (1,2)
 Laryngomalacia (23,24)
 Pachydermia laryngis (2,9)
 Leukoplakia (2)

The etiologic role of gastroesophageal reflux (GER) in some airway diseases remains controversial and is still not accepted by all clinicians. Even among otolaryngologists who have a relatively high index of suspicion for GERD, it appears that reflux laryngitis, specifically called laryngopharyngeal reflux (LPR), is still often underdiagnosed and undertreated. There appears to be a four-part explanation for this phenomenon:

 1. *ORL patients with reflux laryngitis usually deny symptoms of heartburn and/or regurgitation.* LPR may be "silent." Fewer than half of ORL patients with LPR documented by pH monitoring complain of heartburn or regurgitation, symptoms that have traditionally needed to be present in order to diagnose GERD (1,2,5,14,20,29).

 2. *The findings of GERD on laryngeal examination vary considerably.* Laryngeal edema, not erythema, is the hallmark of LPR, and may be overlooked as evidence of reflux laryngitis. Until recently, most otolaryngologists relied solely on the findings of posterior laryngitis (red arytenoids and piled-up, hypertrophic, posterior commissure mucosa) as the diagnostic sine qua non of reflux

Table 2 Some Important Landmarks in the Study of Gastroesophageal Reflux

Year	Person	Ref.	Landmark
1890	C. Jackson	32	Invents the esophagoscope
1899	S. Meltzer	33	Describes esophageal peristalsis
1906	W. Tileson	34	Reports "gastric ulcer" of the esophagus
1921	H. Mosher	35	Reports esophageal stricture
1935	A. Winkelstein	30	Reports peptic esophagitis
1940	F. Ingelfinger	36	Introduces modern manometry
1950	W. Berenberg	31	Reports reflux symptoms in children
1964	F. Miller	37	Introduces prolonged pH monitoring
1968	J. Cherry	15	Reports first reflux-related laryngeal disease
1972	J. Delahunty	4	Reports posterior laryngitis
1976	H. Glanz	9	Reports reflux-related laryngeal cancer
1980	R. Bogdasarian	17	Reports reflux-related subglottic stenosis
1986	G. Weiner	28	Introduces double-probe (pharyngeal and esophageal) pH monitoring
1988	J. Koufman	5	Reports clinical findings and pH results of ORL patients with LPR

laryngitis. Unfortunately, these findings are not present in many LPR patients. Edema, not erythema, is the most prevalent finding of LPR. The edema may be diffuse, or it may create the illusion of sulcus vocalis, an appearance that is the result of subglottic edema (38). Figure 1(a) shows the typical appearance of the larynx of an LPR patient.

3. *Traditional diagnostic tests for GERD lack both sensitivity and specificity for LPR.* The diagnosis of LPR may be confounded by false-negative diagnostic tests. Barium esophagography, radionuclide scanning, the Bernstein acid-perfusion test, and esophagoscopy with biopsy are all usually negative in the ORL patient with LPR (2,20). They are negative because these tests primarily detect esophagitis, which is not commonly present in LPR patients (22,30). In addition, LPR is frequently intermittent, and exacerbations may depend to some extent upon changing dietary and lifestyle factors (2,5).

4. *Therapeutic trials using "traditional" antireflux therapy often fail in ORL patients with LPR-related conditions, so that clinicians may falsely conclude that a diagnosis other than LPR may be the cause of the problem.* The traditional treatment for GERD, particularly in the patient with esophagitis, includes dietary and lifestyle modifications and the use of antacids and H_2 antagonists. Such treatment fails to control LPR in approximately 35% of ORL patients (2,39). In many cases, the intensity of the attempted treatment and the duration of the therapeutic trial are inadequate (2,25). Some clinicians mistakenly believe that a therapeutic trial of antireflux therapy for a few weeks duration is adequate, but that is not the case. Patients with long-standing reflux laryngitis often require months of optimal treatment with near-complete acid suppression to resolve their symptoms (2,16,25).

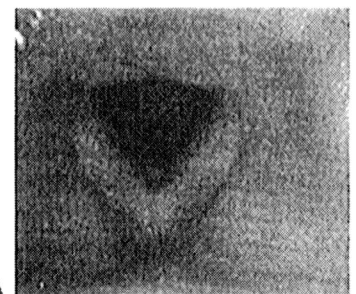 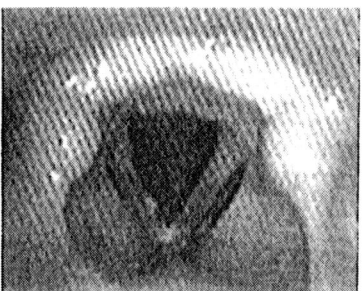

Figure 1 Typical appearance of the larynx of a patient with LPR (A) before and (B) after treatment. (A) The most important findings of LPR are: (1) diffuse laryngeal edema; (2) obliteration of the laryngeal ventricles (the groove between the true and the false vocal cords); (3) pseudosulcus vocalis—due to subglottic edema—giving the true vocal cords the appearance of being thickened with a shallow trench down the middle; and (4) posterior commissure hypertrophy. (B) The same patient after 8 weeks of treatment with a proton pump inhibitor. Note that the vocal cords are thinner, the pseudosulci are gone, the ventricles are open, and the false cord edges are sharply defined. In addition, the patient has small, asymmetrical vocal nodules that were not seen before treatment.

II. Patterns and Mechanisms of Reflux in Otolaryngology Patients

GERD is a common condition, but there appear to be two different populations of patients with GERD. When symptomatic patients with esophagitis seek medical attention, they usually see a gastrointestinal (GI) specialist; however, patients with hoarseness and other reflux-related throat symptoms usually see an ORL specialist. Until relatively recently, it was believed that a majority of patients with LPR presented with esophagitis and its principal symptom, heartburn. This is not the case. Esophagitis patients complain of dysphagia, eructation, regurgitation, and heartburn; symptoms that are frequently absent in patients with reflux laryngitis.

Reflux laryngitis patients usually complain of multiple throat symptoms, including hoarseness, chronic throat clearing and cough, choking episodes, a globus sensation, or sore throat. Ossakow et al. (20) compared the reflux symptoms and findings in two discrete groups: ORL patients with reflux laryngitis ($n = 63$) and GI patients with esophagitis ($n = 36$). They reported that hoarseness was present in 100% of the ORL group and none of the GI group. Heartburn was present in 89% of the GI patients, but in only 6% of the ORL patients. Other authors have reported a low incidence of heartburn as a symptom of reflux laryngitis in ORL patients, ranging from 20 to 43% (1,2,14,29,39).

Usually, ORL patients with reflux laryngitis do not present with the typical diagnostic findings of GI esophagitis patients. Wiener et al. (29) studied ORL patients with hoarseness and found that while 78% had abnormal pH studies, esophageal manometry was normal in 100%, esophagoscopy was normal in 72%, and the Bernstein acid-perfusion test was normal in 66%. Koufman (2) found that only 18% (23/128) of reflux laryngitis patients had findings of esophagitis on barium esophagography.

Several reports of pH-monitoring data in ORL patients and GI patients have emphasized the typical difference in pattern (1,2,5,14,20,25,27–29). ORL patients typically have upright, daytime reflux, but not supine, nocturnal reflux. The pattern in GI patients is typically the opposite, i.e., most of the reflux is nocturnal (2,5,28,29). These same authors have also observed that the total esophageal acid-contact time of supine (GI) refluxers is typically longer than that of upright (ORL) refluxers.

Esophageal acid clearance, the mean time that it takes for the esophageal pH to return to normal (neutral pH) after physiologic or pathologic reflux, is an excellent measure of overall esophageal function (40). Esophageal acid clearance can be calculated from the data of patients who have had ambulatory 24-hour pH monitoring. GI patients with documented erosive esophagitis have prolonged acid clearance due to esophageal dysmotility and sphincter dysfunction. Because ORL patients are predominantly upright refluxers, Koufman et al. (38) calculated the mean esophageal acid clearance in 88 patients with reflux laryngitis and compared the results to data from 10 GI patients with erosive esophagitis. The mean clearance for the ORL group was 0.94 ± 0.23 minutes, while the mean clearance for the GI group was significantly longer ($p < 0.01$) at 2.98 ± 1.23 minutes. It has been postulated that otolaryngology patients with LPR often deny having heartburn and have a relatively low incidence of esophagitis because they are daytime, upright refluxers with relatively normal esophageal motility. These data support this hypothesis and reinforce the belief that most ORL patients with reflux laryngitis experience LPR by different mechanisms than those reported for GI patients with esophagitis.

Experimental instillation of acid in the distal esophagus of normal subjects and patients with esophagitis usually results in a prompt increase in tone of the upper esophageal sphincter (UES) (41). This does not appear to be the case in ORL patients. Our studies have shown that the UES is not an effective barrier to prevent LPR in these patients (26).

In summary, typical GI patients have supine, nocturnal reflux with prolonged esophageal acid clearance. This appears to be due to esophageal dysmotility and lower esophageal sphincter (LES) dysfunction. ORL patients typically have upright, daytime reflux with normal esophageal acid clearance. ORL patients have relatively good esophageal function, but faulty UES function. Thus, it appears that significant differences in the pattern of esophageal dysfunction

Table 3 Differences Between Typical Patients with Reflux Laryngitis and Typical Patients with Esophagitis[a]

	Laryngitis (%)	Esophagitis (%)
Symptoms		
Heartburn	35	89
Hoarseness	85	3
Globus, cough, etc.	64	6
pH Monitoring		
Total abnormal	79	100
Upright	88	46
Supine	45	100
Pharyngeal	50	0
Other Diagnostic Tests	(Abnormal %)	
Esophagoscopy & Bx	27	100
Barium swallow	38	68
Bernstein test	30	89
Esophageal acid clearance	7	70
UES manometry[b]	50	0
H_2-antagonist therapy[c]		
Failure rates	35	10

[a] This table represents a summary of data from many sources. Recognizing that some of the above numbers may not be completely accurate, this table is intended to provide the reader with an overview of the differences between ORL and GI patients with GERD.
[b] J. A. Koufman, unpublished preliminary data (1997), N = 10.
[c] High-dose ranitidine (600–1200 mg/day).

may explain some of the clinical differences between the two patient populations. Table 3 summarizes these differences.

III. Acid and Pepsin

Experimental reflux models in animals have shown that pepsin, and not acid, is responsible for producing tissue injury (2,8). Pepsin, however, requires activation by acid (42). Most animal models have evaluated perfusion of test substances on intact mucosal surfaces, e.g., esophagus, larynx. Using a canine model, Koufman (2) studied the effects of intermittent reflux on the subglottic region of the larynx after a mucosal injury had been created. Following mucosal abrasion, test substances were applied to the subglottic larynges of dogs on alternate weekdays for 2 weeks. The animals were then sacrificed, and the larynges were examined histologically in a blinded manner by a pathologist, who graded the inflammatory findings in a standard fashion. The animals' larynges were painted with: (a) saline; (b) hydrochloric acid alone, pH 1.5, 2.5, and 4.0; or (c) acid and pepsin at the same pH values as the acid-only group. The data reveal that the animals painted with both acid and pepsin had significantly more severe tissue damage than the other two groups ($p < 0.001$).

These experiments show that when a mucosal injury precedes experimental reflux, even intermittent reflux can cause significant tissue injury to the larynx. Even though the animals experienced only three experimental reflux episodes per week for 2 weeks, half of the acid and pepsin animals had frank ulceration of the cricoid cartilage. In addition, these studies confirm that "acid" laryngitis is in reality "peptic" laryngitis, because activated pepsin is needed to produce significant tissue injury (2). These observations may also help explain why effective treatment of reflux laryngitis often requires acid-suppressive doses of a proton pump inhibitor (PPI).

IV. Clinical Manifestations

The larynx, because of its position just above the UES, is a primary target for extraesophageal reflux. LPR may adversely impact other extraesophageal structures, such as the nose, sinuses, and ears (18,43). Since little is known about LPR events, such as the patterns of spread of the refluxate and its clearance, the effect of LPR on structures and organs above and below the larynx remains to be elucidated. Even among otolaryngologists, there is no uniform consensus as to the role of LPR in many diseases of the head and neck. Unfortunately, there are still very few reflux-testing data on the relationship between LPR and conditions such as sinusitis and otitis media. Most of the available clinical data in ORL is related to the relationship between LPR and laryngeal diseases (Table 1).

In a large series of ORL patients with reflux laryngitis and documented LPR, 92% presented with dysphonia (hoarseness) (2). Additional symptoms were experienced by the majority of the patients: chronic throat clearing (50%), chronic cough (44%), globus (sensation of "lump in throat") (33%), and dysphagia (27%). The pattern of dysphonia was either chronic or intermittent. Patients with intermittent dysphonia often complain that they suffer from laryngitis that lasts for days or weeks, several times a year. Half of the patients denied having any heartburn whatsoever; 13% had two or fewer episodes per week, 27% had two to four episodes per week, and only 10% complained of more frequent or daily heartburn (2).

The clinical manifestations of LPR in ORL patients can be divided into three groups, based upon severity: life-threatening, major, and minor. Although most patients with reflux laryngitis present with mild to moderate dysphonia as the primary symptom, some suffer from more serious, even life-threatening, conditions. Less common laryngeal manifestations of LPR include laryngospasm, arytenoid fixation, laryngeal stenosis, and carcinoma. LPR is also associated with the development of polypoid degeneration (Reinke's edema), vocal nodules, and other functional voice disorders.

Table 4 Relative Severity of Symptoms and Sequelae Related to Laryngopharyngeal Reflux

Minor	Major	Life-threatening[a]
Dysphonia[b] (in the "nonvocal professions")	Dysphonia[b] (in a vocalist or professional speaker)	Subglottic stenosis
Ulcer/Granuloma[b] (in the "nonvocal professions")	Ulcer/granuloma[b] (in a vocalist or professional speaker)	Posterior laryngeal stenosis
Globus	Leukoplakia	Arytenoid fixation
Dysphagia	Pachydermia	Carcinoma (especially in nonsmokers)
Chronic throat clearing	Dysplasia	Laryngospasm
Chronic cough	Chronic cough[c]	

[a]The "life-threatening" group is defined by either airway obstruction or malignancy
[b]The purpose of establishing a "difference" between the "severity" (of the same symptom) in the vocalist and the nonvocalist is to emphasize that economic and emotional consequences of a voice disorder depend on the vocal needs and demands of each patient. When a professional vocalist, for example, develops a voice disorder, this may have profound consequences, and thus effective treatment must be maximized (see text).
[c]On occasion, this symptom may be so severe that the patient is relatively incapacitated.
Note: A professional speaker is a person for whom a good voice is essential to his or her profession, e.g., lecturer, minister, telephone operator.

The severity of the clinical manifestations (Table 4) influences the clinician's approach to the diagnosis and treatment of each of the three patient groups. Each group is managed differently. Patients with airway obstruction and malignant neoplasia are considered to have life-threatening reflux. Those with other, less severe symptoms and findings are subgrouped into the major or minor groups. Those subgroup determinations are not only based upon the severity of the clinical situation, but also take into account the vocal needs and occupation of the patient.

A. Functional Voice Disorders

The term functional voice disorder (FVD) applies to a variety of vocal abuse/misuse/overuse syndromes. The FVD conditions are often associated with the development of secondary histopathologic changes in the vocal cords, which include hematomas, nodules, ulcers, granulomas, and Reinke's edema. Available pH-monitoring data suggest that the majority of patients with these functional lesions have LPR in addition to abnormal (or altered) laryngeal biomechanics (22). In many cases, LPR may have precipitated the problem (1).

As part of the evaluation of each patient with a FVD, the clinician should elicit a reflux history. Patients who have posterior laryngeal erythema, edema, or thick mucus in the endolarynx should be suspected of having LPR. Although treatment of LPR alone does not resolve all FVDs, such is the case in some patients. Failure to treat reflux laryngitis, when it is present, may doom what otherwise would be an effective therapeutic intervention.

The laryngeal findings of a patient with a FVD may be subtle, ranging from increased endolaryngeal mucus and subglottic edema to ulceration and granulation. Subglottic edema may give the appearance of a subglottic groove or vocal fold sulcus, i.e., a pseudosulcus. This finding should alert the clinician to the possibility of LPR. Mucus in the larynx is not usually the result of infection or postnasal drip. This finding is generally the result of a local tissue (inflammatory) response to chronic irritation. Ulceration and granulation can be seen in non-LPR patients; however, most patients who present with these findings have both reflux and abnormal vocal usage.

B. Granulomas

Some patients with reflux laryngitis develop granulomas of the arytenoids. The etiology of these lesions is multifactorial; however, LPR should always be suspected. Granulomas often result from the combination of acute mucosal ulceration of the vocal processes, LPR, and chronic vocal trauma due to throat clearing and/or vocal abuse (16). The clinician should, in each case, consider each of the possible contributing etiologic factors and correct each one if therapy is to be effective. Effective antireflux therapy (twice-daily PPI) is sufficient to allow healing in the majority of patients. Surgical removal of granulomas is uncommonly indicated, except when (a) lesions appear suspicious for malignancy (they should be excised for biopsy), (b) large granulomas cause airway obstruction, and (c) granulomas mature and become fibroepithelial polyps (16).

C. Paroxysmal Laryngospasm

Laryngospasm is an uncommon complaint, but patients who experience this frightening symptom are usually able to describe events in vivid detail. If the clinician mimics severe inspiratory stridor, the patient will confirm that his or her breathing during an attack does indeed sound similar. Laryngospasm is sometimes confused with asthma; however, if the patient is asked whether the problem is "getting air in" or "getting it out," the patient with true laryngospasm will always say "in." Laryngospasm is often paroxysmal, and it usually occurs without warning. For some patients, the attacks awake them from sleep. In some cases, the attacks may have a predictable pattern, e.g., postcibal or during exercise. Some patients are aware of a relationship between LPR and the attacks, others are not. Loughlin and Koufman (19) reported that of 12 patients who presented with recurrent paroxysmal laryngospasm, 11 had documented LPR by pH testing and all 12 responded to treatment with a PPI (omeprazole) with a complete cessation of the laryngospasm episodes.

Using a canine model, Loughlin et al. (44) demonstrated that acid stimulation (pH < 2.5) of chemoreceptors, "taste buds," on the epiglottis caused reproducible laryngospasm. The laryngospasm reflex was documented to occur independent of pepsin concentration and tonicity of test substances. This reflex is mediated by the superior laryngeal nerves. This and other studies suggest that reflux-related laryngospasm may be a cause of sudden infant death syndrome (SIDS) (45–48).

D. Polypoid Degeneration (Reinke's Edema)

Polypoid degeneration results from chronic laryngeal irritation over a period of many years. It is almost always bilateral and occurs most frequently in elderly female smokers. Nevertheless, it is also seen is nonsmoking patients with LPR or hypothyroidism. Most patients with polypoid degeneration have abnormal pH testing (1). Consequently, LPR should be considered in the differential diagnosis. Polypoid degeneration may improve with antireflux therapy and cessation of smoking, but most patients with these lesions require surgical treatment as well. Patients undergoing vocal fold surgery for this condition should receive antireflux treatment during the perioperative period.

E. Laryngeal Stenosis

The primary cause of laryngeal stenosis, including subglottic and posterior laryngeal stenosis, is LPR (2,3,8,17). Reflux documented by pH testing has been found in 92% of cases (2). Treatment with PPIs or fundoplication will result in subsequent decannulation of the vast majority of patients with stenosis, in some cases without additional laryngeal surgery. pH monitoring and antireflux therapy are routinely indicated in all cases of laryngeal stenosis, and high-dose PPI treatment and fundoplication are essential adjuncts to laryngeal rehabilitative surgery.

F. Carcinoma of the Larynx

LPR is an important risk factor for the development of laryngeal carcinoma (1,2,6,9–13). Koufman and Cummings (6) reported a prospectively evaluated series of 50 patients with early laryngeal carcinoma in which abnormal reflux was documented in 72%, while only 44% were active smokers. The remaining subjects were 42% ex-smokers (with a median duration of smoking cessation of 8 years) and 14% lifetime nonsmokers. The relationship between LPR and malignant degeneration of the laryngeal mucosa remains to be proven, but the available reflux testing data suggest that most patients who develop laryngeal malignancy both smoke and have LPR (2,6,12,13). For nonsmokers who develop laryngeal cancer, LPR appears to the single most important risk factor (6,11).

Laryngeal carcinogenesis appears to be multifactorial (11). Previously identified risk factors, i.e., tobacco and ethanol, also strongly predispose one to reflux (2,6,49–51). Tobacco and alcohol adversely influence almost all of the body's antireflux mechanisms; they delay gastric emptying, decrease lower esophageal sphincter pressure and esophageal motility, decrease mucosal resistance, and increase gastric acid secretion (49–51).

In a carefully controlled case study, Guenal et al. (52) showed that the major risk factor for the development of supraglottic carcinoma is ethanol consumption and not tobacco. Koufman has reported six patients with apparently premalignant vocal cord lesions (leukoplakia) that resolved, i.e., disappeared, with antireflux therapy alone (2). Routine reflux testing, followed by PPI treatment, is recommended for all patients with laryngeal neoplasia even when other risk factors for the development of carcinoma of the larynx are present.

G. Dysphagia, Globus Pharyngeus, and Other Reflux-Related Cervical Symptoms

Dysphagia (difficulty swallowing), globus pharyngeus (a sensation of a lump in the throat), and chronic sore throat are all symptoms that may be caused by LPR. Reflux commonly causes these symptoms (2,20,21). With this group of symptoms, however, it is incumbent on the clinician to rule out other inflammatory disorders and mass lesions, e.g., hypopharyngeal carcinoma, cervical osteophyte, foreign body, thyroid goiter. With the above symptoms, contrast barium study is recommended as the first diagnostic test after the examination is completed. In addition, if the patient has reflux findings, then manometry and pH monitoring are obtained.

Several mechanisms for dysphagia and globus are reflux-related: (a) patients may have distal esophagitis, without true LPR, and experience these cervical symptoms; (b) patients with LPR may have UES dysfunction, characterized by high resting UES pressure and discoordinated (usually delayed) UES opening; and (c) patients may have sufficient LPR with gastric contents bathing laryngopharyngeal structures, so that throat symptoms are caused by local inflammation and swelling.

Ossakow et al. (20) reported that ORL patients with cervical symptoms usually have actual LPR. The pattern of reflux in this group is similar to that of ORL patients with other LPR symptoms and different from GI patients with esophagitis. The findings of Koufman were somewhat different; he found that ORL patients with globus and dysphagia frequently have esophageal dysfunction, including dysmotility, esophagitis, and stricture formation, more frequently, compared to other ORL patients with LPR (2).

H. Xerostomia and GERD

Xerostomia, dryness of the mouth, commonly encountered in otolaryngologic practice is a major risk factor for the development of GERD. Salivary bicarbonate is needed to restore the intraluminal esophageal pH after a reflux episode. Without normal saliva, the esophageal pH remains very low for an extended period of time (40).

Xerostomia is commonly seen with sicca syndrome, Sjögren's syndrome, scleroderma and most other collagen vascular diseases, cystic fibrosis, and with many medications (e.g., anticholinergics, antihypertensives, antihistamines). Head and neck irradiation also produces xerostomia. Rosman et al. (53) studied seven ORL patients with head and neck irradiation. All had normal esophageal motility; however, six of the seven had abnormal esophageal acid clearance and abnormal pH-monitoring results.

I. Laryngopharyngeal Reflux in Pediatric Patients

Pediatric patients also suffer from LPR; dysphonia, laryngospasm, laryngomalacia, and pulmonary disorders, such as asthma, have been shown to be related to LPR in infants and children (18,23,24,31). A recent report documented LPR in 93% of ORL pediatric patients with airway diseases (23) Double-probe pH monitoring is especially useful in diagnosis of pediatric patients. They seldom complain of symptoms. The double probe is recommended because of its enhanced sensitivity for LPR, the sensitivity of single-probe pH testing being only 47% (23). The treatment algorithms presented herein apply to infants and children; however, it is more difficult to administer and dose PPIs in pediatric patients. Therefore, H_2 antagonists and fundoplication are commonly employed in pediatric patients with LPR.

V. Diagnosis

When a patient presents with symptoms of reflux laryngitis, the clinician should perform a complete otolaryngologic examination. This includes fiberoptic laryngoscopy and photography of the larynx. Ambulatory 24-hour double-probe pH monitoring and barium esophagography should be considered.

Double-probe (simultaneous esophageal and pharyngeal) pH monitoring has a tremendous advantage over any other diagnostic method because it is both highly sensitive and specific (29,54). Furthermore, pH monitoring reveals the pattern of reflux, so that subsequent treatment can be custom-tailored for each patient. For example, if the patient does not have supine nocturnal reflux, elevation of the head of the bed is not necessary. pH monitoring has been available for many years, and standards (normal values) have been established in many laboratories (2,54). The single most important parameter is generally regarded to be the percentage of time that the pH is less than 4. This measurement is usually calculated for time in the upright position, time in the supine position, and the total time of the study. For the upright position, the upper limit of normal is approximately 8.0%, and for the supine position, approximately 2.5% (2,54).

A. The Pharyngeal Probe in ORL Patients with LPR

Detection of pharyngeal reflux episodes during double-probe pH monitoring, with the second probe being placed behind the larynx just above the cricopharyngeus, is indicative of laryngopharyngeal reflux. In our laboratory, none of 20 normal controls had any documented pharyngeal reflux episode (29). Therefore, it may be concluded that even a single pharyngeal reflux episode should be considered diagnostic of LPR (2,26).

Double-probe pH monitoring is particularly important in ORL patients because otherwise the diagnosis might be missed. Recently, it was shown that 37% (28/75) of a consecutive series of ORL patients with abnormal pH testing had normal total acid exposure times in the esophagus, but still had pharyngeal reflux (26). In other words, were it not for the pharyngeal probe findings, these 28 patients would have been falsely presumed not to have reflux. Pharyngeal probe pH monitoring is necessary in ORL patients because it significantly increases the diagnostic yield (sensitivity) of pH monitoring from 50 to 75% (26).

B. Barium Esophagography or Esophagoscopy

It is also advisable to perform a barium swallow/esophagogram or esophagoscopy in ORL patients with LPR to assess the integrity of the esophageal lining (2,55). Although contrast studies are not a sensitive way to diagnose LPR, they may demonstrate significant esophageal abnormalities that might otherwise be missed. In a series of 128 patients, the results of barium study revealed that 18% had esophagitis, 14% had a lower esophageal ring, and 3% had a peptic stricture (2). Since so few ORL patients with LPR have esophagitis, esophagoscopy is not routinely recommended except for elderly Caucasian men, who are at increased risk of developing Barrett's esophagus and esophageal cancer.

VI. Treatment

The larynx is far more susceptible to peptic injury than the esophagus, because it does not have acid-clearance mechanisms (peristalsis and salivary bicarbonate) and because its mucosa is thin, fragile, and poorly adapted to protect against reflux. For some patients with LPR, treatment with lifestyle modifications and an H_2 antagonist is appropriate initial therapy; however, treatment failure can be expected in approximately 35% (2). The problem with H_2 antagonists is that they do not adequately suppress gastric acid. Pepsin, the actual injurious agent in the refluxate, is acid-activated, and at pH 4.5 70% of peptic activity remains (2,56). Since the patient's gastric pH is less than 4 at the therapeutic nadir, activated pepsin is present several times each day and can produce significant injury. In other words, for patients with LPR in whom even infrequent LPR may cause laryngeal damage, H_2 antagonists may be inadequate treatment.

The PPIs (omeprazole and lansoprazole) have revolutionized antireflux treatment for reflux-related esophageal disease (57–61) and for LPR (19,25,39,62,63). However, even when treated with relatively large daily doses of PPI, many patients with LPR will not experience resolution of their symptoms until after several months of treatment. In 1996, a consensus conference of otolaryngologists on LPR suggested that the duration of therapy with PPI should be 6 months (25). In addition, PPI therapy is also useful in difficult-to-diagnose cases. Until the availability of PPIs, a trial of antireflux medication had little validity as a diagnostic test. On the other hand, a therapeutic trial of PPI therapy may be used as a diagnostic test, but again, it is important not to underdose or to treat for too short a period of time.

Treatment of LPR requires considerable individualization with the level of treatment depending on the severity of the patient's condition. Obviously, clinicians have fewer treatment options for patients with life-threatening or major LPR than in patients with minor reflux. In creating treatment algorithms, consideration must be given to both the initial treatment period and long-range therapy (years). Hence, the age and the occupation of the patient must also be considered in formulating treatment plans.

A. Treatment of Life-Threatening LPR

Ideally, all patients with laryngeal carcinoma, stenoses, and laryngospasm should undergo pH monitoring and manometry before antireflux treatment is started. This is not always possible, particularly if the patient requires emergency surgical treatment such as tracheotomy. Nevertheless, every effort should be made to obtain these studies prior to treatment, because (a) it establishes the diagnosis, (b) it determines the severity of the GERD, (c) it establishes baseline manometric parameters, (d) it allows treatment to be individualized, and (e) in selected cases, it justifies unconventional treatment.

Initial treatment in these patients should be with high-dose PPI, e.g., omeprazole 40–60 mg or lansoprazole 60–90 mg, as well as with dietary and lifestyle modification. In the event that the patient is unable to take an orally administered medicine, an intravenous ranitidine drip should be employed, and the gastric contents should be neutralized using antacids and/or continuous enteral alimentation. In selected cases (particularly young patients) with the most severe form of LPR, fundoplication should be considered as an early alternative. If, for example, a young person presents with laryngeal airway obstruction, no prior history of trauma or intubation, and pH evidence of severe reflux with a very low LES pressure on manometry, then fundoplication is probably the first and best antireflux treatment. While this situation is uncommon, it does occur.

For most patients, PPIs are the treatment of choice for at least the first 6 months, or until such time as the clinical situation that prompted the intervention has resolved. It is injudicious to stop or taper PPIs in patients with laryngeal stenosis still undergoing treatment for the stenosis. Since some of these patients present with airway obstruction severe enough to require tracheotomy, PPI treatment should be continued until the patient has been successfully decannulated, and it is clear (by repeat pH testing) that reflux is under control. In practice, most patients with stenosis will require either chronic PPI therapy or fundoplication. The same is true for many patients with carcinoma of the larynx, especially non smokers who develop carcinoma. In this group, the risk of the patient developing new lesions exceeds the risks of definitive long-term antireflux treatment.

In 1989, when omeprazole was introduced in the United States, The Food and Drug Administration recommended that it be used in a dose of 20 mg per day for only 6–8 weeks. It was soon clear that this regimen was woefully inadequate to treat many ORL reflux patients (25,39). Fortunately, long-term omeprazole therapy has been used extensively, and it is now believed to be safe and effective as a long-term therapy (64–66). In patients with life-threatening LPR over the age of 60 years, chronic, long-term PPI treatment is recommended. On the other hand, if the patient has only supine or upright reflux disease, but not both, a single daily dose may suffice for maintenance after the acute phase of the illness has resolved.

For patients under 40 years of age, fundoplication is usually recommended, and for patients between the ages of 40 and 60 years, treatment is selected on an individual basis. In the latter situation, the severity of the LPR and of the underlying ORL condition is considered, as well as the preferences of the patient and his or her overall medical condition.

B. Treatment of Major LPR

The initial phase of treatment for patients in this group is similar to that outlined above, except that fundoplication is rarely considered. As a rule, the first 6 months of treatment should consist of PPI therapy and a program that optimally manages the patient's diet, weight, and lifestyle: (a) smoking cessation (if the patient smokes) (b) weight reduction (if the patient is overweight), (c) avoidance of overeating and night-eating, (d) a low-fat diet, and (e) avoidance of known "refluxogenic" foods, such as coffee, chocolate, mints, and carbonated beverages.

The initial phase of antireflux therapy has two simultaneous goals: to arrest the inflammatory process in the larynx and, if possible, to reconstitute the body's normal antireflux defenses (2,67). After 6 months of PPI therapy, if the patient's larynx has returned to normal, and assuming good patient compliance, the PPI dose may be tapered. The patient may then want to try using an H_2 antagonist. The patient should be followed closely during the therapeutic adjustment period. If the patient appears to be failing medical treatment at any time, repeat pH monitoring should be obtained while the patient is continuing to take the medication to evaluate the efficacy of treatment. In this way, medical treatment failure can be objectively documented. When this situation is encountered, the clinician must consider other therapeutic options.

C. Treatment of Minor LPR

In most ORL practices, the minor reflux group comprises a majority of patients with reflux laryngitis. Minor reflux patients typically have symptoms of intermittent dysphonia, chronic throat clearing, globus pharyngeus, and dysphagia and findings such as laryngeal edema and posterior laryngitis. It is appropriate for the clinician to adopt a less aggressive and more conventional approach to the management of patients in this group. Clearly, it is not essential to obtain pH monitoring in all of these patients prior to treatment. Furthermore, conventional antireflux therapy is sufficient for many patients in this group. If initial therapy fails, the medication type and dosage should be escalated in a stepwise fashion.

Patients who fall into the minor reflux group, based upon the symptoms and findings, should be managed conservatively if they do not have laryngeal lesions for which surgery is contemplated. It is prudent to treat all patients undergoing laryngeal surgery with PPIs. The PPI should be started prior to, and continued after, surgery, until healing of the larynx is complete. The routine use of perioperative omeprazole appears to decrease postoperative complications of laryngeal surgery and enhance the results (1,6).

VII. Reflux, the Internal Environment, and a New Paradigm of Airway Disease

We are at a crossroads in terms of our understanding of LPR/GERD. It is the likely cause of, or a primary catalyst for, many inflammatory and neoplastic diseases of the airway, including some occurring apart from the laryngopharynx. Reflux may also influence regulatory functions and vagal reflexes, both normal and maladaptive (e.g., the possible relationship between LPR and SIDS).

Based upon clinical and double-probe pH-monitoring data, the sensitivity of pH testing using the current state-of-the-art instrumentation for the diagnosis of LPR is at best 80% (1,2,5,6). The problem, however, is not the instrumentation, but rather that LPR is frequently intermittent. In addition, demonstration of a LPR event by pH testing does not prove causality, i.e., that LPR is the cause of disease. Until recently, the medical community may have underestimated the impact of LPR/GERD on airway diseases, because LPR is often silent, intermittent, and therefore, sometimes difficult to diagnose.

Research is needed in three areas. The first is epidemiology. Little is known about the prevalence and incidence of premorbid and symptomatic LPR. In a study of a community-based cohort of 100 adults, Reulbach et al. (68) found that 70% of people over the age of 40 years had symptoms and findings of reflux laryngitis. Subclinical LPR may be ubiquitous, and its impact on airway diseases may be profound.

The second area is vagal physiology, including (a) normal and abnormal vagal reflexes, (b) relationships and interactions between the regulatory functions of different organs supplied by the vagus, and (c) the impact of exogenous diseases, e.g., viral infection or trauma, on vagal function and LPR/GERD.

The third area is related to the impact of reflux on a cellular level, including (a) humoral responses of airway mucosa, (b) cell membrane permeability and damage, and (c) metaplasia, neoplasia, and carcinogenesis.

It seems reasonable to propose that a multitude of interrelated factors (genetic, anatomic, neuromuscular, and inflammatory) may influence LPR/GERD and that LPR/GERD, even when ubiquitous and silent, may adversely influence the internal environment in significant ways. Development of such a new paradigm of LPR/GERD will require a multidisciplinary approach.

VIII. Conclusion

Laryngopharyngeal reflux is an illusive, ubiquitous, and pernicious cause of laryngopharyngeal inflammatory and neoplastic disorders. Frequently underdiagnosed and undertreated, LPR is believed to be an etiologic factor in approximately half of patients with laryngeal and voice disorders. The pervasive and serious nature of LPR in laryngology demands that clinicians caring for patients with laryngeal and voice disorders consider this diagnosis in almost every case. The most important advances in the management of LPR are ambulatory 24-hour double-probe pH monitoring and the proton pump inhibitors. These have revolutionized the diagnosis and treatment of reflux in otolaryngology.

References

1. Koufman JA, Cummins MM. The prevalence and spectrum of reflux in laryngology. a prospective study of 132 consecutive patients with laryngeal and voice disorders. Presented at the Meeting of the Southern Section of the American Laryngological, Rhinological and Otological Society, Inc., Naples, FL, January 10, 1996.
2. Koufman JA. The otolaryngologic manifestations of gastroesophageal reflux disease. Laryngoscope 1991; 101(Suppl 53):1–78.
3. Bain WM, Harrington JW, Thomas LE, et al. Head and neck manifestations of gastroesophageal reflux. Laryngoscope 1983; 93:175–179.
4. Delahunty JE. Acid laryngitis. J Laryngol Otol 1972; 86:335–342.
5. Koufman JA, Wiener CJ, Wu W, et al. Reflux laryngitis and its sequelae: the diagnostic role of ambulatory 24-hour pH monitoring. J Voice 1988; 2:78–89.
6. Koufman JA, Cummins MM. Reflux and early laryngeal carcinoma: a prospective study using pH monitoring. Presented at the Meeting of the Southern Section of the American Laryngological, Rhinological and Otological Society, Inc., Key West, FL, January 7, 1995.
7. Jindal JR, Milbrath MM, Shaker R, et al. Gastroesophageal reflux disease as a likely cause of "idiopathic" subglottic stenosis. Ann Otol Rhinol Laryngol 1994; 103: 186–191.

8. Little FB, Koufman JA, Kohut RI, et al. Effect of gastric acid on the pathogenesis of subglottic stenosis. Ann Otol Rhinol Laryngol 1985; 94:516–519.
9. Glanz H, Kleinsasser O. Chronische Laryngitis und Carcinom (with English abstract). Arch Otorhinolaryngol 1976; 212:57–75.
10. Freije JE, Beatty TW, Campbell BH, et al. Carcinoma of the larynx in patients with gastroesophageal reflux. Am J Otol 1996; 17:386–390.
11. Koufman JA, Burke AJ. The etiology and pathogenesis of laryngeal carcinoma. Oto Clin NA 1997; 30:1–19.
12. Morrison MD. Is chronic gastroesophageal reflux a causative factor in glottic carcinoma? Otolaryngol Head Neck Surg 1988; 99:370–373.
13. Ward PH, Hanson DG. Reflux as an etiological factor of carcinoma of the laryngopharynx. Laryngoscope 1988; 98:1195–1199.
14. Olson NR. Laryngopharyngeal manifestations of gastroesophageal reflux disease. Otol Clin NA 1991; 24:1201–1213.
15. Cherry J, Margulies SI. Contact ulcer of the larynx. Laryngoscope 1968; 78:1937–1940.
16. Koufman JA. Contact ulcer and granuloma of the larynx. In: Gates GA, ed. Current Therapy in Otolaryngology—Head and Neck surgery. 5th ed. St. Louis: Mosby, 1993:456–459.
17. Bogdasarian RS, Olson NR. Posterior glottic laryngeal stenosis. Otolaryngol Head Neck Surg 1980; 88:765–772.
18. Contencin P, Narcy P. Gastropharyngeal reflux in infants and children. A pharyngeal pH monitoring study. Arch Otol Head Neck Surg 1992; 118:1028–1030.
19. Loughlin CJ, Koufman JA. Paroxysmal laryngospasm secondary to gastroesophageal reflux. Laryngoscopy 1996; 106:1502–1505.
20. Ossakow SJ, Elta G, Colturi T, et al. Esophageal reflux and dysmotility as the basis for persistent cervical symptoms. Ann Otol Rhinol Laryngol 1987; 96:387–392.
21. Woo P, Noordzij P, Ross JA. Association of esophageal reflux and globus symptom: comparison of laryngoscopy and 24-hour pH manometry. Otol Head Neck Surg 1996; 115:502–507.
22. Koufman JA, Blalock PD. Functional voice disorders. Oto Clin NA 1991; 24:1059–1073.
23. Little JP, Matthews BL, Glock MS, et al. Extraesophageal pediatric reflux: 24-hour double-probe pH monitoring of 222 children. Ann Otol Rhinol Laryngol 1997; 106:1–16.
24. Roger G, Denoyelle F, Triglia JM. Severe laryngomalacia: surgical indications and results in 115 patients. Laryngoscope 1995; 105:1111–1117.
25. Koufman J, Sataloff RT, Toohill R. Laryngopharyngeal reflux: consensus conference report. J Voice 1996; 10:215–216.
26. Koufman JA. Unpublished data.
27. Shaker R, Milbrath M, Ren J, et al. Esophagopharyngeal distribution of refluxed gastric acid in patients with reflux laryngitis. Gastroenterology 1995; 109:1575–1582.
28. Wiener GJ, Cooper JB, Wu WC, et al. Is hoarseness an atypical manifestation of gastroesophageal reflux (GER)? An ambulatory 24 hour pH study. Gastroenterology 1986; 90A:1691.
29. Wiener GJ, Koufman JA, Wu WC, et al. Chronic hoarseness secondary to gastro-

esophageal reflux disease: documentation with 24-h ambulatory pH monitoring. Am J Gastro 1989; 84:1503–1508.
30. Winkelstein A. Peptic esophagitis: a new clinical entity. JAMA 1935; 104:906–909.
31. Berenberg W, Neuhauser EBD. Cardio-esophageal relaxation (chalasia) as a cause of vomiting in infants. Pediatrics 1950; 5:414–420.
32. Jackson C. The Life of Chevalier Jackson: An Autobiography. New York: Macmillan Co., 1938:229.
33. Meltzer SJ. On the causes of the orderly progress of peristaltic movements in the oesophagus. Am J Physiol 1899; 2:266–272.
34. Tileson W. Peptic ulcer of the oesophagus. Am J Med Sci 1906; 132:240–265.
35. Mosher HP. The liver tunnel and cardiospasm. Ann Otol Rhinol Laryngol 1921; 30:1065–1067.
36. Ingelfinger FJ, Abbott WO. Intubation studies of human small intestine: diagnostic significance of motor disturbances. Am J Dig Dis 1940; 7:468–474.
37. Miller FA, DoVale J, Gunther T. Utilization of inlying pH probe for evaluation of acid-peptic diathesis. Arch Surg 1964; 89:199–203.
38. Koufman JA, Postma GN, Panetti M, Nowak L. Esophageal acid clearance in otolaryngology patients with laryngopharyngeal reflux. Presented at the Annual Meeting of the American Academy of Otolaryngology—Head and Neck Surgery, San Francisco, September 19, 1997.
39. Hanson DG, Kamel PL, Kahrilas PJ. Outcomes of antireflux therapy for the treatment of chronic laryngitis. Ann Otol Rhinol Laryngol 1995; 104:550–555.
40. Helm JF, Dodds WJ, Riedel DR, et al. Determinants of esophageal acid clearance in normal subjects. Gastroenterology 1983; 85:607–612.
41. Gerhardt DC, Schuck TJ, Bordeaux EA, et al. Human upper esophageal sphincter response to volume, osmotic, and acid stimuli. Gastroenterology 1978; 75:268–274.
42. Wolfe MM, Soll AH. The physiology of gastric acid secretion. NEJM 1988; 319:1707–1715.
43. Gibson WS Jr, Cochran W. Otalgia in infants and children—a manifestation of gastroesophageal reflux. Int J Ped Otorhinolaryngol 1994; 28:213–218.
44. Loughlin CJ, Koufman JA, Averill DB, et al. Acid-induced laryngospasm in canine model. Laryngoscope 1996; 106:1506–1509.
45. Bauman NM, Sander AD, Schmidt C, et al. Reflex laryngospasm induced by stimulation of distal esophageal afferents. Laryngoscope 1994; 104:209–214.
46. Denoyelle F, Garabedian EN, Roger G, et al. Laryngeal dyskinesia as a cause of stridor in infants. Arch Otol Head Neck Surg 1996; 122:612–616.
47. Shatz A, Hiss J, Arenberg B. Basement-membrane thickening of the vocal cords in sudden infant death syndrome. Laryngoscope 1991; 101:484–486.
48. Wetmore RF. Effects of acid on the larynx of the maturing rabbit and their possible significance to the sudden infant death syndrome. Laryngoscope 1993; 103:1242–1254.
49. Dennish DW, Castell DO. Inhibitory effect of smoking on the lower esophageal sphincter. N Engl J Med 1971; 284:1136–1137.
50. Vitale GC, Cheadle WG, Patel B, et al. Effect of alcohol on nocturnal gastroesophageal reflux. JAMA 1987; 258:2077–2079.
51. Vitale GC, Cheadle WF, Patel B, et al. Smoking delays gastric emptying of solids. Gut 1989; 30:50–53.

52. Guenel P, Chastang J-F, Luce D, et al. A study of the interaction of alcohol drinking and tobacco smoking among French cases of laryngeal cancer. J Epidemiol Commun Health 1988; 42:350–354.
53. Rosman AS, Goldberg H, Federman Q, et al. Chronic xerostomia alters 23 hour pH and is associated with esophageal inflammation. Gastroenterology 1988; 94:A387.
54. Richter JE, ed. Ambulatory Esophageal pH Monitoring: Practical Approach and Clinical Applications. Tokyo: Igaku-Shoin, 1991.
55. Ott DJ, Cowan RJ, Gelfand DW, et al. The role of diagnostic imaging in evaluating gastroesophageal reflux disease. Postgrad Radiol 1986; 6:3–14.
56. Piper DW, Fenton BH. pH stability and activity curves of pepsin with special reference to their clinical importance. Gut 1965; 6:506–508.
57. Klinkenberg-Knol EC. Recent Advances in the Diagnosis and Management of Gastro-oesophageal Reflux Disease: The Role of Omeprazole in Clinical Practice. Amsterdam: VU University Press, 1990.
58. Klinkenberg-Knol EC, Meuwissen SG. Medical therapy of patients with reflux oesophagitis poorly responsive to H2-receptor antagonist therapy. Digestion 1992; 1:44–48.
59. Klinkenberg-Knol EC. The role of omeprazole in healing and prevention of reflux disease. Hepato-Gastroenterology 1992; 1:27–30.
60. Langtry HD, Wilde MI. Lansoprazole. An update of its pharmacological properties and clinical efficacy in the management of acid-related disorders. Drugs 1997; 54:473–500.
61. Sontag SJ, Hirschowitz BI, Holt S, et al. Two doses of omeprazole versus placebo in symptomatic erosive esophagitis: the U.S. Multicenter Study. Gastroenterology 1992; 102:109–118.
62. Kamel PL, Hanson D, Kahrilas PJ. Omeprazole for the treatment of posterior laryngitis. Am J Med 1994; 96:321–326.
63. Shaw GY, Searl JP, Young JL, et al. Subjective, laryngoscopic, and acoustic measurements of laryngeal reflux before and after treatment with omeprazole. J Voice 1996; 10:410–418.
64. Heudebert GR, Marks R, Wilcox CM, et al. Choice of long-term strategy for the management of patients with severe esophagitis: a cost-utility analysis. Gastroenterology 1997; 112:1078–1086.
65. Hillman AL, Bloom BS, Fendrick M, et al. Cost and quality effects of alternative treatments for persistent gastroesophageal reflux disease. Arch Intern Med 1992; 152:1467–1472.
66. Klinkenberg-Knol EC, Festen HPM, Jansen JBMJ, et al. Long-term treatment with omeprazole for refractory reflux esophagitis: efficacy and safety. Ann Intern Med 1994; 121:161–166.
67. Katz PO, Knuff TE, Benjamin SB, et al. Abnormal esophageal pressures in reflux esophagitis: cause or effect? Am J Gastroenterol 1986; 81:744–746.
68. Reulbach TR, Postma GN, Koufman JA. Unpublished data.

5

GERD
A Major Factor in Chronic Cough

CURTIS J. MELLO

Brown University School of Medicine
Providence, Rhode Island

I. Introduction

Cough is a common symptom for which patients seek medical attention. Approximately 30 million visits to primary care physicians occur each year because of cough (1). Cough is the third leading cause for seeing an office-based internist (2,3). The economic impact of cough is significant. Over $500 million are spent each year on cough and cold preparations (1).

Cough can be caused by a multiplicity of factors. Although it is beyond the scope of this chapter to discuss every cause of cough, and it is important for the reader to become familiar with some of the most frequent causes of cough and to consider gastroesophageal reflux as a cause of cough. There are three important distinguishing considerations when evaluating the cause of cough: duration, smoking status, and findings on chest roentgenogram. Cough can be acute or chronic. Chronic cough is defined most frequently as a cough lasting longer than 3 or 4 weeks (3–8). The most frequent cause of an acute cough is the common cold (3). The presence or absence of cigarette smoking is the single most important consideration in assessing the cause of persistent cough. Smoke-induced airway inflammation is the most common cause of chronic cough in cigarette smokers (1,10,11). The consideration of causes of chronic cough differs depending on the presence or absence of a normal chest roentgenogram. Puolijoki and Lahdensuo (12) studied 198 patients with cough lasting longer than 2 months. Among the 51 patients with abnormal chest roentgenograms, lung cancer and sarcoidosis were the two most frequent causes of cough. Asthma and postnasal drip were most commonly implicated as the etiologies of cough in the 147 patients with a normal chest roentgenogram. Asthma and postnasal drip have been found to be among the most frequent causes of cough in nonsmokers with a normal chest roentgenogram in a number of other studies as well (4,5,7,8,13–17).

Gastroesophageal reflux has been implicated as a cause of chronic cough in numerous studies (4,5,7,9,14,17–32). Depending on the clinical setting, i.e., primary care setting or referral center, GER-induced cough accounts for 4–24% of the cases of chronic cough (4,5,14,17,18). In nonsmokers with normal chest roentgenograms who are not using angiotensin-converting enzyme inhibitors and in whom asthma and postnasal drip have been ruled out, gastroesophageal reflux is the most frequent cause of chronic cough (5,7,12,13,16). Irwin et al. (5) demonstrated that GER was the third most frequent cause of cough in 102 consecutive and unselected patients evaluated for chronic cough, with only postnasal drip and asthma being more prevalent, respectively (Fig. 1). Furthermore, gastroesophageal reflux was found to be the cause of cough in 21% of patients. Hoffstein (6) obtained similar results when he evaluated 228 patients with persistent cough. Gastroesophageal reflux was found to be involved in causing cough in 24% of patients and again was only less common than postnasal drip and asthma as the etiology of persistent cough in nonsmokers with normal chest roentgenograms. Smyrnios (9) also found that gastroesophageal reflux was the most common cause of cough in patients who fit the aforementioned clinical profile. Fitzgerald et al. (24) was able to control cough in 14 of 20 patients with a 3-month course of medical antireflux therapy in whom no cause of cough could be found. In 5 of the remaining 6 patients, a more invasive evaluation confirmed gastroesophageal reflux. Four of these five patients underwent fundoplication and were asymptomatic 3 months after surgery. The relationship between gastroesophageal reflux and persistent cough is not limited to any particular age group. Smyrnios et al. (16) demonstrated that gastroesophageal reflux is a common cause of cough in the elderly, while Holinger and Sanders (13) obtained similar results in 72 infants and children under the age of 16 years.

There are some who are skeptical of gastroesophageal reflux playing a causative role in cough. Laukka et al. (33) studied 10 patients with chronic cough using pH probe monitoring. Eighty-two percent of cough episodes had no correlation with gastroesophageal reflux. Of those episodes where cough and gastroesophageal reflux were felt to be related, only 30% of coughs followed episodes of gastroesophageal reflux. The authors concluded that gastroesophageal reflux

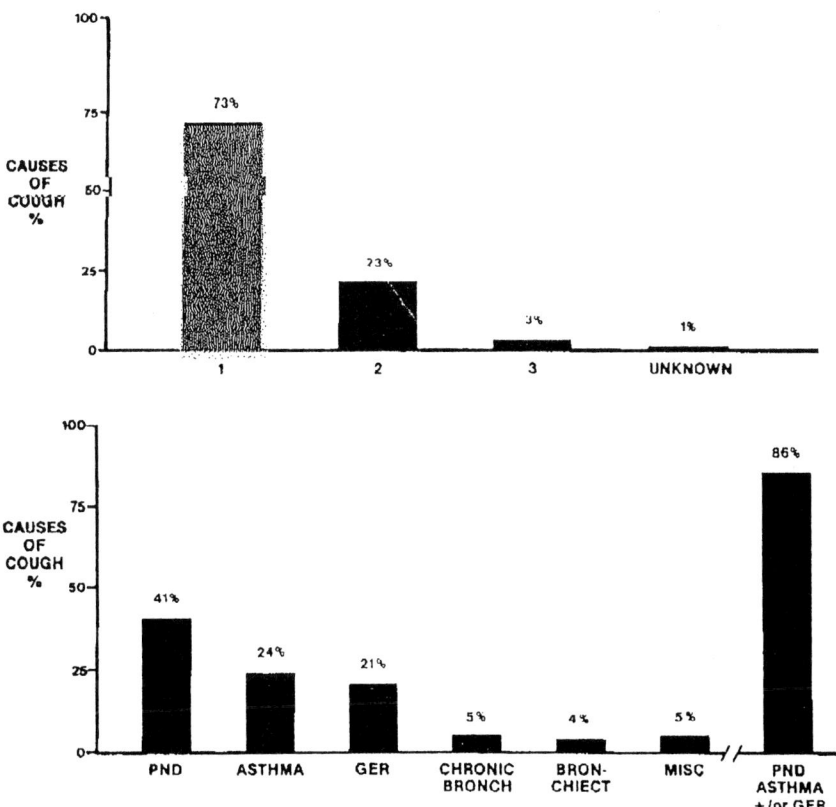

Figure 1 The causes of chronic cough. Top panel. The cause was determined in 99% of patients; it was due to a single condition in 73% of patients and to multiple disorders in 26%. Bottom panel. The spectrum and frequency of the 131 causes (PND = postnasal drip syndrome; GER = gastroesophageal reflux; Bronch = bronchitis; bronchiect = bronchiectasis; misc = miscellaneous). Reprinted with permission from Ref. 5.

is not a frequent cause of chronic cough. In another study, instillation of 0.1 N HCl into the esophagi of anesthetized cats failed to induce cough (34). It should be emphasized, however, that despite these two studies there is a preponderance of evidence linking gastroesophageal reflux to cough.

Cough can be caused by a multitude of factors in any one patient. The suspicion that cough may be caused, at least in part, by GER should be raised if cough has only partially improved with treatment directed at the other more common causes of cough, i.e., postnasal drip and asthma. Irwin et al. (5) demonstrated that cough may have multiple causes in a study of 102 patients with chronic cough, while Mello et al. (7) found that the cause of cough was multifactorial in 59% of 88 patients with persistent cough. Smyrnios et al. (9) concluded that cough was caused by two or more etiologies in 62% of patients with chronic cough with excessive sputum production. In all three studies, gastroesophageal reflux was determined to be a major cause of cough, frequently in combination with other disorders. Euler et al. (28) studied 30 children with recurrent pulmonary disease and gastroesophageal reflux disease proven by esophagram, esophageal manometry, pH probe testing, or esophagoscopy with biopsy. Nineteen of the 30 children studied had a history of nocturnal cough, and all had a history of asthma or previous pneumonia. Sixty-three percent of subjects were found to have underlying gastroesophageal reflux.

II. Pathophysiology

In order to understand how gastroesophageal reflux may cause cough, one needs to have a basic understanding of the cough reflex. The involuntary cough reflex is a vagally mediated function. Cough can only be initiated from structures innervated by the vagus (35). Afferent cough receptors are located in the laryngeal and tracheal mucosa, the mucosa of large bronchi, the tympanic membrane and external auditory canal, and possibly throughout the mucosa of the esophagus. Receptors in the laryngeal and tracheobronchial tree belong to a class of receptors called rapidly adapting irritant receptors (3,36–40). These receptors are activated by a number of mechanical and chemical stimuli including mucus, dust, foreign bodies, tobacco smoke, acid and alkaline solutions, as well as inflammatory mediators (3). Impulses from afferent receptors travel via various neural pathways to the medulla oblongata within the brainstem, where synapses with motor outputs occur (13). Motor outputs to the respiratory muscles originate in the nucleus retroambigualis, whereas motor neurons to the larynx and tracheobronchial tree begin in the nucleus ambiguus. It is important to note that these same afferents may also stimulate submucosal glands within the airways to secrete mucus (3,38,39). It is not clear, however, whether these same afferents also cause bronchial smooth muscle contraction or if another class of afferents is responsible for bronchoconstriction following exposure to various stimuli that are known to cause both cough and bronchospasm (40). In addition to the tracheobronchial cough reflex, several investigators also have postulated a vagally mediated tracheobronchial-esophageal reflex (19,20,41–44). It is believed that there are afferent receptors within the esophageal mucosa that, when stimulated by exposure to acid and possibly alkali, send impulses to the previously described cough center within the brainstem, triggering outputs along motor neurons to the respiratory muscles and tracheobronchial tree and resulting in cough. Finally, the esophagoglottal and phyaryngoglottal reflexes promote closure of the vocal cords and introitus to the trachea, protecting against retrograde aspiration of gastroesophageal contents (45).

As one can envision, gastroesophageal reflux can cause cough via two basic mechanisms: aspiration and/or neural reflex arcs. Gross or microaspiration of gastric/esophageal contents is a well-known cause of cough. Chernow et al. (23) studied six patients with chronic respiratory symptoms suspected of having nocturnal aspiration from gastroesophageal reflux using pH monitoring and gastric instillation of technetium 99m sulfur colloid. Lung scans were performed 8 hours after placement of technetium in the stomachs of subjects. Three of the six subjects were found to have radioactive uptake within the lungs by lung scanning, and all three had prolonged episodes of gastroesophageal reflux on pH monitoring. Fujimori et al. (46) reported a patient with nocturnal cough and frequent heartburn. Upper gastrointestinal roentgenogram demonstrated reflux of barium into the proximal esophagus, while esophageal endoscopy revealed reflux esophagitis. Bronchial biopsy specimens showed chronic inflammatory changes. The patient's cough improved after a course of therapy directed at gastroesophageal reflux. Nussbaum et al. (47) demonstrated the presence of lipid-laden macrophages in 85% of 74 children with chronic respiratory tract symptoms and proven gastroesophageal reflux. Grading the number of lipid-laden alveolar macrophages seen on tracheal aspirates has also been shown to correlate with the presence of gastroesophageal reflux in children (48). Gastroesophageal reflux with resultant microaspiration of gastric contents has been implicated in the development of pulmonary dysfunction in patients with progressive systemic sclerosis (49). Tracheotomized patients are at risk for aspiration (50) even in the presence of a gastrostomy tube (51). Therefore, gastroesophageal reflux with occult aspiration should be considered in these individuals, especially if they are experiencing chronic cough and/or recurrent pneumonias. In a study of gastroesophageal reflux in asthmatics and chronic bronchitics, Ducolone et al. (52) demonstrated that pulmonary aspiration was present in 21% of patients with reflux.

The second mechanism by which gastroesophageal reflux causes cough is through neural reflex arcs. As previously stated, several investigators have suggested a reflex arc between the esophagus and trachebronchial tree (see Chap. 2) (19,20,41–44,53). It is believed that the esophageal mucosa contains afferent receptors, which, when stimulated by mechanical and chemical stimuli, send impulses to the cough center, which, in turn, generates motor outputs along efferents to the respiratory muscles involved in the generation of cough. It is critical to understand that under this mechanism, aspiration of gastroesophageal contents is not required for the precipitation of cough. Irwin and colleagues (42) studied nine patients with chronic cough using prolonged esophageal pH monitoring. Both the proximal and distal portions of the esophagus were monitored. Coughs simultaneously occurred with a pH < 4 in the distal esophagus 35% of the time and only 8% of the time in the proximal esophagus. Furthermore, coughs only correlated with distal esophageal events, suggesting that microaspiration was not necessary for developing cough. In another study (20), 12 individuals with chronic cough were evaluated. All subjects were nonsmokers and no one was taking an angiotensin-converting enzyme inhibitor. Methacholine inhalational challenge was negative in all. Treatment directed at postnasal drip syndrome failed to resolve chronic cough. Twenty-four hour, double-probe, esophageal pH monitoring with event recorders was performed in all subjects. Significantly more gastroesophageal reflux–induced coughs were recorded from the distal esophagus than from the proximal esophagus. Two subjects who were found to have distal gastroesophageal reflux–induced cough failed to cough during reflux events in the proximal esophagus. Finally, pH monitoring failed to detect proximal gastroesophageal reflux in one individual with cough induced by distal esophageal reflux. Schnatz et al. (21), using dual-probe esophageal pH monitoring, also found that chronic cough could be induced by distal esophageal reflux alone and that symptoms responded to therapy directed at gastroesophageal reflux. Ing and colleagues (64) studied the role of distal esophageal acid exposure in 22 subjects with chronic cough and gastroesophageal reflux determined by esophageal pH monitoring and 12 matched controls. In a double-blind controlled fashion, 0.1 N HCl and 0.9% saline were instilled in random order into the esophagi of all subjects. Coughs were monitored using a microphone and computer analysis. Study subjects had statistically significant more coughs (36.5) during acid infusion compared to controls (0.0). The inhibition of acid-induced cough was then evaluated. Repeat acid perfusion was performed 15 minutes after the application of 4% lignocaine or ipratropium bromide. Subjects who received lignocaine had a significant reduction in the frequency of cough, while individuals who received the instilled ipratropium bromide had no significant reduction in any cough parameter. However, a significant reduction in cough frequency was observed when ipratropium bromide was administered by the inhalational route. The authors concluded that these observations provided indirect evidence of the tracheobronchial-esophageal reflex since instilled lignocaine acted locally, presumably on the afferent limb of the cough reflex, while inhaled ipratropium inhibited the efferent limb in suppressing cough.

Gastroesophageal reflux may lower the cough threshold. Ferrari and coworkers (55) studied 29 patients with digestive symptoms but no cough using esophageal manometry and pH monitoring. Fifteen subjects were thought to be refluxers based upon abnormally high total esophageal acid-exposure time. The cough threshold was then evaluated in both refluxers and nonrefluxers using methacholine and capsaicin inhalational challenge. The dosage of methacholine causing a 20% fall in the forced expiratory volume in 1 second (provocative dose or PD_{20}) was similar in refluxers and nonrefluxers. Capsaicin's ability to cause cough was evaluated in a similar fashion. The concentration of inhaled capsaicin in a dosimeter was gradually increased until five coughs were produced (PD_5) or the maximal dosage of capsaicin was reached. Refluxers were found to have a much lower PD_5 (0.51 nmol) than nonrefluxers (19.8 nmol). Based upon these observations, the investigators concluded that acid reflux appears to lower the cough threshold.

There is also a considerable amount of data in asthmatics supporting the existence of the tracheobronchial-esophageal reflex. Intraesophageal perfusion of 0.1 N HCL has been shown to decrease vital capacity and the forced expiratory volume in one second in asthmatics (56,57). Esophageal acid instillation also has been shown to increase respiratory airway resistance and the degree of bronchoconstriction produced by methacholine provocation testing in asthmatics (58,59). Similar observations have been seen in anesthetized cats (60). Increased airway resistance following intraesophageal acid perfusion has been seen in dogs and can be abolished by vagotomy (61). It should be noted, however, that gastric acid may not be the only stimulus of afferent receptors within the esophagus. Intraesophageal perfusion of acid has not reliably produced cough in patients with proven gastroesophageal reflux-induced cough (20,42). Irwin et al. observed cough induced by alkaline reflux events (20). In a study of 29 patients with digestive symptoms but without respiratory complaints, acid reflux was evaluated using pH monitoring and esophageal manometry (55). Acid reflux was observed to induce cough in only one individual. Furthermore, the severity of gastroesophageal acid reflux in individuals with enhanced sensitivity to capsaicin but free of respiratory symptoms was similar to that reported by others where gastrocsophageal reflux was found to cause cough (19,42,62). Other constituents of gastric secretions, particularly pepsin and trypsin, have been shown in animal models to be more damaging to the esophageal mucosa than acid (63,64). Mechanical forces may also be important triggers of afferent receptors within the esophagus. Mansfield and coworker (61) observed that, in addition to esophageal acid instillation, esophageal distention by balloon inflation increased airway resistance in dogs. Again, this observation did not occur once the animals were vagotomized. Further studies are needed to elucidate the exact mediators of gastroesophageal reflux–induced cough.

Some researchers believe that reflux is provoked by a pumping effect imposed on the stomach by exaggerated respiratory efforts in patients with respiratory disease, while others have postulated the existence of a positive feedback cycle between cough and gastroesophageal reflux (41,54,65–68). Allen and colleagues (69) demonstrated that reflux is unlikely to be provoked by respiratory efforts or that cough induces further reflux. Inspiratory loading during tidal breathing failed to induce reflux in patients with reflux disease and in control subjects. Furthermore, inspiratory loading and coughing appeared to terminate reflux events. Increases in transdiaphragmatic pressure during coughing have not been shown to promote gastroesophageal reflux in patients with normal basal lower esophageal sphincter tone (41).

Intraesophageal pH is typically around 7 (70). Johnson and colleagues (71) defined reflux as an intraesophageal pH less than 4. Gastroesophageal reflux is a normal physiologic process. It occurs in every individual many times each day without causing signs or symptoms of injury. Physiologic reflux is defined as rapidly cleared upright reflux episodes occurring primarily after meals (70,71). The total time at pH < 4, sometimes referred to as the acid-exposure time, is felt to be the single best indicator of abnormal reflux (70–74). The upper limit of normal for acid-exposure time in the distal esophagus is felt to be between 5 and 7% (72,74,75). Gastroesophageal reflux becomes pathologic, however, when it produces symptoms or signs of injury within the digestive or respiratory tracts (76). In patients with chronic cough felt to be secondary to gastroesophageal reflux, the number and duration of reflux episodes, total acid-exposure time, and the temporal relationship between reflux episodes and cough are important considerations in establishing causality. Ing et al. (19) observed that patients with reflux-induced cough experienced more reflux events per 24 hours and longer reflux episodes. Furthermore, significantly more time was spent with an intraesophageal pH < 4.0 in patients with gastroesophageal reflux–induced cough than in control subjects. Irwin et al. (42) observed that the number of coughs was significantly correlated with the number of refluxes, the longest reflux, and the percentage of time that the intraesophageal pH was <4.0. These findings were duplicated in a study of 30 patients with cough thought to be due to gastroesophageal reflux (62). These characteristics, however, are not universal in patients with reflux-induced cough. Patients with proven gastroesophageal reflux–induced cough sometimes have a normal number of reflux events and percentage of time with an intraesophageal pH < 4.0 (20). In some patients, the only significant finding is a correlation between an episode of reflux and the initiation of cough (20). Gastroesophageal reflux should be considered as a potential cause of cough in patients with normal standard reflux parameters if a definite temporal relationship is observed (41). It should also be noted that gastroesophageal reflux may be the cause of cough even if the temporal correlation between reflux and cough episodes is low. In a study of 15 patients with chronic, unexplained cough, esophageal manometry and pH monitoring were used to evaluate the temporal relationship between reflux and cough episodes (77). Gastroesophageal reflux was found to precede coughing in only 9% of the total cough episodes.

III. Clinical Presentation

Cough due to gastroesophageal reflux does not have any unique qualities. The duration of cough due to gastroesophageal reflux can be quite variable. It is not uncommon for patients to present with cough that has been present for a number of years. In our study of the characteristics of cough (7), the mean duration of cough was 6.6 years with a range of 1 month to 44 years, while in two other studies of cough due to gastroesophageal reflux, the mean duration of cough was 33 and 39 months, respectively (20,42).

Reflux-induced cough has varying degrees of sputum production. The spectrum and frequency of the causes of cough, based on the quantity of sputum production, were evaluated in our study of the predictive values of the character, timing, and complications of chronic cough (7). Of those subjects with reflux-induced cough, 50.7% had dry cough, while 15.9% had more than 60 ml per day of sputum. Smyrnios et al. (9) studied 71 patients who complained of cough productive of greater than 30 ml of sputum per day. Gastroesophageal reflux was the third most common cause of cough in this cohort and was the etiologic factor in 15% of patients overall. That gastroesophageal reflux can produce mucus, even in the absence of gross or microaspiration, should not come as a surprise since laboratory studies have demonstrated that gastric irritation is capable of causing a vagally mediated increase in the secretion of tracheal mucus in cats (78). Furthermore, when gastroesophageal reflux results in aspiration syndromes, tracheobronchitis with fevers, wheezing, and purulent sputum production may develop (52).

While it has been stated in the literature that nocturnal cough is typical of gastroesophageal reflux disease, this relation has not been seen consistently in detailed studies that have evaluated this issue (52,79). In fact, nocturnal cough has been found to occur as frequently in patients with gastroesophageal reflux as it does in individuals with asthma and postnasal drip–induced cough (7). In addition, Irwin et al. (42), using prolonged esophageal pH monitoring, demonstrated that cough due to gastroesophageal reflux most commonly occurs while patients are awake and upright.

It is important to emphasize that symptoms suggestive of gastroesophageal reflux are frequently lacking in patients with reflux-induced cough, and their absence should not sway one away from considering reflux as a potential cause of cough. Ing and colleagues have reported that between 50 and 75% of patients with reflux-induced cough deny reflux symptoms (54,62). Irwin et al. (42) demonstrated that cough can be the only symptom of gastroesophageal reflux disease proven by 24-hour esophageal pH monitoring.

Gastroesophageal reflux–induced cough, however, can be accompanied by prominent classic reflux symptoms such as heartburn, waterbrash, regurgitation, and sour taste (81). Furthermore, some individuals may present with reflux-induced cough and atypical symptoms such as chest pain, globus sensation intractable nausea, intermittent wheezing and stridor, dental erosion, hoarseness, and sore throat (52,81–86).

IV. Diagnosis

A high degree of clinical suspicion must exist if one is to diagnose gastroesophageal reflux–induced cough. A carefully taken history is probably not helpful in diagnosing gastroesophageal reflux as the cause of cough. Our group evaluated the clinical utility of a carefully taken history and physical examination in predicting the cause of chronic cough (7). Eighty-eight patients with chronic cough were evaluated prospectively in a tertiary care, pulmonary, outpatient clinic that specializes in the diagnosis and treatment of chronic cough. Gastroesophageal reflux was determined to be the cause of cough in 40% of subjects. Patients were provided a fixed, alternative yes-or-no questionnaire that assessed the character, timing, and complications of cough. Descriptors included paroxysmal, honking, barking, postprandial, nocturnal, and associated with meals. No descriptor or characteristic of cough was found to be helpful in predicting the cause of cough. In addition, as previously stated, typical accompanying symptoms of gastroesophageal reflux are commonly absent (54,62).

Air-contrast barium swallow has been employed widely in the diagnosis of gastroesophageal reflux. Traditionally, movement of barium from the stomach into the esophagus is considered diagnostic for gastroesophageal reflux (76). Cough is believed to be likely due to reflux when other, more common, causes of cough have been ruled out and there is evidence of reflux on barium esophagram (9,20). The precipitation of cough with reflux of barium into the esophagus is not required for the presumptive diagnosis of gastroesophageal reflux–induced cough. Hence, barium swallow only confirms the presence of reflux but does not establish the cause of the patient's cough. In this setting, causality is established only when therapy for gastroesophageal reflux results in resolution of the patient's cough. Upper gastrointestinal series have been shown to produce a high rate of false-positive and false-negative results. Several studies have demonstrated that approximately 20% of normal control subjects will have abnormal barium esophagrams (87,88). Irwin and colleagues have reported extensively on the reliability of barium swallow in diagnosing reflux-induced cough (9,10,20). The sensitivity and specificity of barium swallow in diagnosing gastroesophageal reflux–induced cough ranges from 48 to 92% and 42 to 76%, respectively. The clinical usefulness of barium esophagography in diagnosing cough in this clinical setting has been reported to be as low as 17% (9). Barium esophagography, however, may have a role as a noninvasive study when local anatomic disorders or complications of gastroesophageal reflux such as hiatal hernia, strictures, and ulcerations are suspected (76).

Esophageal endoscopy is another diagnostic modality by which the presence of gastroesophageal reflux can be established. As is the case with barium swallow, endoscopy only confirms the presence of reflux but does not establish that reflux is the etiology of the patient's cough. Again, causality is established retrospectively after a course of therapy for gastroesophageal reflux abolishes the cough. The sensitivity of esophageal endoscopy in diagnosing gastroesophageal reflux is limited to the presence of mucosal damage. Endoscopic and histologic mucosal changes are found in only 30–50% of individuals with symptomatic reflux (70,89–91). In one study of gastroesophageal reflux–induced cough (20), histologic evidence of esophagitis was found in only 25% of patients. Endoscopy, however, is very useful (and mandatory) in patients with longstanding reflux symptoms and in those with warning symptoms suggestive of malignant disease (92).

The Bernstein test is another method of evaluating acid-related symptoms. This test is performed by instilling either 0.1 N HCl or normal saline into the esophagus and is considered positive when symptoms are reproduced with the instillation of acid but not saline. The reported sensitivity of the Bernstein test for gastroesophageal reflux disease has been reported to average around 78–80% (76,93,94). The test's sensitivity, however, appears to be much lower (7–27%) when attempting to ascertain the cause of atypical chest pain (95,96). Similar disappointing results have been obtained when attempting to reproduce cough and nausea in patients with proven gastroesophageal reflux–induced cough and nausea (20,42,82).

Prolonged esophageal pH monitoring appears to be the single best test in screening for gastroesophageal reflux disease. Esophageal pH monitoring has a sensitivity and specificity of approximately 96% in patients with typical reflux symptoms (70,93,97,98). The distal pH electrode is usually placed 5–6 cm above the gastroesophageal junction (5,42,70). A second, proximal pH sensor can be placed in the hypopharynx or proximal esophagus at least 2 cm above the thoracic inlet (5,42,99). Two types of data are obtained from esophageal pH monitoring. First, intraesophageal pH is recorded in real-time fashion. Second, symptoms are time-logged using an event marker and diary. Data from the event marker, diary, and pH probes can then be evaluated for temporal relations between symptoms and changes in intraesophageal pH. Ambulatory esophageal pH monitoring appears to have its greatest utility in diagnosing atypical symptoms caused by gastroesophageal reflux. Furthermore, the American College of Gastroenterology has stated that patients with pulmonary symptoms may benefit from ambulatory pH monitoring (93). The utility of pH-metry in evaluating unexplained pulmonary symptoms has now been demonstrated by a number of investigators (5,7,16,19–21,24,28,42,54,77,85,99). Esophageal pH monitoring is felt to be the "gold standard" in the evaluation of reflux-induced cough and may be the only method of diagnosing gastroesophageal reflux in up to 32% of patients with reflux-induced cough (5). The sensitivity and specificity of esophageal pH monitoring in diagnosing reflux-induced cough are felt to approximate 92% (20). The importance of using a dual-probe esophageal pH-monitoring system cannot be overemphasized because both proximal as well as distal reflux events can trigger cough. In a study of gastroesophageal reflux and cough, Vaezi and Richter (100) found a statistically significant increase in the number of distal, supine, and upright reflux events, as well as proximal reflux episodes in the upright position in patients with GER-related cough compared to patients with cough due to other causes (Figs. 2, 3) The importance of proximal reflux events was further documented by Shaker and colleagues (101) in a study of the esophageal distribution of gastric acid refluxate in patients with reflux-induced laryngitis. These investi-

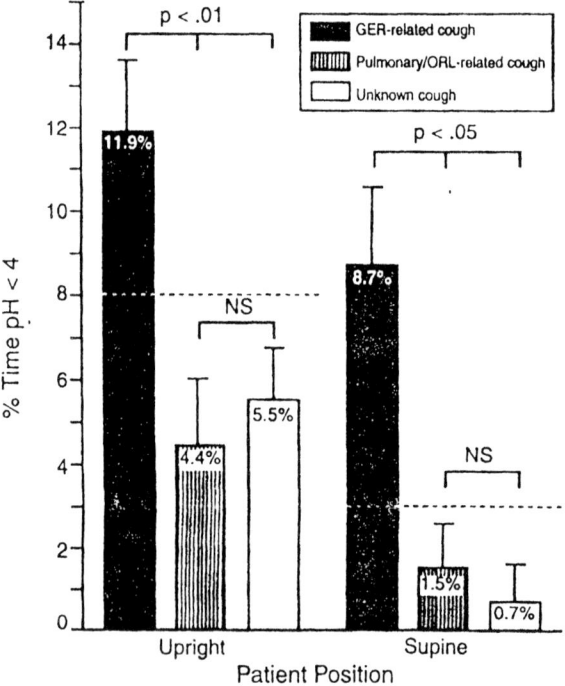

Figure 2 Mean distal esophageal acid reflux values (upright and supine positions) for patients with cough due to gastroesophageal reflux (GER), pulmonary/otorhinolaryngologic (ORL) causes, and unknown causes. Broken lines indicates upper limits of normal. (NS = not significant.) Reprinted with permission from Ref. 100.

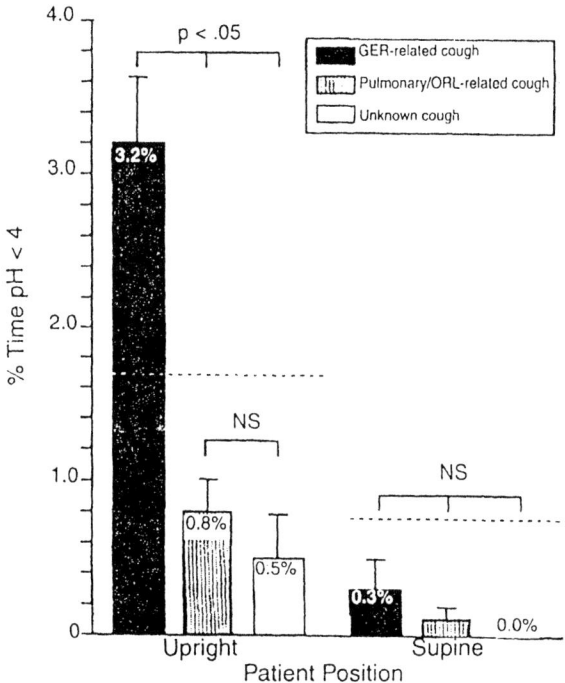

Figure 3 Mean proximal esophageal acid reflux values (upright and supine positions) for patients with cough due to gastroesophageal reflux (GER), pulmonary/otorhinolaryngologic (ORL) causes, and unknown causes. Broken lines indicate upper limits of normal (NS = not significant). Reprinted with permission from Ref. 100.

gators found that more proximal reflux events occurred in patients with laryngitis than in controls (Table 1). As previously stated, the temporal relationships between reflux episodes and symptoms, the number and duration of reflux events, and the total acid-exposure time are felt to be important diagnostic parameters obtained from esophageal pH monitoring. More specifically, gastroesophageal reflux is felt to be the cause of cough based upon a pH-monitoring study when the following indicators are also present: (a) reflux events appear to induce cough, (b) there are more than four reflux events lasting more than 4 minutes, (c) percent of time that pH is <4.0 is longer than 4.4%, and (d) the number of reflux events is greater than 50 (20,80). Caution must be used, however, in attempting to establish a causal relationship between reflux and cough when the total number or duration of reflux events is extremely high and only a few reflux episodes are temporally related to coughing. Any temporal relationship in this particular set-

Table 1 Comparison of Regional Distribution of Refluxed Gastric Acid Between Distal and Proximal Esophageal and Pharyngeal Sites

Ratio	Groups			
	Normal controls (%)	ENT controls (%)	GERD (%)	Laryngitis (%)
Total study duration				
Proximal/distal	23 ± 6.5	16 ± 6.8	32 ± 5.4	51 ± 7.0[a]
Pharynx/proximal	1.2 ± 1.0	0	0.2 ± 0.21	30 ± 10[a]
Upright duration				
Proximal/distal	1.9 ± 5.6	11 ± 5.6	27 ± 5.5	49 ± 7.4[b]
Pharynx/proximal	1.0 ± 0.006	0	2.0 ± 0.05	30 ± 14[a]
Supine duration				
Proximal/distal	11 ± 7.0	28 + 12	30 + 7.0	25 + 7.6
Pharynx/proximal	0	0	0.1 ± 0.1	13 ± 8.0[a]

Note: Results are expressed as mean ± SE.
[a] $p < 0.05$, laryngitis vs. all other groups.
[b] $p < 0.05$, laryngitis vs. ENT and normal controls.
Source: Ref. 101.

ting may be coincidental, and, as a result, one can only be certain that a pH-monitoring study is truly positive if specific antireflux therapy results in resolution of cough.

Finally, an empiric trial of antireflux therapy is an alternative and reasonable diagnostic tool. This approach is particularly attractive when esophageal pH monitoring is not available. If an empiric therapeutic trial is chosen, it should be noted that treatment should be continued for 3–4 months before one can declare treatment failure, based upon observations from four prospective studies on gastroesophageal reflux–induced cough (5,42). However, laboratory confirmation of the presence of gastroesophageal reflux, preferably by pH monitoring, should be obtained whenever possible for two major reasons. First, patient acceptance of reflux-induced cough in the absence of laboratory confirmation of the presence of underlying reflux can be difficult, especially if typical gastrointestinal symptoms of gastroesophageal reflux are absent. Second, since the negative predictive value of pH-metry is high, documenting the absence of reflux prevents the use of unnecessary, costly, and prolonged therapeutic trials and expedites the diagnostic process.

In the appropriate clinical setting, that is, a nonsmoker with a normal chest roentgenogram who is not using an angiotensin-converting enzyme inhibitor and in whom asthma and postnasal drip have been excluded as the cause of chronic cough, gastroesophageal reflux should be considered the most likely etiology of the patient's cough (5–9,13,16). Several studies have confirmed that cough often can be caused by multiple, simultaneously contributing factors (4–9,13,14,17, 102). Given this observation, gastroesophageal reflux also should be considered as a cause of cough in individuals in whom specific treatment directed at asthma and postnasal drip results in partial improvement. In this setting, esophageal pH monitoring is indicated to assess for the possibility that gastroesophageal reflux also may be contributing to the patient's cough.

V. Treatment

The management of gastroesophageal reflux–induced cough involves both lifestyle modifications and pharmacotherapy. Occasionally, under certain circumstances, surgical intervention is needed. It is important to note that the cough caused by gastroesophageal reflux tends to respond very slowly to therapy, and, as a result, a prolonged course of therapy is required. The duration of therapy may be as long as 179 ± 205 days before a significant response to treatment is obtained (5).

The concept of lifestyle modifications stresses the avoidance of foods, drinks, and practices known to make reflux worse and is the mainstay of therapy for reflux-induced cough. While lifestyle modifications have not been systematically studied as monotherapy for gastroesophageal reflux–induced cough, they have been evaluated in combination with H_2 blockers and/or prokinetic agents (5,20,24,42). Physiologic studies have demonstrated that reduction of fat intake, elevation of the head of the bed, and avoidance of food and drink 3 hours prior to recumbancy decrease distal gastroesophageal reflux (93,103–106). It is recommended that patients be placed on a diet which is high in protein and low in fat (80). Total daily fat intake should not exceed 45 grams. Chocolate, peppermint and spearmint, onions, coffee, tea, cola beverages, and citric fruit juices should be avoided because these substances have been shown to promote gastroesophageal reflux (76,107–109). Smoking cessation is also important because smoking has been shown to provoke acid reflux and may reduce lower esophageal sphincter pressure (110).

H_2-receptor antagonists most commonly have been employed in the treatment of gastroesophageal reflux–induced cough (5,7,20,24,42). These agents work by decreasing acid secretion and gastric volume by inhibiting histamine-2 receptors. In gastroesophageal reflux disease, 60% (range 32–82%) of patients experience symptom improvement with the use of H_2 antagonists (93). Response rates of reflux-induced cough treated with H_2 blockers, either alone or in combination with prokinetic agents, range between 70 and 84% (5,24). It should also be noted that no one H_2 receptor antagonist has been shown to be superior in the management of reflux-induced cough. Given the extensive data on the use of these agents, histamine-2 receptor antagonists should be considered first-line therapy, along with lifestyle modifications, for the treatment of reflux-induced cough.

The proton pump inhibitors have been shown to be effective in the treatment of gastroesophageal reflux disease. These agents have been shown to be more efficacious than H_2 antagonists in healing erosive esophagitis and alleviating the symptoms of gastroesophageal reflux (111–113). It is important to note that there is little data on the use of proton pump inhibitors in treating gastroesophageal reflux–induced cough. Kamel and colleagues (112) reported that omeprazole may be effective in treating acid laryngitis. In another study, Harding et al. (113) investigated the role of omeprazole in 30 asthmatics with gastroesophageal reflux documented by esophageal pH probe monitoring. Patients were started on 20 mg of omeprazole per day, and the dose was titrated until acid suppression was demonstrated by esophageal pH monitoring. Once acid suppression had been attained, subjects were then treated with the adjusted dose of omeprazole for 3 months. These investigators found that at the end of the 3-month trial, omeprazole improved asthma symptoms and/or peak expiratory flow rates by >20% in 73% of subjects. Depla et al. (114) reported a case where a 25-year-old male with severe nocturnal asthma who had failed a course of high-dose ranitidine experienced a dramatic improvement in asthma symptoms after treatment with omeprazole was instituted. In a double-blind placebo crossover study by Ford and colleagues (115), omeprazole failed to improve asthma symptoms and peak expiratory flow rates in 11 asthmatics. It should be noted, however, that, unlike the study by Harding et al. (113), where subjects were treated with omeprazole for 3 months, Ford et al. (115) treated patients for only 4 weeks. This observation suggests that the duration of therapy with proton pump inhibitors, as with other forms of therapy for gastroesophageal reflux–induced cough, may need to be prolonged as well, i.e., 3 months or longer. Until further data on the efficacy of proton pump inhibitors in the treatment of reflux-induced cough is obtained, H_2 antagonists should be considered as first-line therapy.

Prokinetic agents, such as metoclopramide and cisapride, work by increasing lower esophageal sphincter pressure and gastric emptying. These agents, in combination with H_2 blockers, are useful in the treatment of reflux-induced cough. In a study of 20 patients with reflux-induced cough, metoclopramide, in combination with a H_2 blocker and antireflux diet, was successful in stopping cough in 70% of subjects (24). Combination therapy with a H_2 antagonist and cisapride has also been shown to be effective at ameliorating asthma symptoms in asthmatics with gastroesophageal reflux (116). Prokinetic agents may also be useful as monotherapy for reflux-induced cough. Most of the studies that have used a prokinetic agent alone have been performed in children. Saye and Forget

(117) studied 19 children with reflux-associated bronchopulmonary disease. Subjects were treated with cisapride 0.3 mg/kg three times a day for 1 month. Esophageal pH monitoring was performed before and at the end of the treatment period. Of the 13 children with nocturnal cough fits, 12 experienced complete resolution of nocturnal coughing by the completion of the treatment period. Furthermore, these investigators demonstrated that cisapride significantly reduces the percentage of the total time the pH was <4, the duration of the longest reflux event, and the duration of reflux at night. Similar results were obtained in a study of 38 children with severe chronic pulmonary disease, including chronic cough (118). Twenty-four subjects were found to have abnormal gastroesophageal reflux by pH monitoring. These children were then treated with cisapride 0.3 mg/kg for a total of 6 months. Cisapride was effective at producing resolution of respiratory symptoms in 82% of subjects. The combination of a prokinetic agent and a proton pump inhibitor may also be effective in the management of reflux-associated pulmonary symptoms. Vigneri et al. (119) demonstrated that omeprazole in combination with cisapride is more effective than ranitidine and cisapride in the maintenance treatment of reflux esophagitis. It is important to note that until studies that specifically evaluate the efficacy of prokinetic agents and/or proton pump inhibitors either alone or in combination are completed, H_2 antagonists, with or without a prokinetic agent, and behavior modification should be considered first-line therapy for the medical management of gastroesophageal reflux–induced cough.

Nissen's and Belsey's fundoplications and Hill's posterior gastroplexy are surgical procedures that can be used in cases of refractory gastroesophageal reflux (76). The superiority of antireflux surgery over standard medical therapy in preventing relapse of the signs and symptoms of gastroesophageal reflux is well established (120,121). A number of studies have evaluated the efficacy of antireflux surgery in the management of reflux-associated respiratory symptoms (122–126). In a study of 13 patients with symptomatic asthma and chronic cough who responded to H_2 antagonists, respiratory symptoms were controlled in 11 subjects following antireflux surgery (121). Lomasney (124) produced relief of respiratory symptoms, including cough, in 74% of 129 consecutive patients who underwent antireflux surgery for respiratory complaints associated with gastroesophageal reflux. DeMeester (123) has suggested that only those patients with normal esophageal motility are likely to benefit from antireflux surgery to control respiratory symptoms. The efficacy of fundoplication in children with reflux-induced respiratory disease is also well established (125,126). Surgical intervention is indicated when there are gastrointestinal complications of gastroesophageal reflux such as stricture, hemorrhage, and Barrett's esophagus despite maximum medical therapy (65,76). Fundoplication should also be considered when refractory gastroesophageal reflux results in ongoing damage to the respiratory system or if persistent coughing adversely affects one's lifestyle or poses a significant risk of injury. Puetz and Vakil (127) reported a case of refractory reflux-induced cough that resulted in frequent cough-induced syncope. Nissen fundoplication resulted in resolution of both cough and syncope. In another study, four patients with refractory reflux-induced cough who underwent fundoplication experienced total resolution of cough 3 months after surgery (24). Recurrent aspiration with resultant pneumonia, bronchiectasis, and interstitial fibrosis, despite maximum medical therapy, also should be considered an indication for surgery.

VI. Conclusion

Gastroesophageal reflux is a well-known cause of chronic cough. Reflux-induced cough is thought to occur either by aspiration or stimulation of the tracheobronchial-esophageal reflex. Symptoms of gastroesophageal reflux, such as heartburn, are frequently absent in patients with reflux-induced cough. The single best test for the diagnosis of reflux-induced cough is esophageal pH monitoring. Lifestyle modifications and H_2 antagonists, sometimes in combination with a prokinetic agent, are the mainstay of treatment for cough due to gastroesophageal reflux. If complications develop, surgical intervention is sometimes warranted.

References

1. Braman SS, Corrao WM. Chronic cough: diagnosis and treatment. Prim Care 1988; 12:217–225.
2. Office Visits to Internists: The National Ambulatory Medical Care Survey, United States 1975, Washington, DC: Department of Health, Services, and Welfare; U.S. DHEW publication PHS 79-1787. Vital and Health Statistics Series 13 No. 36, 1978, pp. 4–29.
3. Irwin RS, Widdicombe J. In: Murray JF, Nadel JA, eds. Textbook of Respiratory Medicine. 2d ed. Philadelphia: W.B. Saunders Co., 1996:529–544.
4. Irwin RS, Corrao WM, Pratter MR. Chronic persistent cough in the adult: the spectrum and frequency of causes and successful outcome of specific therapy. Am Rev Respir Dis 1981; 123:413–417.
5. Irwin RS, Curley FJ, French CL. Chronic cough. The spectrum and frequency of causes, key components of the diagnostic evaluation, and outcome of specific therapy. Am Rev Respir Dis 1990; 141:640–647.
6. Hoffstein V. Persistent cough in nonsmokers. Can Respir J 1994; 1:40–46.
7. Mello CJ, Irwin RS, Curley FJ. Predictive values of the character, timing, and complications of chronic cough in diagnosing its cause. Arch Intern Med 1996; 156: 997–1003.

8. Pratter MR, Bartter T, Akers S, Dubois J. An algorithmic approach to chronic cough. Ann Intern Med 1993; 119:977–983.
9. Smyrnios NA, Irwin RS, Curley FJ. Chronic cough with a history of excessive sputum production. Chest 1995; 108:991–997.
10. Sackner MA. In: Murray JF, Nadel JA, eds. Textbook of Respiratory Medicine. Philadelphia: W.B. Saunders Co., 1988:397–408.
11. Phillips AM, Phillips RW, Thompson JL. Chronic cough: analysis of etiologic factors in a survey of 12,743 men. Ann Intern Med 1956; 45:216–231.
12. Puolijoki H, Lahdensuo A. Causes of prolonged cough in patients referred to a chest clinic. Ann Med 1989; 21:425–427.
13. Holinger LD, Sanders AD. Chronic cough in infants and children: an update. Laryngoscope 1991; 101:596–605.
14. Poe RH, Israel RH, Utell MJ, Hall WJ. Chronic cough: bronchoscopy of pulmonary function testing. Am Rev Respir Dis 1982; 126:160–162.
15. Cloutier MM, Loughlin GM. Chronic cough in children: a manifestion of airway hyperreactivity. Pediatrics 1981; 67:6–12.
16. Smyrnios NA, Curley FJ, French CL, Irwin RI. Chronic cough in the elderly: causes and outcome of diagnostic evaluation and specific therapy. Am Rev Respir Dis 1993; 147(pt 2, suppl):A-381.
17. Poe RH, Harder RV, Israel RH, Kallay MC. Chronic persistent cough: experience in diagnosis and outcome using an anatomic diagnostic protocol. Chest 1989; 95:723–728.
18. Holinger LD. Chronic cough in infants and children. Laryngoscope 1986; 96:316–322.
19. Ing AJ, Ngu MC, Breslin ABX. Chronic persistent cough and gastro-oesophageal reflux. Thorax 1991; 46:479–483.
20. Irwin RS, French CL, Curley FJ, Zawacki JK, Bennet FM. Chronic cough due to gastroesophageal reflux: clinical, diagnostic, and pathogenetic aspects. Chest 1993; 104:1511–1517.
21. Schnatz PF, Castell JA, Castell DO. Pulmonary symptoms associated with gastroesophageal reflux: use of ambulatory pH monitoring to diagnose and to direct therapy. Am J Gastroenterol 1996; 91:1715–1718.
22. Stulbarg M. Evaluating and treating intractable cough-Medical Staff conference, University of California, San Francisco. West J Med 1985; 143:223–228.
23. Chernow B, Lawrence LF, Janowitz WR, Castell DO. Pulmonary aspiration as a consequence of gastroesophageal reflux. A diagnostic approach. Dig Dis Sci 1979; 24:839–844.
24. Fitzgerald JM, Allen CJ, Craven MA, Newhouse MT. Chronic cough and gastroesophageal reflux. Can Med Assoc J 1989; 140:520–524.
25. Johnston BT, Gideon RM, Castell DO. Editorial: excluding gastroesophageal reflux disease as a cause of chronic cough. J Clin Gastroenterol 1996; 22:168–169.
26. Nishi K, Amemiya T, Mizuguchi M, Ooka T, Fujimura M, Matsuda T. A case of chronic persistent cough caused by gastro-esophageal reflux. Nippon Kyobu Shikkan Gakkai Zasshi 1995; 33:652–659.
27. Bel A, Labarre JF, Thivolle P, Passot E. Broncho-pulmonary manifestations and gastroesophageal reflux. Poumon Coeur 1977; 33:345–350.

28. Euler AR, Byrne WJ, Ament ME, Fonkalsrud EW, Strobel CT, Siegel SC, Katz RM, Rachelefsky GS. Recurrent pulmonary disease in children: a complication of gastroesophageal reflux. Pediatrics 1979; 63:47–51.
29. Hoyoux C, Forget P, Lambrechts L, Geubelle F. Chronic bronchopulmonary disease and gastroesophageal reflux in children. Pediatr Pulmonol 1985; 1:149–153.
30. Thomson HG, Batch AJ. Acid reflux presenting as a persistent cough (letter). Ear Nose Throat J 1989; 68:881–882.
31. Bret P, Meraud P, Saubier E. The nocturnal cough, symptomatic of certain esophageal diseases (apropos of 2 cases). J Radiol Electrol Med Nucl 1968; 49:87.
32. Fujimori K, Satch M, Sasagawa M, Suzuki E, Arakawa M. A case of chronic persistent cough (CPC) caused by gastroesophageal reflux (including a study of CPC caused by suspected GER). Arerugi 1992; 41:454–458.
33. Laukka MA, Cameron AJ, Schei AJ. Gastroesophageal reflux and chronic cough: which comes first? J Clin Gastroenterol 1994; 19:100–104.
34. Tatar M, Pecova R. The effect of experimental gastroesophageal reflux on the cough reflex in anesthetized cats. Bratisl Lek Listy 1996; 97:284–288.
35. Korpas J, Tomori Z. Cough and Other Respiratory Reflexes. Basel: Karger, 1977.
36. Widdicombe, JG. Reflexes from the upper respiratory tract. In: Cherniak NS, Widdicombe JG, eds. Handbook of Physiology. Section 3: Respiration. Vol. 2. Control of Breathing. Bethesda, MD: American Physiological Society, 1986:363–394.
37. Sant'Ambrogio G. Afferent pathways for the cough reflex. Clin Resp Physiol 1987; 23(suppl):19s–23s.
38. Coleridge HM, Coleridge JCG. Reflexes evoked from tracheobronchial tree and lungs. In: Cherniack NS, Widdicombe JG, eds. Handbook of Physiology. Section 3: Respiration. Vol. 2. Control of Breathing. Bethesda, MD: American Physiological Society, 1986:395–429.
39. Sant'Ambrogio G. Nervous receptors in the tracheobronchial tree. Annu Rev Physiol 1987; 49:611–627.
40. Karlsson JA, Sant'Ambrogio G, Widdicombe JG. Afferent neural pathways in cough and reflex bronchoconstriction. J Appl Physiol 1988; 55:1007–1023.
41. Ing AJ. Cough and gastroesophageal reflux. Am J Med 1997; 103(SA):915–965.
42. Irwin RS, Zawacki JK, Curley FJ, French CL, Hoffman PJ. Chronic cough as the sole presenting manifestation of gastroesophageal reflux. Am Rev Respir Dis 1989; 140:1294–1300.
43. Benjamin SB. Extraesophageal complications of gastroesophageal reflux. J Clin Gastroenterol 1986; 8(suppl 1):68–71.
44. Mansfield LE, Stein MR. GE reflux and asthma: a possible reflex mechanism. Ann Allergy 1978; 41:224–226.
45. Shaker R. Airway protective mechanisms: current concepts. Dysphagia 1995; 10: 216–227.
46. Fujimori K, Suzuki E, Arakawa M. A case of chronic persistent cough caused by gastroesophageal reflux. Nippon Kyobu Shikkan Gakkai Zasshi 1993; 1:1303–1307.
47. Nussbaum E, Maggi JC, Mathis R, Galant SP. Association of lipid-laden alveolare macrophages and gastroesophageal reflux in children. J Pediatr 1987; 110:190–194.

48. Collins KA, Geisinger KR, Wagner PH, Blackburn KS, Washburn LK, Block SM. The cytologic evaluation of lipid-laden alveolar macrophages as an indicator of aspiration pneumonia in young children. Arch Pathol Lab Med 1995; 119:229–231.
49. Johnson DA, Drane WE, Curran J, Cattau EI, Ciarleglio C, Khan A, Cotelingam J, Benjamin SB. Pulmonary disease in progressive systemic sclerosis. A complication of gastroesophageal reflux and occult aspiration? Arch Intern Med 1989; 149:589–593.
50. Nash M. Swallowing problems in the tracheotomized patient. Otolaryngol Clin North Am 1988; 21:701–709.
51. Coben RM, Weintraub A, DiMartino AJ Jr, Cohen D. Gastroesophageal reflux during gastrostomy tube feeding. Gastroenterology 1994; 106:13–18.
52. Ducolone A, Vandevenne A, Jouin H, Grob J-C, Coumars D, Meyer C, Burghard G, Methlin G, Hollender L. Gastroesophageal reflux in patients with asthma and chronic bronchitis. Am Rev Respir Dis 1987;135:327–332.
53. Deschner WK, Benjamin SB. Extraesophageal manifestations of gastroesophageal reflux disease. Am J Gastroenterol 1989; 84:1–5.
54. Ing AJ, Ngu MC, Breslin AB. Pathogenesis of chronic persistent cough associated with gastroesophageal reflux. Am J Respir Crit Care Med 1994; 149:160–167.
55. Ferrari M, Olivieri M, Sembenini C, Benini S, Zuccali V, Bardelli E, Bovo P, Cavallini G, Vantini I, Lo Cascio V. Tussive effect of capsaicin in patients with gastroesophageal reflux without cough. Am J Respir Crit Care Med 1995; 557–561.
56. Perpina M, Pellicer C, Marco V, Maldonado J, Ponce J. The significance of the reflex bronchoconstriction provoked by gastroesophageal reflux in bronchial asthma. Eur J Respir Dis 1985; 66:91–97.
57. Ekstrom T, Tibbling L. Esophageal acid perfusion, airway function, and symptoms in asthmatic patients with marked bronchial hyperreactivity. Chest 1989; 96:995–998.
58. Andersen LI, Schmidt A, Bundgaard A. Pulmonary function and acid application in the esophagus. Chest 1986; 90:358–363.
59. Herve P, Denjean A, Jian R, Simonneau G, Duroux P. Intraesophageal perfusion of acid increases the bronchomotor response to methacholine and to isocapnic hyperventilation in asthmatic subjects. Am Rev Respir Dis 1986; 134:986–989.
60. Tuchman DN, Boyle JT, Pack AI, Scwartz J, Kokonos M, Spitzer AR, Cohen S. Comparison of airway responses following tracheal or esophageal acidification in the cat. Gastroenterology 1984; 87:872–881.
61. Mansfield LE, Hameister HH, Spaulding HS, Smith NJ, Glab N. The role of the vagus nerve in airway narrowing caused by intraesophageal hydrochloric acid provocation and esophageal distention. Ann Allergy 1981; 47:431–434.
62. Ing AJ, Ngu MC, Breslin AB. Chronic persistent cough and clearance of esophageal acid. Chest 1992; 102:1668–1671.
63. Lillemoe KD, Johnson LF, Harmon JW. Role of the components of the gastroduodenal contents in experimental acid esophagitis. Surgery 1982; 92:276–284.
64. Johnson LF, Harmon JW. Experimental esophagitis in a rabbit model: clinical relevance. J Clin Gastroenterol 1986; 8(suppl 1):26–44.

65. Allen CJ, Craven MA, Waterfall WE, Newhouse MT. Gastroesophageal reflux and chronic respiratory disease. In: Baum G, Wolinksy E, eds. Textbook of Pulmonary Diseases. 4th ed. Boston: Little, Brown and Co., 1989:1471–1486.
66. Boyle JT, Tuchman DN, Altschuler SM, Nixon TE, Pack AI, Cohen S. Mechanisms for the association of gastroesophageal reflux and bronchospasm. Am Rev Respir Dis 1985; 131:S16–20.
67. Hughes DM, Spier S, Rivlin J, Levison H. Gastroesophageal reflux during sleep in asthmatic patients. J Pediatr 1983; 102:666.
68. Allen CJ, Varry M, Waterfall WE. Is gastroesophageal reflux induced by increased respiratory efforts? First International Symposium on gastro-esophageal reflux and respiratory disorders, Brussels 1988. Abstract P2.
69. Allen CJ, Waterfall WE. The effect of respiratory loading on the lower esophageal sphincter in normal subjects. Dig Dis Sci 1984; 29:567.
70. Mattox HE, Richter JE. Prolonged ambulatory esophageal pH monitoring in the evaluation of gastroesophageal reflux disease. Am J Med 1990; 89:345–356.
71. Johnson LF, DeMeester TR. Twenty-four-hour pH monitoring of the distal esophagus. Am J Gastroenterol 1974; 62:325–332.
72. de Caestecker JS, Heading RC. Esophageal pH monitoring. Gastroenterol Clin North Am 1990; 19:645–669.
73. Weiner GJ, Morgan TM, Copper JB, Wu WC, Castell DO, Sinclair JW, Richter JE. Ambulatory 24-hour esophageal pH monitoring. Reproducibility and variability of pH parameters. Dig Dis Sci 1988; 33:1127–1133.
74. Schindlbeck NE, Heinrich C, Konig A et.al. Optimal thresholds, sensitivity and specificity of long term pH-metry for the detection of gastroesophageal reflux disease. Gastroenterology 1987; 93:85–90.
75. Netzer P, Hammer B. Indications for, results and consequences of 24-hour pH monitoring. Schweiz Med Wochenschr Suppl 1996; 79:53S–57S.
76. Orlando RC. Reflux esophagitis. In: Yamada T, Alpers DH, Owyang C, Powell DW, Silverstein FE, eds. Textbook of Gastroenterology. 2d ed. Philadelphia: J.B. Lippincott Co., 1995:1214–42.
77. Paterson WG, Murat BW. Combined ambulatory esophageal manometry and dual-probe pH-metry in evaluation of patients with chronic unexplained cough. Dig Dis Sci 1994; 39:1117–1125.
78. German VF, Corrales R, Ueki If, Nadel JA. Reflex stimulation of tracheal mucus gland secretion by gastric irritation in cats. J Appl Physiol 1982; 52:1153–1155.
79. Huxley EJ, Viroslav J, Gray WR, Pierce AK. Pharyngeal aspiration in normal adults with depressed consciousness. Am J Med 1978; 644:564–568.
80. Irwin RS, Mello CJ. Chronic cough as a symptom of GERD. Contemp Intern Med 1995; 7:15–25.
81. Janssens J, Vantrappen G, Ghillebert G. Twenty-four hour recording of esophageal pressure and pH in patients with non-cardiac chest pain. Gastroenterology 1986; 90:1978–1984.
82. Brzana RJ, Koch KL. Gastroesophageal reflux disease presenting with intractable nausea. Ann Intern Med 1997; 126:704–707.

83. Orenstein SR, Orenstein DM, Whitington PF. Gastroesophageal reflux causing stridor. Chest 1983; 84:301–302.
84. Schroeder PL, Filler SJ, Ramirez B, Lazarchik DA, Vaezi MF, Richter JE. Dental erosion and acid reflux disease. Ann Intern Med 1995; 122:809–815.
85. Koufman JA, Wiener GJ, Wu WC, Castell DO. Reflux laryngitis and its sequelae: the diagnostic role of ambulatory 24-hour pH monitoring. J Voice 1988; 2:78–89.
86. Putnam PE, Orenstein SR. Hoarseness in a child with gastroesophageal reflux. Acta Paediatr 1992; 81:635–636.
87. Ott DJ, Gelfand DW, Wu WC. Reflux esophagitis: radiographic and endoscopic correlation. Diagn Radiol 1979; 130:583.
88. Kaul B, Petersen H, Grette K, Myrvold HE. Reproducibility of gastroesophageal reflux scintigraphy and the standard acid reflux test. Scand J Gastroenterol 1986; 21:795–798.
89. Schindlbeck NE, Wiebecke B, Klauser AG, Voderholzer WA, Muller-Lissner SA. Diagnostic value of histology in non-erosive gastro-oesophageal reflux disease. Gut 1996; 39:151–154.
90. Richter JE, Castell DO. Gastroesophageal reflux:pathogenesis, diagnosis and therapy. Ann Intern Med 1982; 97:93–103.
91. Robinson MG, Orr WC, McCallum R, Nardi R. Do endoscopic findings influence response to H2 antagonist therapy for gastroesophageal reflux? Am J Gastroenterol 1987; 82:519–522.
92. Freston JW, Malagelada JR, Petersen H, McCloy RF. Critical issues in the management of gastroesophageal reflux disease. Eur J Gastroenterol Hepatol 1995; 7:577–586.
93. DeVault KR, Castell DO. Guidelines for the diagnosis and treatment of gastroesophageal reflux disease. Arch Intern Med 1995; 155:2165–2173.
94. Bernstein LM, Baker LA. A clinical test for esophagitis. Gastroenterology 1958; 34:760–781.
95. Katz PO, Dalton CB, Richter JE, Wu WC, Castell DO. Esophageal testing in patients with noncardiac chest pain or dysphagia: results of three years' experience with 1161 patients. Ann Intern Med 1987; 106:593–597.
96. Janssens J, VantrappenG, Ghillebert G. 24-hour recording of esophageal pressure and pH in patients with noncardiac chest pain. Gastroenterology 1986; 90:1978–1984.
97. Fuchs KH, DeMeester TR, Albertucci M. Specificity and sensitivity of objective diagnosis of gastroesophageal reflux disease. Surgery 1987; 102:575–580.
98. Rosen SN, Pope CE II. Extended esophageal pH monitoring. An analysis of the literature and assessment of its role in the diagnosis and management of gastroesophageal reflux. J Clin Gastroenterol 1989; 11:260–270.
99. Conley SF, Werlin SL, Beste DJ. Proximal pH-metry for diagnosis of upper airway complications of gastroesophageal reflux. J Otolaryngol 1995; 24:295–298.
100. Vaezi MF, Richter JE. Twenty-four-hour ambulatory pH monitoring in the diagnosis of acid reflux-related chronic cough. South Med J 1997; 90:305–311.
101. Shaker R, Milbrath M, Ron J, Toohill R, Hogan WJ, LiQ, Hofman CL. Esophago-

pharyngeal distribution of refluxed gastric acid in patients with reflux laryngitis. Gastroenterology 1995; 109:1575–1582.
102. O'Connell F, Thomas VE, Pride NB, Fuller RW. Capsaicin cough sensitivity decreases with successful treatment of chronic cough. Am J Respir Crit Care Med 1994; 150:374–380.
103. Becker DJ, Sinclair J, Castell DO, Wu WC. A comparison of high and low fat meals on postprandial esophageal acid esposure. Am J Gastroenterol 1989; 84:782–786.
104. Johnson LF, DeMeester TR. Evaluation of elevation of the head of the bed, bed, bethanechol, and antacid foam tablets on gastroesophageal reflux. Dig Dis Sci 1981; 26:673–680.
105. Stanciu C, Bennett JR. Effects of posture on gastro-oesophageal reflux. Digestion 1977; 15:104–109.
106. Hamilton JW, Boisen RJ, Yamamoto DT, Wagner JI, Reichelderfer M. Sleeping on a wedge diminishes exposure of the esophagus to refluxed acid. Dig Dis Sci 1988; 33:518.
107. Murphy DW, Castell DO. Chocolate and heartburn: evidence of increased esophageal acid exposure after chocolate ingestion. Am J Gastroenterol 1988; 93:633–636.
108. Sigmund CJ, McNally EF. The action of a carminative on the lower esophageal sphincter. Gastroenterology 1969; 56:13–18.
109. Allen ML, Mellow MH, Robinson MG, Orr WC. The effect of raw onions on acid reflux and reflux symptoms. Am J Gastroenterol 1990; 85:377–380.
110. Kahrilas PJ, Guptu RR. Mechanisms of acid reflux associated with cigarette smoking. Gut 1990; 31:4–10.
111. Dent J, Yeomans ND, Mackinnon M, Reed W, Narielvala FM, Hetzel DJ, Solcia E, Shearman DJC. Omeprazole v ranitidine for prevention of relapse in reflux oesophagitis. A controlled double blind trial of their efficacy and safety. Gut 1994; 35:590–598.
112. Kamel P, Kahrilas PJ, Hanson DG, McMahan J, Brenic S. Prospective trial of omeprazole in the treatment of ''reflux laryngitis.'' Gastroenterology 1992; 102:A93.
113. Harding SM, Richter JE, Guzzo MR, Schan CA, Alexander RW, Bradley LA. Asthma and gastroesophageal reflux: acid suppressive therapy improves asthma outcome. Am J Med 1996; 100:395–405.
114. Depla AC, Bartelsman JF, Roos CM, Tytgat GN, Jansen HM. Beneficial effect of omeprazole in a patient with severe bronchial asthma and gastro-oesophageal reflux. Eur Respir J 1988; 1:966–968.
115. Ford GA, Oliver PS, Prior JS, Butland RJ, Wilkinson SP. Omeprazole in the treatment of asthmatics with nocturnal symptoms and gastro-oesophageal reflux: a placebo-controlled cross-over study. Postgrad Med J 1994; 70:350–354.
116. Sienra-Monge JJ, Rio-Navarro BE, Ponce-Castro H, Arciniega-Olvera RM, Mercado-Ortiz VM. Evolution of asthma in patients treated for gastroesophageal reflux. Adv Ther 1996; 13:20–28.
117. Saye Z, Forget PP. Effect of cisapride on esophageal pH monitoring in children with reflux-associated bronchopulmonary disease. J Pediatr Gastroenterol Nutr 1989; 8:327–332.

118. Malfroot A, Vandenplas Y, Verlinden M, Piepsz A, Dab I. Gastroesophageal reflux and unexplained chronic respiratory disease in infants and children. Pediatric pulmonol 1987; 3:203–213.
119. Vigneri S, Termini R, Leandro G, Badalamenti S, Pantalena M, Savarino V, Di Mario F, Battaglia G, Sandro Mela G, Pilotto A, Plebani M, Davi G. A comparison of five maintenance therapies for reflux esophagitis. N Engl J Med 1995; 333: 1106–1110.
120. Behar J, Sheahan GG, Biancani P. Medical and surgical management of reflux esophagitis. N Engl J Med 1975; 293:263–268.
121. Spechler SJ. Comparison of medical and surgical therapy for complicated gastroesophageal reflux disease in veterans. N Engl J Med 1992; 326:786–792.
122. Giudicelli R, Dupin B, Surpas P, Badier M, Charpin D, Lapicque JC, Fuentes P, Reboud E. Gastroesophageal reflux and respiratory manifestations: diagnostic approach, therapeutic indications and results. Ann Chir 1990; 44:552–554.
123. DeMeester TR, Bonavina L, Iascone C, Courtney JV, Skinner DB. Chronic respiratory symptoms and occult gastroesophageal reflux. A prospective clinical study and results of surgical therapy. Ann Surg 1990; 211:337–345.
124. Lomasney TL. Hiatus hernia and the respiratory tract. Ann Thorac Surg 1977; 24: 448–450.
125. Foglia RP, Fonkalsrud EW, Ament ME, Byrne WJ, Berquist W, Siegel SC, Katz RM, Rachelefsky GS. Gastroesophageal fundoplication for the management of chronic pulmonary disease in children. Am J Surg 1980; 140:72–79.
126. Eizaguirre I, Tovar JA, Arana J, Garay J. Results of gastroesophageal reflux with respiratory manifestations. Chir Pediatr 1987; 28:20–23.
127. Puetz TR, Vakil N. Gastroesophageal reflux-induced cough syncope. Am J Gastroenterol 1995; 90:2204–2206.

6

The Prevalence of GERD in Asthma

STEPHEN J. SONTAG

Veterans Affairs Hospital
Hines, Illinois and
Loyola University Stritch School of Medicine
Maywood, Illinois

> And God formed the human, of dust from the soil
> And blew into his nostrils the breath of life
> And the human became a living being.
>
> Genesis 2:7 (1)

According to the Hebrew Bible, the human body was first constructed, then life was added by the acquisition of Holy breath. *And so began the cycle of respirations.* It was immediately clear, however, that the respirations could be sustained only by energy. *And so from a Garden called Eden came the source of that energy—food. There was life and there was the source of life . . . and there was asthma and GER.*

I. Introduction

The relationship between gastroesophageal reflux (GER) and asthma has been pondered since the beginning of time. We are not told whether Adam feared the first night in the garden because he had never before seen darkness or because he was worried about nocturnal wheezing. Readers of Genesis are left to their own interpretation. In time, great thinkers began to use food for certain medicinal purposes. In the Talmud (the vast collection of third- to sixth-century commentaries on the Hebrew Bible), the treatment for unwanted pulmonary symptoms usually involved some type of food. Coughing was treated with a fish oil drink (2), and asthma was treated with three wheat cakes soaked in honey followed by a drink of undiluted wine (3). Meanwhile, the fifth-century Roman physician Aurelianus Caelius, who was considered second only to Galen in the line of Greco-Roman physicians, offered detailed descriptions of night-time wheezing and noted the frequent nocturnal occurrence of asthma attacks (4). By the twelfth century, the great physician-philosopher, Moses Maimonides, strongly warned against overeating (5). Writing of an association between eating, lying down, and wheezing, Maimonides suggested in his *Treatise on Asthma* that sleep was dangerous during an attack:

> One should not sleep face downwards, nor on one's back, but lying on the side; at the beginning, on the left side, and the close of one's rest, on the right side. One should not go to sleep immediately after a meal, but only when three or four hours have elapsed. One should not sleep during the day.

During the eighteenth century, Nicholas Rosen von Rosenstein, the First Physician to His Swedish Majesty, discussed in his 1776 textbook *The Diseases of Children and Their Remedies* what he terms "the stomachic cough" of children: "Such a cough is caused by the natural proclivity of children to ingest huge quantities of disgusting food, that cannot be digested or changed as it ought" (6). Twenty-six years later, in his 1802 textbook *The History and Cure of Diseases*, William Heberden wrote, "in most persons, the breath is shorter and more difficult after a meal" (7).

Almost a century later, in 1892, Sir William Osler published *The Principles and Practice of Medicine* in which he prepared for the twentieth century with an emphasis on eating habits: "Diet, too has an important influence and in persons subject to this disease severe paroxysms may be induced by overloading the stomach, or by taking certain articles of food" (8). Osler also suggested that particular attention be paid to the diet of the asthmatic: "A rule of which experience generally compels them to make is to take the heavy meal in the early part of the day and not retire to bed before gastric digestion is completed."

Despite the emphasis on diet and the strong references to a relationship between food, eating habits, and asthma, the GER/asthma concept remained difficult to swallow. For the next 50 years, only a few scattered wheezes were heard amidst the competing voices of subspecialty medicine's bellowing burps and clamoring coughs. One of these scattered wheezes was G. W. Bray, who in 1934, at the height of the world depression, reported that dietary indiscretion in some patients could lead to asthmatic attacks (9). Bray's comments, however, went relatively unnoticed until Belsey, in a review on pulmonary complications of esophageal disease, reported that patients with GER were liable to severe, progressive, and disabling pulmonary damage (10). Within 2 years, J. H. Kennedy aroused not only the medical community's hearts and minds, but its guts and lungs as well by suggesting that "silent" GER may be an important but poorly recognized cause of pulmonary complications (11). In 1967 Urschel and Paulson reported their experience in a highly selected population referred for repair of hiatal hernia (12). Figure 1 shows the results of their 5-year experience (1961–1966) in 636 patients, ranging in age from 7 months to 94 years, who were referred for surgical correction of GER. Thirty-nine percent had classic reflux symptoms consisting of heartburn, indigestion, and postural aggravation without respiratory symptoms, 45% had both reflux symptoms and respiratory symptoms, and 16% had respiratory symptoms only. Thus, more than 60% of these patients, who were being referred for surgery to correct a gastroesophageal abnormality, actually had respiratory symptoms. Within a year of Urschel's publication, Cherry and Margulies vocalized their findings and reported that laryngeal contact ulcers, as well as other abnormalities of the voice box, might be a result of chronic GER (13).

By the 1970s, the stage had been set for serious and meaningful research on the relationship between GER and asthma. In the ensuing 27 years, investigators fondled the GER/asthma concept as if they were trying to atone for the previous

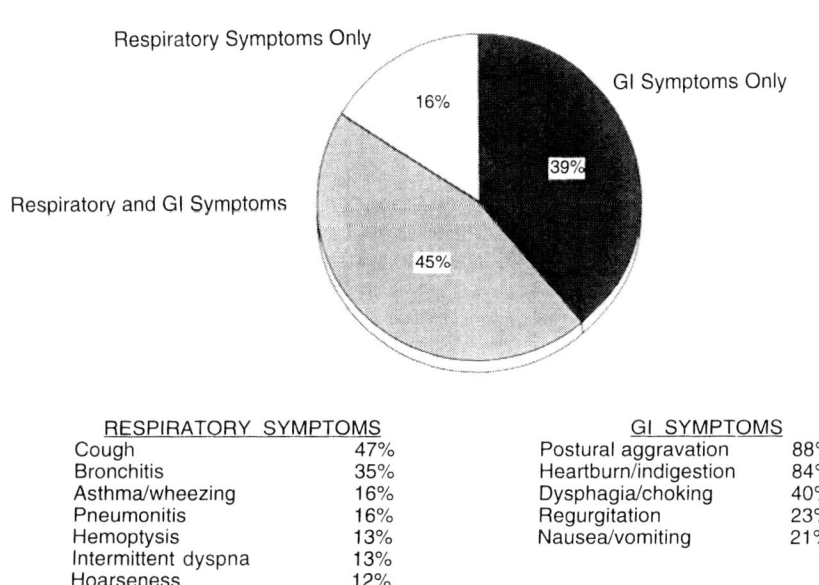

Figure 1 Symptoms in patients referred for antireflux surgery.

2000 years of neglect. Indeed, a MEDLINE search using the terms GER and asthma revealed no fewer than 177 English language publications between 1966 and 1997. Figure 2 shows the types of publications in both the adult and pediatric literature. Of the 177 articles published, half were actual studies in which some type of diagnostic procedure or intervention was undertaken, and almost 80% were published in the adult literature. Indeed, the widespread belief that the GER-asthma relationship pertains mainly to the pediatric, not the adult, population has no basis in fact. Figure 3 shows the percentage of adult and pediatric publications for each 5-year period since 1966. From 1966 to 1970 there were virtually no pediatric publications. From 1971 to 1985 the articles in the pediatric literature remained at approximately 33–42% of the total. At no time, however, did the number of pediatric articles surpass the number of adult articles. In fact, for every 5-year period, the number of publications in the adult literature was numerically greater than that in the pediatric literature. The burst of enthusiasm among pediatric investigators from 1971 to 1985 was followed by a 12-year wane that continues to the current day.

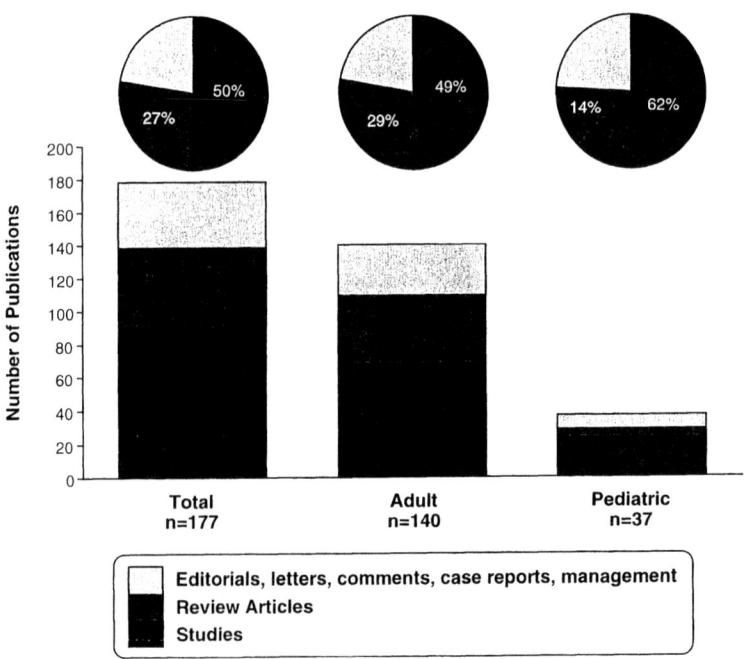

Figure 2 The GER/asthma relationship: types of publications (1966–1997).

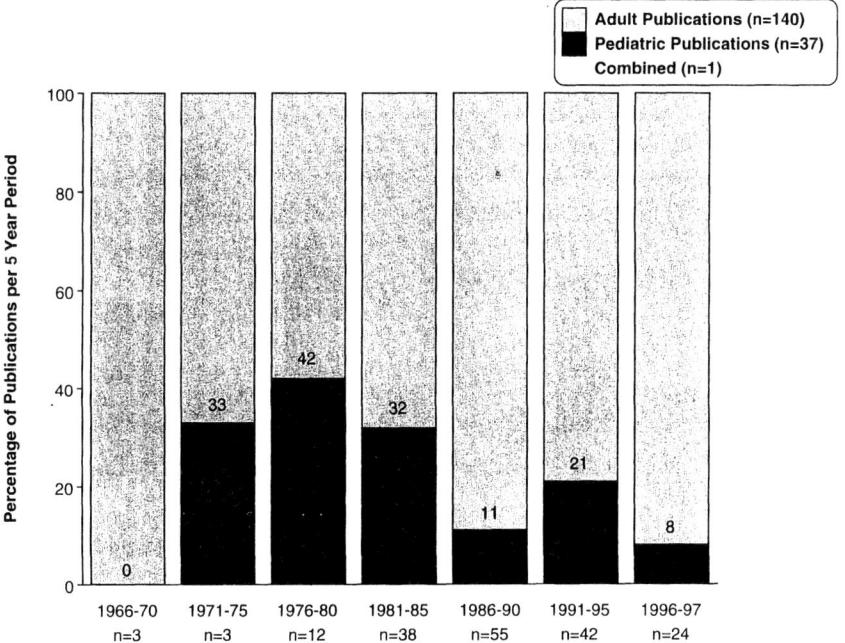

Figure 3 The GER/asthma relationship: adult vs. pediatric publications (1966–1997).

In general, the number of GER/asthma publications appears to be on the increase. Figure 4 shows the incidence of publications for each 5-year period. The average number of publications increases dramatically each year from 1980 to 1985 and then modestly for the next decade. The number of review articles parallels the number of total publications. Interestingly, in the 18-month period from January 1996 through June 1997, there was approximately one review article for every two publications.

II. Coexistence

Numerous authors have studied potential GER-induced asthma mechanisms and reported on the coexistence of GER and asthma in both children (14–16) and adults (17–20). Although these studies strongly suggest a dependent relationship between GER and asthma, they were designed for the most part to clarify the mechanism by which GER might cause asthma. They were not designed to determine the prevalence of GER in the asthmatic population.

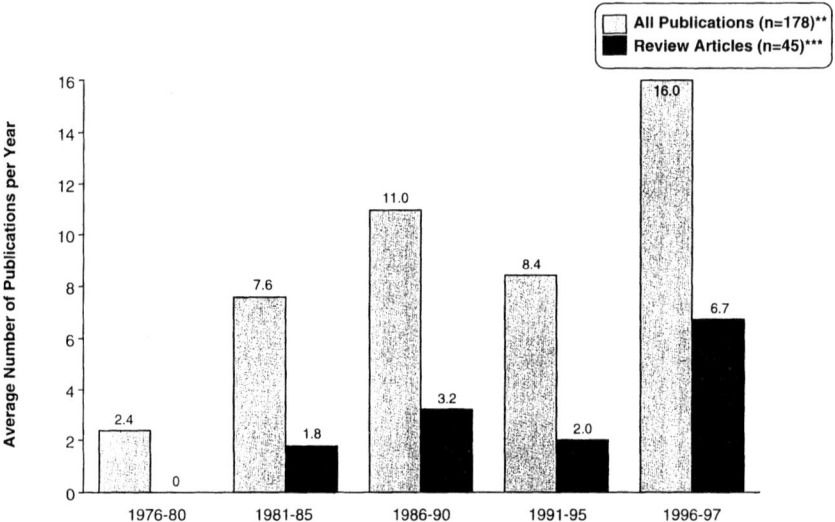

Figure 4 The GER/asthma relationship: incidence of publications (1996–1997).

III. Definitions

Of the 177 articles published, we identified 18 (7 children, 11 adult) with sufficient information from which prevalence data could be extracted. In general, the definitions of asthma were uniform, but the definitions of GER differed considerably. For the most part, however, the definition of GER did reflect the presence of pathological reflux. The terms *prevalence* and *incidence* were often confused and used interchangeably. We took the liberty of switching the terms when incidence was mistakenly used for prevalence.

A. Asthma

Most of the prevalence studies originate from pulmonary referral centers. The definition of asthma was not always defined in the reports. The occurrence of wheezing and reversible airway disease, as well as the requirement for classical asthmatic therapy, indicates that almost all if not all of the patients enrolled in these studies truly met the accepted criteria for asthma. A few of the studies, reported by groups with a focus in gastroenterology, actually documented the asthmatic state with the methacholine bronchoprovocation test and/or the measurement of airway reversibility after bronchodilator administration.

B. GER Disease

The prevalence studies varied in their methods for determining the presence or absence of GER. The documentation of GER was based on either direct or indirect evidence. The number of methods used to document the occurrence of GER disease by any given center varied from 1 to 5. Table 1 shows the methods used to document the presence of GER.

C. Prevalence and Incidence

The term *incidence*, which is one of the most misused terms in the medical literature today (21), is often used erroneously in place of *prevalence*. Indeed, a number of the GER/asthma publications unintentionally used the word incidence in the title, although they actually reported the prevalence. In the clinical setting, for example, the term incidence refers to the number of new cases of a disease (e.g., GER) that surface in a defined population (e.g., asthmatics) over a specific period (e.g., 10 years) of time (22). Since incidence is always expressed in terms of time (cases per year), the true incidence of GER symptoms in asthma could be determined only by following a large group of asthmatics who do not now have GER and identifying those that develop GER over time. The total absence of data on the true incidence of GER in asthma, therefore, is understandable, since determining incidence would be an undertaking of almost impossible dimensions.

Prevalence, on the other hand, refers to the number of cases of a disease (e.g., GER) that exist at a specific period of time (today) in a defined population (e.g., asthmatics) (22). Since prevalence is expressed in terms of current numbers (cases per thousand people), the true prevalence of GER symptoms in asthma could be determined by identifying a large group of asthmatics and identifying those who have GER now. Determining the prevalence is a feasible task and within the reach of many academic centers. It is not difficult to understand, therefore, why all the epidemiological data on the relationship between GER and

Table 1 Methods Used to Document the Presence of GER

Direct Evidence	Indirect Evidence
Short-duration esophageal pH testing	Symptoms of GER
Long-duration (24-h) esophageal pH testing	Esophageal manometry and motility
Esophagoscopy	Presence of hiatal hernia on standard barium radiography
Cine barium radiography	
Scintigraphy	

Table 2 Differences Between Incidence and Prevalence

Incidence	Prevalence
Define a group of asthmatics	Define a group of asthmatics
Select those without GER	Select entire group
Follow for years	Workup now
Identify those that develop GER each year	Identify those that have GER now
Example: 10 new GER cases/yr/1000 asthmatics followed	Example: 80 current GER cases/1000 asthmatics now

asthma are limited to reporting the prevalence rates. Table 2 demonstrates the major differences between prevalence and incidence.

The differences between incidence and prevalence are important to both the physician and the patient, with the patient usually interested in the incidence. For example, an asthmatic patient might be less interested in knowing the number of patients who have GER at any particular moment (the prevalence rate), and more interested in knowing how frequently asthmatics like himself, who do not currently have GER, will develop GER at some point in the future (incidence rate).

IV. Study Design and Sampling Procedures

Accurate prevalence studies rely on accurate recruitment of patients. For data to be meaningful and generally applicable, the population of asthmatics studied should represent the population of asthmatics at large. Most of the epidemiological studies originate in large academic teaching hospitals. Since teaching hospitals and clinics are dependent on the referral of patients for treatment, the studies that report on prevalence rates are subject to two types of selection bias: subject selection bias and spectrum bias (23–26). In subject selection bias, patients are unintentionally selected who have both asthma and GER or who have neither asthma nor GER. The importance of such selection bias cannot be overemphasized since the bias (although unintentional) can produce seriously misleading results. In the available studies on prevalence rates, the difficulty in recruiting consecutive patients was clearly an issue. Indeed, selection bias, which could not be avoided, remains a real problem in the interpretation of the results.

Spectrum bias, the second type of bias, may occur when more patients with GER than without GER volunteer for a study. Again, such a bias may be unintentional on the part of both the investigators and patients. Spectrum bias, however, rather than create an association when none exists, is more likely to lessen associations between variables. Thus, in studies reporting an association between GER and asthma, the presence of spectrum bias is more likely to lessen that association. Selection bias and spectrum bias are considered common problems in clinical samples.

A third type of bias is the hidden bias of Berkson's fallacy—the possibility of spurious associations between diseases (GER associated with asthma) in specific studies. Because of the nature of most referral centers, it is likely that the results of prevalence studies do show Berkson's fallacy, which states that the interplay of differential admission rates "from an underlying population to a particular study group" can result in an artificial association in the study group (27). For instance, many patients are likely to have GER and many patients are likely to have asthma. In tertiary hospitals and referral centers, therefore, GER and asthma are likely to occur together in the same patient merely by chance. Such an occurrence may represent a spurious association between GER and asthma. Unfortunately, the nature of tertiary hospitals and referral centers is such that Berkson's fallacy is difficult to avoid.

In a few of the 18 studies, the investigators actually attempted to eliminate bias from the study sample by confining the study to consecutive asthmatics and eliminating from the data any asthmatics who were referred for work-up because of gastrointestinal symptoms. Even in this population, however, Berkson's fallacy could not entirely be ruled out.

V. Prevalence of GERD in Adults with Asthma

A. GERD Defined as the Presence of Reflux Symptoms

Figure 5 shows the prevalence of GER symptoms in adult asthmatics in three studies with sufficient interpretable data. In the first study, Perrin Foyalle et al. (28) found evidence of reflux symptoms in 65% of 150 consecutive asthmatics. In the second study, O'Connell et al. (29) reported that 72% of 189 consecutive asthmatics had heartburn. Almost half of the 189 had supine nocturnal heartburn, and 18% had nocturnal burning in the throat. In the third study, Field et al. (30) studied 109 asthmatics and 135 controls in a questionnaire-based, cross-sectional analytic study. Seventy-seven percent of the asthmatics had heartburn, 55% had regurgitation, and 24% had difficulty with swallowing; 37% of the group required at least one antireflux medication, and 41% during the prior week had reflux-associated respiratory symptoms. Pulmonary symptoms occurred significantly more frequently in the asthmatics than in the controls.

The results of these three studies, which together comprise a group of 448 asthmatics from France, Canada, and the United States, are remarkably similar. Taken as a group, 318 of the 443 patients had reflux symptoms, indicating that 72% of asthmatics have reflux symptoms. Despite some weaknesses in the pa-

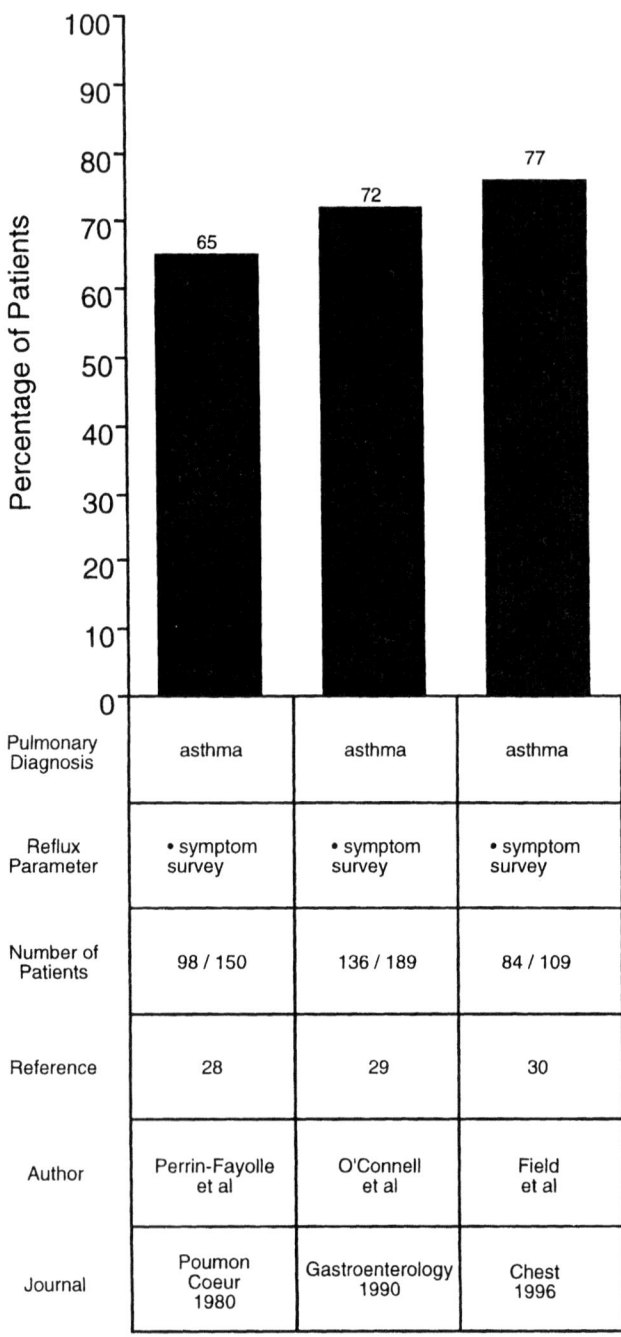

Figure 5 GER symptoms: prevalence in adult asthmatics.

tient-selection methods in all three studies, these reports present the most reliable data in the medical literature on GER symptoms in consecutive asthmatics.

B. GERD Defined as the Presence of Abnormal Acid Reflux

Figure 6 shows the prevalence of abnormal acid reflux in adult asthmatics in six studies comprising 527 patients from six centers in four countries (France, Chili, Great Britain, and United States). The prevalence of abnormal acid reflux, as determined by pH testing, ranged from 33 to 90% (31–36). In two of the studies (31,36), short-term acid reflux testing was used to determine the presence of GER. These studies were conducted in the 1980s before the availability of ambulatory 24-hour pH testing. The remaining four studies (32–35), comprising 365 patients, utilized ambulatory 24-hour pH testing to determine abnormal GER. In all six studies, recruitment of consecutive asthmatics was suboptimal in that all depended on referral centers to enroll their patients. Nevertheless, the studies represent the most reliable data found in the literature on pH testing and the prevalence of GER in asthma. When the results of these six studies are combined, 362 of the 527 (69%) enrolled patients had evidence of acid reflux, suggesting that up to 70% of asthmatics have GER as defined by abnormal acid pH testing.

C. GERD Defined as the Presence of Esophageal Mucosal Damage

Figure 7 shows the prevalence of esophageal mucosal damage in adult asthmatics (37). Esophageal erosions or ulcerations as seen on endoscopy were present in 39% of consecutive asthmatics, and 13% had Barrett's esophagus. In this study, Sontag et al. limited the recruitment to consecutive asthmatics who were referred for endoscopy in an approved study on the prevalence of GER abnormalities in consecutive asthmatics. The authors eliminated from their study any patients who were referred for workup because of gastrointestinal symptoms and who were not part of the consecutive asthmatic protocol. Thus, this study appears to be one of the few that reports the prevalence of GER as it relates to esophageal mucosal damage in consecutive asthmatics.

D. GERD Defined as the Presence of Hiatal Hernia

Figure 8 shows three studies that used the presence of hiatal hernia as indirect evidence of the presence of GER (37–39). In the first study, Mays reported on 28 patients with severe asthma, 64% of whom had hiatus hernia and 46% of whom had barium reflux (38). These studies were criticized by Chernow and Castell (40) because of the lack of data demonstrating aspiration, the reliance on upper gastrointestinal series to determine GER, and the abnormally low prevalence of hiatus hernia and barium reflux in the control group. Despite the criticisms, however, they concluded that the postulated relationship between GER

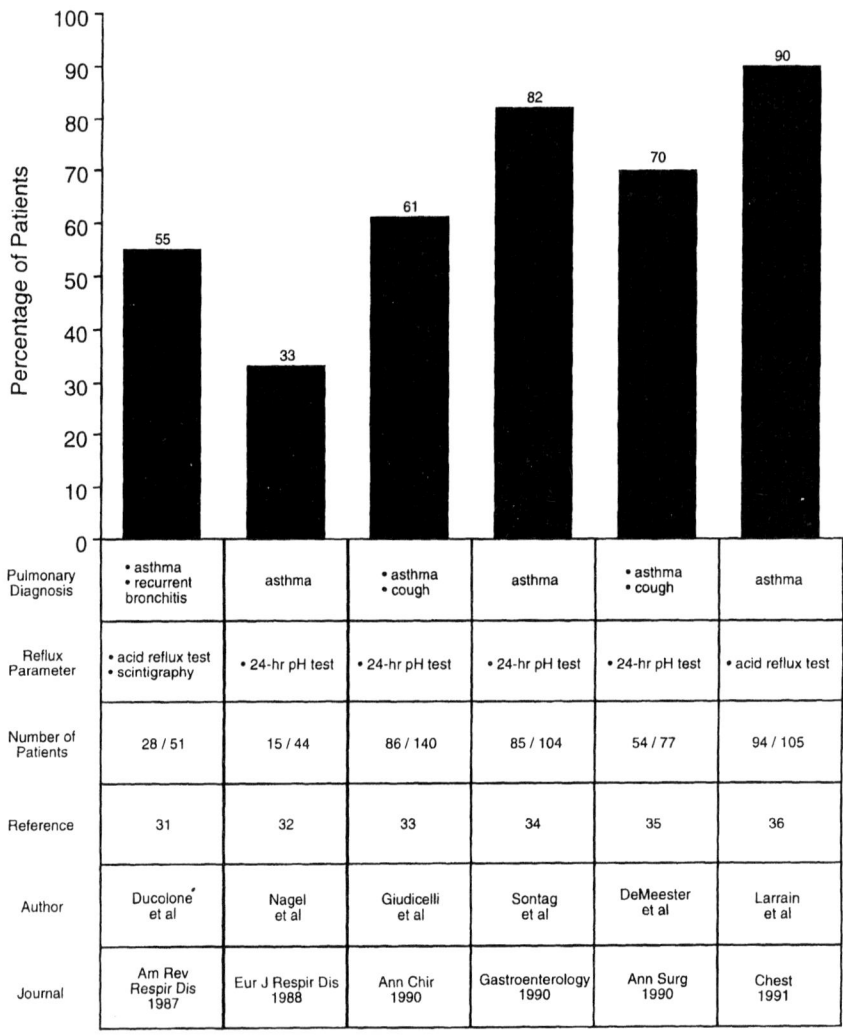

Figure 6 Abnormal acid reflux: prevalence in adult asthmatics.

and asthma most likely existed, but that it was premature to suggest cause and effect. In the second study, which included 15 patients with nocturnal asthma (39), Rodriguez-Villarrel reported a 73% prevalence rate of reflux based on a combination of barium x-ray studies, endoscopy, and technetium scintigraphy. In his report, 11 of 15 patients had abnormal barium x-rays, indicating a 73%

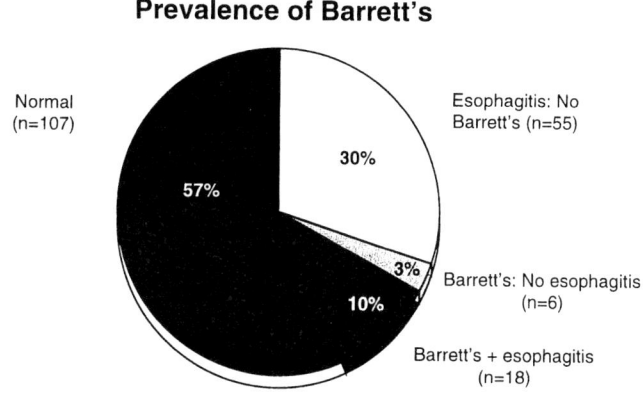

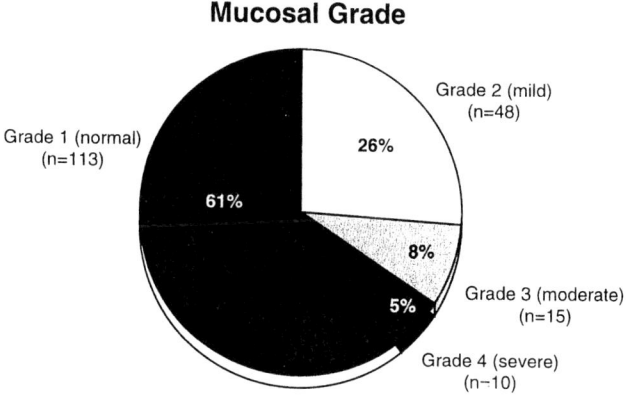

Figure 7 Esophageal mucosal damage: prevalence in adult asthmatics.

prevalence rate of reflux in asthmatics. In the third study, Sontag et al. (37) showed that hiatal hernia was present in 58% of consecutively chosen asthmatics using predetermined endoscopic criteria for hiatal hernia and esophagitis. In this study, all endoscopies were performed by one of two endoscopists using the same criteria for esophageal mucosal disease and the presence of hiatal hernia. In asthmatics with esophagitis, the hiatal hernia occurred seven times more frequently than in asthmatics without esophagitis, indicating that hiatal hernia in asthmatics is associated with more severe esophageal disease. When all three studies are combined, the prevalence of GER as defined by abnormal barium reflux on fluoroscopy or the presence of a hiatal hernia was 50%.

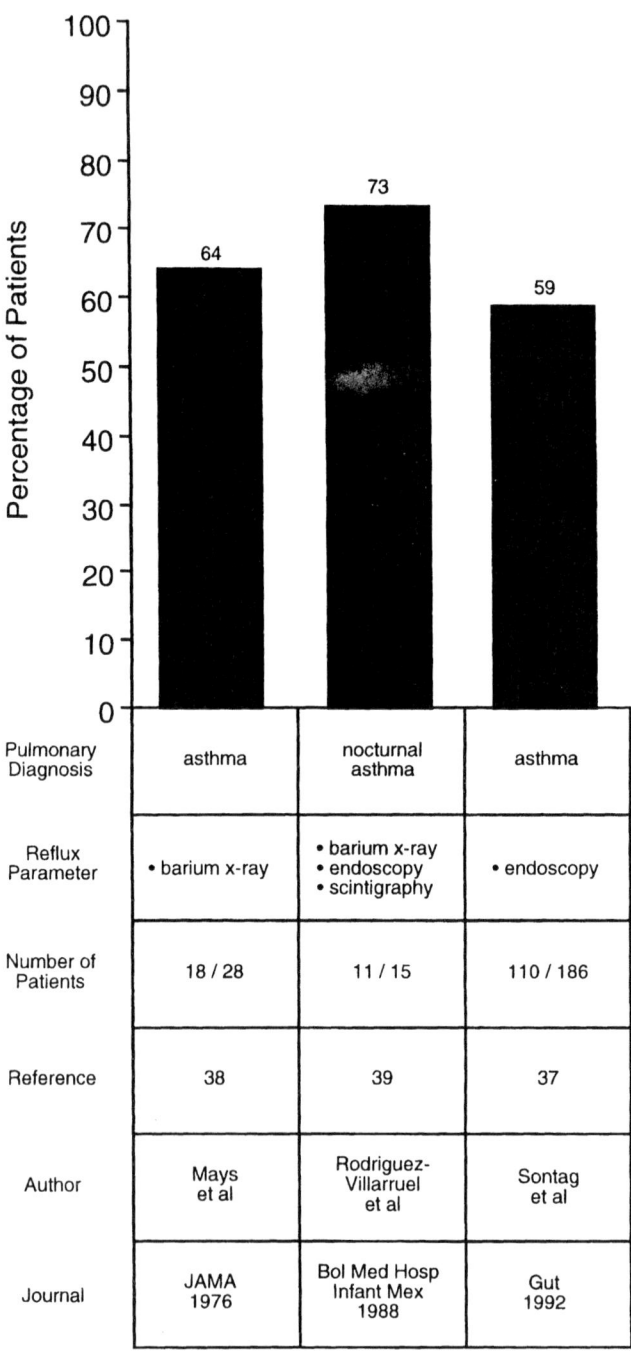

Figure 8 Hiatal hernia: prevalence in adult asthmatics.

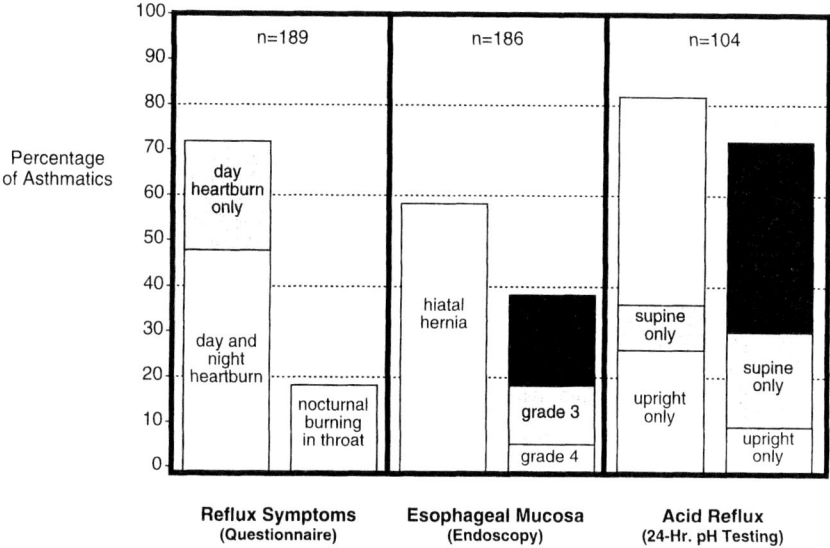

Figure 9 Abnormal reflux parameters: prevalence in consecutive adult asthmatics.

Taken together, the results of the retrospective studies, with their highly selected referral patterns, agree to a great extent with the results of the prospective epidemiological and cross-sectional studies, which clearly demonstrate that GER is highly prevalent in asthmatic patients.

Figure 9 summarizes the three prospective studies, which are part of the 12 adult prevalent studies. Approximately 75% of the asthmatics have heartburn, and almost 20% awaken with nocturnal burning in the throat (29), 80% of consecutive asthmatics have pathologic acid GER in either the upright or supine position, and 75% have increased frequency of reflux episodes (34). In addition, almost 60% of consecutive asthmatics have hiatal hernias (37), almost 40% have esophageal mucosal damage from reflux (37), and 90% of asthmatics have either reflux symptoms or esophageal mucosal disease or abnormal acid reflux. These data strongly indicate that GER is highly prevalent in consecutive adult asthmatics.

VI. Prevalence of GERD in Children with Asthma

Figure 10 shows the prevalence of GER in child asthmatics (41–48). The eight studies, with a total of 783 patients, report prevalence rates of GER ranging from 47 to 64%, with a mean prevalence of 56%. Although these studies suffer from the same biases in selection process as the adult studies, they provide the most

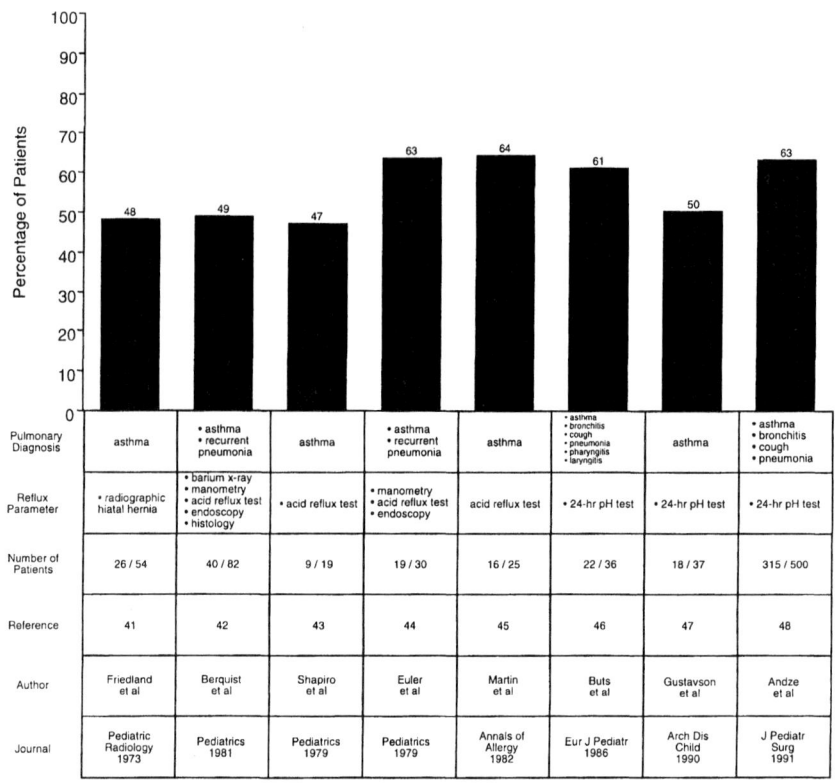

Figure 10 Prevalence of GER in child asthmatics.

reliable data available. In the first study, which is a retrospective radiographic review of 54 children with unremitting asthma, Friedman reported a 48% prevalence rate of hiatal hernia (41). The prevalence rate was significantly higher than the 19% prevalence of hiatus hernias seen in the matched control group. Despite the well-known limitations of such retrospective radiographic reviews, the finding that almost 50% of the patients had a hiatal hernia is powerful evidence in support of the GER/asthma relationship. In the remaining seven studies (42–48), pH testing was used to define the presence of GER. Four of the studies used the short-term acid reflux test, while three used 24-hour esophageal pH testing. Taken together, 439 of the 783 child asthmatics had evidence of GER by either short-term pH testing, long-term pH testing, or radiographic evidence of hiatal hernia. Thus, the GER prevalence rate of 56% in child asthmatics is similar to that reported in adult asthmatics.

VII. Bronchodilators and GER in Asthmatics

Support for the bronchodilator-induced GER concept comes from the numerous reports suggesting that asthma drug therapy relaxes the LES (14,49–51). Such an effect might be expected to promote GER, and asthmatics who require continuous bronchodilators would likely have more GER than those who do not require bronchodilators. In addition, bronchodilators might increase the risk of nocturnal asthma because of the loss of bronchodilating effect as the drug is eliminated throughout the night.

Recent studies argue against the bronchodilator-induced GER concept. When asthmatic subjects who received bronchodilators were compared with those who did not receive bronchodilators, the reflux patterns were similar in both groups of asthmatics, indicating that the reflux was indeed intrinsic to the asthma and not a result of the bronchodilator therapy (34). Figure 11A shows the effect of asthma medications on the LES pressure, the total acid-contact time and the total reflux frequency in asthmatics taking bronchodilators and asthmatics taking

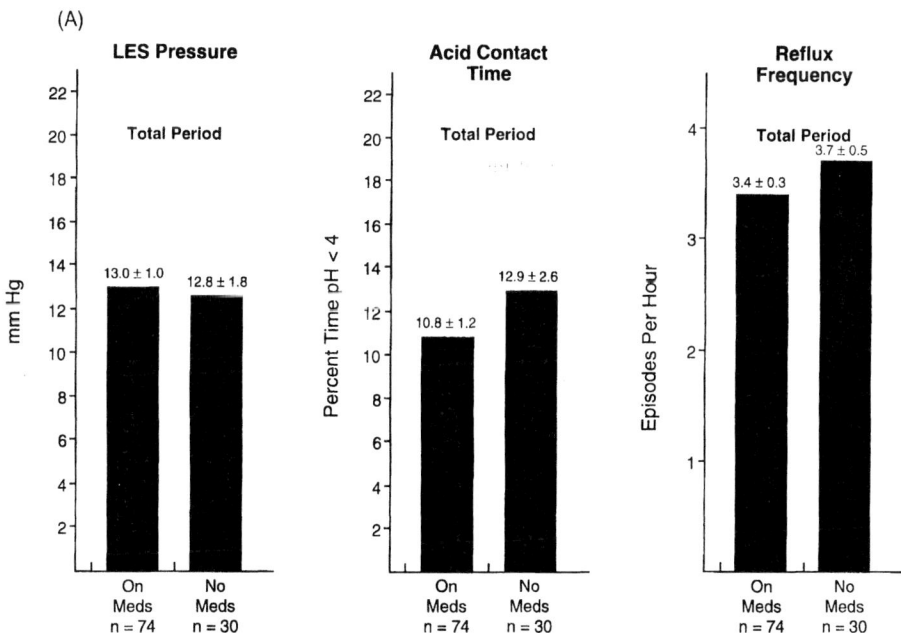

Figure 11 Effect of asthmatic medicine (A) on reflux parameters during the total 24-hour period; (B) on reflux frequency before and after eating and daytime and nighttime;(C) on acid contact time before and after eating and daytime and nighttime.

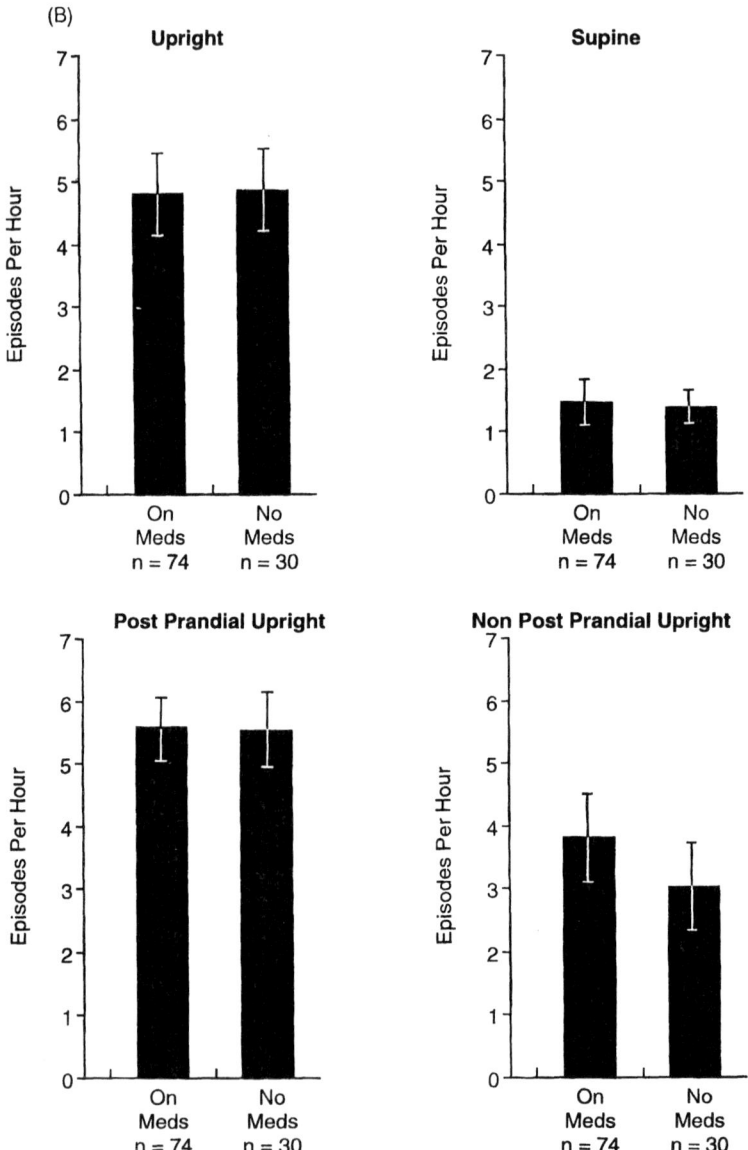

Figure 11 Continued

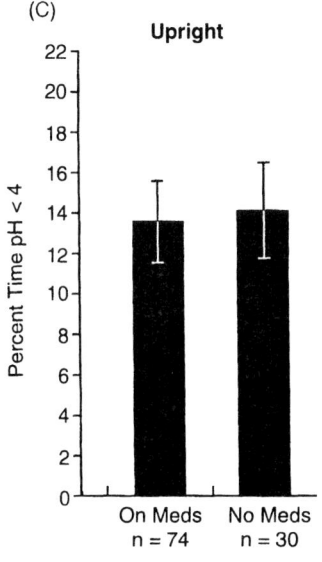
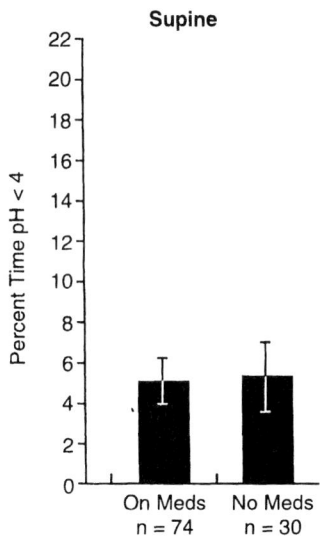
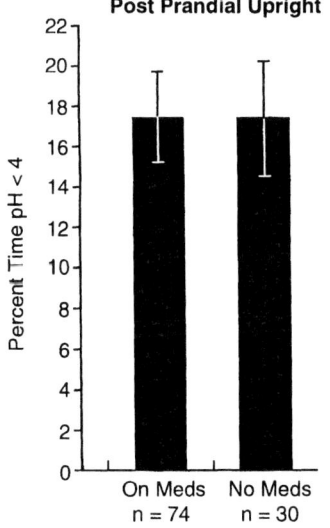
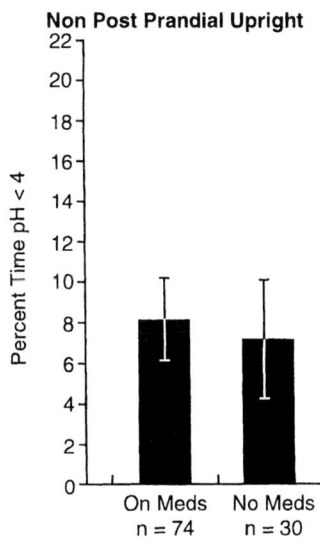

no bronchodilators. Asthma medications clearly had no adverse effect on any of the three reflux parameters. Figures 11B and 11C demonstrate the effect of asthma medications, positions, and eating on the acid-contact time and frequency of reflux episodes in the same two groups of asthmatics—those receiving bronchodilators and those receiving no bronchodilators. The results clearly show that bronchodilators do not influence any of the GER parameters during the upright, supine, postprandial, or nonpostprandial periods (52). Asthmatic subjects receiving bronchodilators had no worse reflux than those not receiving bronchodilators, suggesting that bronchodilators do not promote postprandial or nocturnal GER.

In summary, these 24-hour esophageal pH test results obtained during the normal, everyday positions in asthmatics receiving bronchodilator therapy and those receiving no bronchodilator therapy clearly suggest that GER is an intrinsic abnormality of asthma and not a result of bronchodilator-induced smooth muscle relaxation of the LES.

VIII. Incidence

The true incidence of GER in asthma is unknown. Since incidence (Table 2) can be determined only by following a large group of asthmatics who do not now have GER and identifying those that develop GER over time—a formidable task—the total absence of such data is understandable.

Despite the lack of data on the incidence of GER, data on the prevalence raise an important issue: if the prevalence of GER in adult asthmatics is similar to the prevalence of GER in child asthmatics, what is the true incidence of GER? There are two explanations: (a) all the child asthmatics with GER grow up to become the adult asthmatics with GER (GER incidence = 0%), or (b) some child asthmatics with GER outgrow either the GER or the asthma; some adults with asthma develop GER while others with GER develop asthma (low, medium, or high incidence depending on the numbers). It is not unreasonable to suspect that some child asthmatics with GER become adult asthmatics with GER, or that children with GER who apparently ''outgrow'' their asthma later surface as adults with both asthma and GER. Since most children leave their pediatricians after adolescence, the information required to demonstrate continued asthma or GER is lost. As a result, the medical community sees two completely different populations, each with very similar conditions: childhood asthma with GER and adult asthma with GER.

IX. The High Prevalence of GER and the GER/Asthma Theory

If the high prevalence of GER in asthmatics is clinically relevant, it should be readily explainable. We suggest that the GER-asthma relationship consists of a self-propagating situation whereby reflux aggravates asthma, which in turn induces further reflux. In the early course of the disease, asthma may not be apparent, as aspiration-induced pulmonary symptoms may occur very infrequently—perhaps once or twice a year. With time, however, aspiration may become more frequent, and the pulmonary tree may become hypersensitive. The individual may be diagnosed as having asthma. The pulmonary tree becomes increasingly hypersensitive to a variety of stimuli. In such a scenario, the initial contribution of acid aspiration is no longer apparent, as the primary focus is on the asthma. In any individual patient, the emphasis may be placed on the GER if reflux symptoms predominate or on asthma if pulmonary symptoms predominate. The result is confusion over whether a patient with severe reflux has pulmonary symptoms or whether a patient with asthma has reflux symptoms. The unending debate about whether GER is a cause of the asthma or a result of the asthma becomes the focus of attention. At such a point, the question of whether GER exists in asthmatics or whether pulmonary symptoms exist in refluxers is irrelevant. For the individual patient, gastric contents refluxed into the pulmonary tree is an undesirable event, whether cause or effect, and it is up to the physician to determine how such events can be stopped.

X. Summary

Despite the 178 published studies on the relationship between GER and asthma, the true prevalence of GER in asthmatics must be estimated from fewer than 20 of the studies. The estimated prevalence is between 60–80% in adults and 50–60% in children. The studies comprise highly selected referred populations that may not reflect the overall populations with asthma. Despite the limitations, however, we believe that the data reflect the general asthma population as much as can be expected.

XI. Conclusion

GER and asthma occur together frequently. The prevalence of GER is significantly increased both in children with asthma and in adults with asthma. Almost every study on the relationship between GER and asthma emphasizes the high prevalence of GER. A relationship between GER and asthma has been recognized for more than 2000 years, but has not been appreciated until recently—or perhaps it really once was appreciated, but lost to memory. It was King Solomon who once described in the Hebrew Book of Ecclesiastes the paradox of memory:

Only that shall happen
Which has happened,
Only that occur
Which has occurred;
There is nothing new
Beneath the sun!

Sometimes there is a phenomenon
  of which they say,
"Look, this one is new!"
It occurred long since,
  in ages that went by before us.

The earlier ones are not remembered;
So too those that will occur later
Will no more be remembered
Than those that will occur at the very end.

Ecclesiastes 1:9–11

References

1. The Hebrew Bible. Genesis 2:7.
2. The Talmud: Divrei Chayyim II, 52.
3. The Talmud: Gittin, 69b.
4. Aurelianus Caelius. In: De Morbis Acutis et Chronicis. Amsterdam: Wetstenland, 1709.
5. Maimonides M. Treatise on asthma. In: Munter S, ed. Medical Writings of Moses Maimonides. Philadelphia: Lippincott, 1963.
6. Nicholas Rosen von Rosenstein. On the cough of children. In: The Diseases of Children and Their Remedies. Birmingham, AL: LB Adams, 1776:183–190.
7. Heberden W. Asthma. In: The History and Cure of Diseases. Birmingham, AL: LB Adams, 1802:62–69.
8. Sir William Osler. Bronchial asthma. In: The Principles and Practice of Medicine. Birmingham, AL: LB Adams, 1776:497–503.
9. Bray GW. Recent advances in the treatment of asthma and hay fever. Practitioner 1934; 34:368–371.
10. Belsey R. The pulmonary complications of oesophageal disease. Br J Dis Chest 1960; 54:342–348.
11. Kennedy JH. "Silent" gastroesophageal reflux: an important but little known cause of pulmonary complications. Dis Chest 1962; 42:42–45.
12. Urschel HC, Paulson DL. Gastroesophageal reflux and hiatal hernia: complications and therapy. J Thorac Cardiovasc Surg 1967;53:21–32.
13. Cherry J, Margulies SI. Contact ulcer of the larynx. Laryngoscope 1968; 78:1937–1940.
14. Berquist WE, et al. Quantitative gastroesophageal reflux and pulmonary function in

asthmatic children and normal adults receiving placebo, theophylline, and metaproterenol sulfate therapy. J Allergy Clin Immunol 1984; 73:253–258.
15. Davis RS, Larsen GL, Grunstein MM. Respiratory response to intraesophageal acid infusion in asthmatic children during sleep. J Allergy Clin Immunol 1983; 72:393–398.
16. Hughes DM, Spier S, Rivlin J, Levison H. Gastroesophageal reflux during sleep in asthmatic patients. J Pediatr 1983; 102:666–672.
17. Overholt RH, Voorhees RJ. Esophageal reflux as a trigger in asthma. Dis Chest 1966; 49:464–466.
18. Davis MV. Relationship between pulmonary disease, hiatal hernia, and gastroesophageal reflux. NY State J Med 1972; 72:935.
19. Bretza J, Novey HS. GE reflux and asthma. West J Med 1979; 131:320.
20. Perrin-Fayolle M, Gormand F, Braillon G, et al. Long-term results of surgical treatment for gastroesophageal reflux in asthmatic patients. Chest 1989; 96:40–45.
21. Colton T. Statistics in Medicine. Boston: Little, Brown and Company, 1974: 46–47.
22. Stedman's Medical Dictionary. Baltimore: Williams & Wilkins, 1990.
23. Ransohoff DF, Feinstein AR. Problems of spectrum and bias in evaluating the efficacy of diagnostic tests. N Engl J Med 1978; 299:926–930.
24. Philbrick JT, Horowitz RI, Feinstein AR, Langou RA, Chandler JP. The limited spectrum of patients studied in exercise test research: analyzing the tip of the iceberg. JAMA 1982; 248:2467–2470.
25. Feinstein AR. On blind men, elephants, spectrums, and controversies: lessons from rheumatic fever revisited. J Chronic Dis 1986; 39:337–342.
26. Miller TQ, Turner CW, Tinsdale RS, Posavac EJ. Disease based spectrum bias in referred samples and the relationship between type A behavior and arteriosclerosis. J Clin Epidemiol 1988; 41:1139–1149.
27. Berkson J. The statistical study of association between smoking and lung cancer. Mayo Clin Proc 1955; 30:319–324.
28. Perrin-Foyalle M, Bel A, Kofman J, et al. Asthma and gastroesophageal reflux. Results of a survey of over 150 cases. Poumon Coeur 1980; 36:225–230.
29. O'Connell S, Sontag SJ, Miller T, Kurucar C, Brand L, Reid S. Asthmatics have a high prevalence of reflux symptoms regardless of the use of bronchodilators. Gastroenterology 1990; 98(2):A97.
30. Field SK, Underwood M, Brant R, Cowie RL. Prevalence of gastroesophageal reflux symptoms in asthma. Chest 1996; 109:316–322.
31. Ducolone A, Vandevenne A, Jouin H, Grob JC, Coumaros D, Meyer C. Gastroesophageal reflux in patients with asthma and chronic bronchitis. Am Rev Respir Dis 1987; 135: 327–332.
32. Nagel RA, Brown P, Perks WH, Wilson RSE, Kerr GD. Ambulatory pH monitoring of gastro-oesophageal reflux in ''morning dipper'' asthmatics. Br Med J 1988; 297: 1371–1373.
33. Giudicelli R, Dupin B, Surpas P, Badier M, Charpin D, Lapicque JC, Fuentes P, Reboud E. Reflux gastro-oesophagien et manifestations respiratoires: attitute diagnostique, indications therapeutiques et resultats. Ann Chir 1990; 44:552–554.
34. Sontag S, O'Connell S, Khandelwal S, Miller T, Nemchausky B, Serlovsky R,

Schnell T. Most asthmatics have gastroesophageal reflux with or without bronchodilator therapy. Gastroenterology 1990; 99:613–620.
35. DeMeester TR, Bonavina L, Iascone C, Courtney JV, Skinner DB. Chronic respiratory symptoms and occult gastroesophageal reflux. Ann Surg 1990; 11:337–345.
36. Larrain A, Carrasco E, Galleguillos F, Sepulveda R, Pope C. Medical and surgical treatment of non-allergic asthma associated with gastroesophageal reflux. Chest 1991; 99:1330–1336.
37. Sontag SJ, Schnell TG, Miller TQ, Khandelwal S, O'Connell S, Chejfec G, Greenlee H, Seidel UJ, Brand L. Prevalence of oesophagitis in asthmatics. Gut 1992; 33:872–876.
38. Mays EE. Intrinsic asthma in adults, association with gastroesophageal reflux. JAMA 1976; 36:2626–2628.
39. Rodriguez-Villarrel H, et al. Reflujo gastroesofagico associado a asthma bronquial. Bol Md Hosp Infant Mex 1988; 45:442.
40. Chernow B, Castell DO. Asthma and gastroesophageal reflux (letter). JAMA 1977; 37:2379.
41. Friedland GW, Yamate M, Marinkovich VA. Hiatal hernia and chronic unremitting asthma. Pediatr Radiol 1973; 1:156–160.
42. Berquist WE, et al: Gastroesophageal reflux-associated recurrent pneumonia and chronic asthma in children. Pediatrics 1981; 68:29–35.
43. Shapiro GG, Christie DL. Gastroesophageal reflux in steroid-dependent asthmatic youths. Pediatrics 1979; 63:207–212.
44. Euler AR, Byrne WJ, Ament ME, et al. Recurrent pulmonary disease in children: a complication of gastroesophageal reflux. Pediatrics 1979; 63:47–51.
45. Martin ME, Grunstein MM, Larsen GL. The relationship of gastroesophageal reflux to nocturnal wheezing in children with asthma. Ann Allergy 1982; 49:318–322.
46. Buts JP, Barudi C, Moulin D, Calus D, Cornu G, Otte JB. Prevalence and treatment of silent gastro-oesophageal reflux in children with recurrent respiratory disorders. Eur J Pediatr 1986; 145:396–400.
47. Gustafsson PM, Kjellman N-IM, Tibbling L. Bronchial asthma and acid reflux into the distal and proximal oesophagus. Arch Dis Child 1990; 65:1255–1258.
48. Andze GO, Brandt ML, St Vil D, et al. Diagnosis and treatment of gastroesophageal reflux in 500 children with respiratory symptoms: the value of pH monitoring. J Pediatr Surg 1991; 26:295–300.
49. DiMarino AJ, Cohen S. Effect of an oral beta 2-adrenergic agonist on lower esophageal sphincter pressure in normals and in patients with achalasia. Dig Dis Sci 1982; 27:1063–1066.
50. Johannesson N, Andersson KE, Joelsson B, Persson CG. Relaxation of lower esophageal sphincter and stimulation of gastric secretion and diuresis by antiasthmatic xanthines. Role of adenosine antagonism. Am Rev Respir Dis 1985; 131:26–30.
51. Stein MR, Towner TG, Weber RW, et al. The effect of theophylline on the lower esophageal sphincter pressure. Ann Allergy 1980; 45:238–239.
52. Sontag S, O'Connell S, Khandelwal S, Miller T, Nemchausky B, Schnell T, Serlovsky R. Effect of positions, eating and bronchodilators on gastroesophageal reflux in asthmatics. Dig Dis Sci 1990; 35:849–856.
53. The Hebrew Bible. Ecclesiastes 1:9–11.

7

GERD, Airway Disease, and the Mechanisms of Interaction

SUSAN M. HARDING

University of Alabama at Birmingham
Birmingham, Alabama

Asthma is exacerbated by triggers that ignite an inflammatory response. There is an increased prevalence of gastroesophageal reflux in asthmatics and antireflux therapy can improve asthma outcome in selected patients. The mechanisms whereby esophageal acid induces bronchoconstriction have been examined extensively on a physiological basis. These mechanisms were first described by Sir William Osler, who stated that "attacks may be due to direct irritation of the bronchial mucosa or . . . indirectly, too, by reflex influences from stomach . . ." (1). These two mechanisms, microaspiration of esophageal acid into the upper airway and a vagally mediated reflex, are still thought to play a major role in acid-induced bronchoconstriction. However, to date, there are no studies evaluating molecular mechanisms of acid-induced bronchoconstriction. As discussed in Chapter 2, the autonomic nervous system plays a role in inducing neurogenic inflammation. This chapter will review data supporting a vagal reflex mechanism and data supporting a microaspiration model. Next, pulmonary mechanisms predisposing asthmatics to develop gastroesophageal reflux disease (GERD) are discussed including the role of the crural diaphragm in lower esophageal sphincter (LES) pressure generation, heightened thoraco-abdominal pressure differential predisposing to reflux development, and the effects of asthma medications on GERD. Finally, data examining predictors of asthma response from clinical trials will be reviewed, since these predictors provide insight into the underlying mechanisms of acid-induced bronchoconstriction.

I. Pathophysiology of Esophageal Acid-Induced Bronchoconstriction

There are three mechanisms in which GERD induces or exacerbates airflow obstruction in asthmatics, including first, a vagally mediated reflex where acid in the esophagus stimulates acid-sensitive receptors resulting in bronchoconstriction. Second, esophageal acid causes heightened bronchial reactivity, so that when an asthmatic is exposed to a trigger, there is a heightened bronchoconstrictive response. Third, microaspiration of gastric contents into the upper airway causes bronchoconstriction. These three mechanisms may interact and further augment airway responses. The vagus nerve is involved in all three mechanisms, including microaspiration.

A. Vagal Reflex Mechanism

The tracheobronchial tree and the esophagus share embryonic foregut origins and share autonomic innervation through the vagus nerve. Airway reflexes may be protective in order to avoid exposure to noxious agents by causing apnea, laryngeal narrowing, and bronchoconstriction, or defensive, aiming to remove noxious agents by sneezing or coughing (2). Stimulation of the upper aerodigestive tract leads to clinically significant respiratory responses (3). Osler was the first to propose that a vagally mediated reflex could exacerbate asthma (1). Vagal innervation of the esophagus includes both sensory and motor fibers. Sensory nerves in the esophagus respond to irritation and esophageal distention. Sensory information from the esophagus is conveyed through the vagus nerve to the nucleus of the solitary tract in the dorsomedial medulla. Interneurons then project from the nucleus of the solitary tract to motor neuron pools in the ventrolateral medulla just dorsal to the inferior olives in the region of the nucleus ambiguus. Motor efferents in the vagus nerve then travel to nerve endings in the tracheobronchial tree, resulting in bronchoconstriction (Fig. 1) (3).

Reflux-induced bronchoconstriction was extensively investigated by Mansfield et al. (4). Using a dog model, they produced esophagitis by instilling hydrochloric acid (HCl) into the esophagus for a week (4). On testing day, anesthetized dogs sequentially had 100 ml of normal saline infused into their esophagii over 15 minutes, followed by an infusion of 0.1 N HCl, followed by lower esophageal distention using a 60-ml air-filled balloon. Total respiratory resistance and functional residual capacity (FRC) were measured at the conclusion of each procedure. In another group of experimental animals, bilateral vagotomy was performed before the esophageal manipulations (4). Esophageal acid caused a

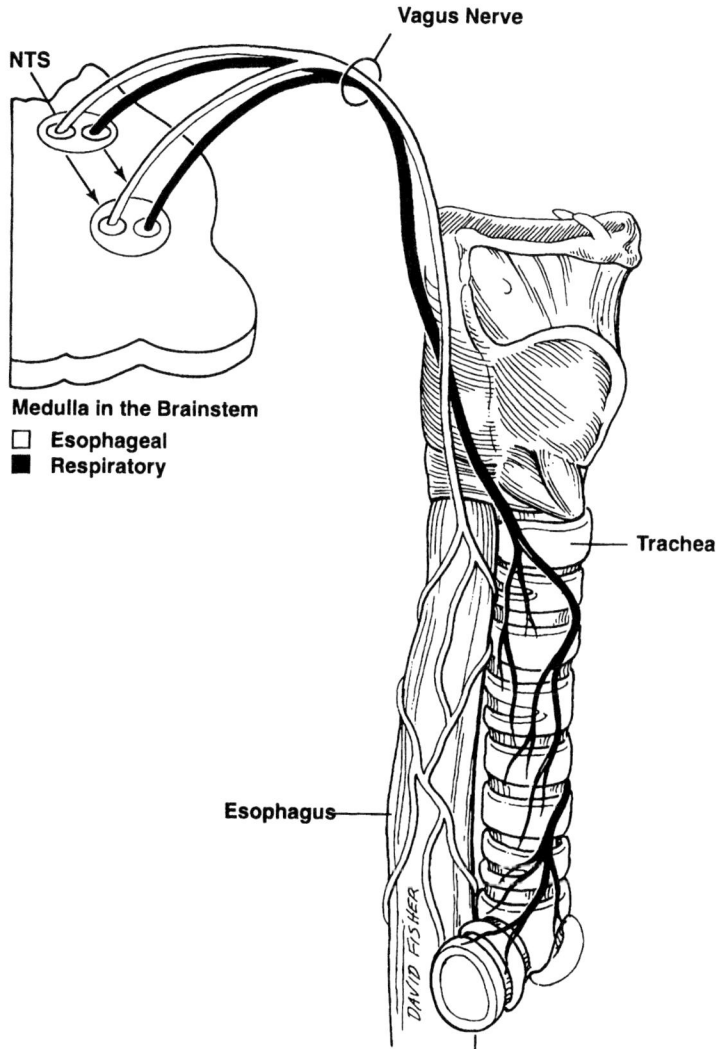

Figure 1 Central neural control of the esophagus and tracheobronchial tree through the vagus nerve. Sensory information from the esophagus is conveyed by the vagus nerve to the nucleus of the solitary tract (NTS) in the dorsomedial medulla. Interneurons project to the motor neuron pools in the ventrolateral medulla, after which motor efferents located in the vagus nerve project to the tracheobronchial tree. (Modified from Ref. 3.)

significant fall in respiratory conductance, the reciprocal of total respiratory resistance. Esophageal distention also caused a similar fall in respiratory conductance. In the dogs who had bilateral vagotomy, the previously described fall in respiratory conductance did not occur, thus showing that the vagus nerve was involved in esophageal acid–induced bronchoconstriction. Esophagitis was found in all dogs. These findings support that esophageal acid or balloon distention of the distal esophagus in dogs with esophagitis causes bronchoconstriction (4).

There are also human studies that support a vagally mediated reflex. Mansfield and Stein examined 15 asthmatics with GERD and monitored spirometry and total respiratory resistance at baseline, after 15 minutes of a normal saline esophageal infusion, and after an esophageal acid infusion of 0.1 N HCl for 30 minutes or until symptoms of esophagitis occurred (pyrosis) (5). Normal saline infusions caused no change in pulmonary function. When symptoms of esophagitis appeared with esophageal acid, there was an increase in total respiratory resistance and a decrease in airflow at 25% of vital capacity. Pulmonary function returned to baseline values after symptom relief with antacids. Since testing was performed in the upright position, the authors concluded that microaspiration was unlikely and that a reflex mechanism was responsible for the bronchoconstriction (5).

The same group of investigators performed a double-blind esophageal acid infusion study in four subject groups: asthmatics with GERD, asthmatics without GERD, subjects with GERD, and normal control subjects (6). Esophageal acid infusion resulted in no change in pulmonary function in the asthmatics without GERD, with GERD, and the normal control groups. The asthmatics with a positive Bernstein test group had a 10% increase in total respiratory resistance when reflux symptoms occurred, which returned to baseline when reflux symptoms abated with antacids ($p < 0.01$). The changes in total respiratory resistance were even more pronounced (72% over baseline) in asthmatics with GERD who associated asthma attacks with reflux symptoms ($p < 0.0001$) (6). They concluded that a positive symptom response in an acid-sensitive esophagus of an asthma patient was required and that the rapid fall in total respiratory resistance after antacid treatment makes it likely that a reflex mechanism was involved (6).

Other investigators, however, have found that the presence of reflux symptoms was not necessary to evoke airway responses with esophageal acid. Ducoloné et al. monitored pulmonary function in 13 asthmatics with GERD and 7 asthmatics without GERD during esophageal acid infusions (7). There was a significant change in maximal expiratory flow at 50% and 25% of vital capacity after esophageal acid infusion in both the asthmatics with and the asthmatics without GERD without a significant change in FEV_1 (7) Pulmonary function changes were not observed in patients with chronic bronchitis with or without GERD or in normal controls (7).

To further examine the role of the vagus nerve in acid-induced bronchoconstriction, investigators used atropine to block the parasympathetic reflex responses. Andersen et al. performed esophageal acid infusions in three groups: patients with esophagitis without asthma, patients with asthma without esophagitis, and asthmatics with esophagitis (8). Pulmonary function tests, including total lung capacity, airway resistance, residual volume, and peak expiratory flow rates were measured after esophageal infusions of 50 ml of normal saline and 50 ml of 0.1 N HCl. Esophageal infusions were also performed after an intravenous injection of atropine (0.01 mg/kg of body weight). There was a significant decrease in peak expiratory flow rate and an increase in airway resistance after HCl infusion seen only in the asthmatics with esophagitis. Six patients with asthma and esophagitis also received atropine pretreatment, and esophageal acid failed to produce changes in peak expiratory flow rate or airway resistance (8). They concluded that there is modest bronchoconstriction with esophageal acid in asthmatics with endoscopy-proven esophagitis. This response was inhibited with intravenous atropine, indicating vagal mediation (8).

To further study acid-induced esophagobronchial-cardiac reflexes in humans, Wright et al. examined 136 unselected individuals with esophageal infusions of water, normal saline, and 0.1 N HCl (9). Highly significant reductions in airway flow measured by FEV_1 (<0.0001) and oxygen saturation (<0.0001) were noted with esophageal acid. A positive Bernstein test was not necessary for these airway responses. Also, the previously noted decrements in airflow and oxygen saturation with esophageal acid infusion were absent in atropine-pretreated (0.6 mg intramuscular) patients (9). These data indicate that the cholinergic reflex is universal, present not only in subjects with bronchospasm, but also in subjects without pulmonary symptoms. Also, an acid-sensitive esophagus (as defined by a positive Bernstein test) was not required to evoke the bronchoconstriction response (9).

To further evaluate the pulmonary effects of esophageal acid, Kjellen et al. studied three study groups—15 patients with asthma and GERD, 5 patients with asthma and a negative Bernstein test, and 5 patients without asthma with GERD (10). Pulmonary function tests including vital capacity, closing volume, and slope of alveolar plateau were measured during esophageal acid infusion. There was a decrease in vital capacity of 0.2 liters and an increase in alveolar plateau of 0.9% in asthmatics with GERD, but not in the two other groups. All patients in the group with asthma and GERD had a positive Bernstein test, suggesting that an inflammatory reaction in the esophageal mucosa was necessary to elicit airflow obstruction with esophageal acid (10).

Many asthmatics with GERD have nocturnal bronchospasm. Davis et al. studied respiratory responses with esophageal acid infusion in eight asthmatic children during sleep (11). On the basis of the Bernstein test, two groups were identified: those with and those without heartburn during the Bernstein test. Esophageal saline and acid infusions were administered at midnight and at 4:00

a.m. Only asthmatics with a positive Bernstein test had a decrease in respiratory time fraction (40% decrease) and an increase in mean respiratory flow with esophageal acid. They concluded that there is an active reflex mechanism initiated from an inflamed esophagus causing bronchial smooth muscle contraction (11).

Despite many studies showing evidence of acid-triggered bronchoconstriction, there are also studies that fail to show alterations in pulmonary function. Ekström et al. studied eight moderate to severe asthmatics with GERD, with four patients having reflux-associated respiratory symptoms (12). Subjects underwent histamine-inhalation testing to measure airway hyperresponsiveness: 2–3 hours later, esophageal acid infusions were performed with FEV_1 measurements. They found that patients with reflux-associated respiratory symptoms had greater histamine reactivity than those without. A more negative change in FEV_1 with esophageal acid was seen in patients with a positive Bernstein test (12). However, clinically significant bronchospasm and significant changes in FEV_1 were not seen (12). Furthermore, Wesseling et al. studied 12 asthmatics with GERD and monitored spirometry and respiratory impedance after esophageal acid infusions and found no statistically significant difference in peak expiratory flow rate or impedance of the respiratory system with esophageal acid (13). They concluded that there was no evidence for a direct causal relationship between esophageal acid and increased bronchomotor tone (13).

Since autonomic regulation is altered during sleep and airway responses may be augmented during sleep, Tan et al. monitored spontaneous esophageal acid events and performed esophageal acid infusions in 15 sleeping asthmatics (14). Respiratory parameters measured included airflow, tidal volume, and pulmonary resistance. Subjects were divided into those with a positive Bernstein test and those without. Lower airway resistance did not change on the night that the subject was exposed to esophageal acid. The presence of esophagitis, as defined by a positive Bernstein test, did not influence the pulmonary response to esophageal acid. Although meticulously executed, one potential problem with the study design is that the investigators combined data from spontaneous acid events and events during esophageal acid infusions. Their study population combined asthmatics with GERD and asthmatics without GERD (14). Previous studies have shown that a bronchoconstrictive effect is only present in asthmatics with GERD.

There are many factors that could explain conflicting data. Studies show that esophageal acid may produce a modest bronchoconstrictive response, which may not be present in all subjects tested. In selected asthmatics, sensitive measurements of bronchoconstriction, including peak expiratory flow rate and airway resistance, were found. The magnitude of the change in these parameters was in the range of 10–20% with esophageal acid (15). Esophageal acid resulted in these changes more commonly in subjects with positive Bernstein tests or evidence of esophagitis than in subjects without evidence of GERD. Another problem with most of the studies is that the population size was small, especially in the control groups. Also, study group definitions and entrance criteria were poorly defined in some of the studies. No study reviewed thus far investigated the possibility of microaspiration of acid into the larynx or trachea.

In order to further investigate the role of a vagally mediated reflex causing bronchoconstriction, our laboratory performed a series of studies, which included strictly defined patient populations. In the first study, 47 nonsmoking adult subjects were divided into four groups. The first group included 20 asthmatics with GERD (with asthma being defined by American Thoracic Society criteria) and evidence of airway hyperresponsiveness. GERD was defined by reflux symptoms including heartburn and/or regurgitation and abnormal esophageal acid contact times on 24-hour esophageal pH test (16). The second group included seven asthmatics without GERD. The third group included 10 patients with GERD, without pulmonary symptoms, and the fourth group included 10 normal controls who had normal esophageal pH tests, no pulmonary symptoms, and normal pulmonary function studies. To evaluate for microaspiration, dual esophageal pH monitoring was performed during esophageal infusions. The proximal esophageal pH probe measured pH just below the upper esophageal sphincter (UES), assuming that patients with proximal esophageal reflux have increased potential for microaspiration.

Patients presented after an overnight fast and the dual esophageal pH probe was placed with pH electrodes 5 cm above a manometrically defined LES and just below the UES. Esophageal infusions of normal saline, 0.1 N HCl, and normal saline were performed in an order blinded to the patient at the rate of 7 ml per minute for 15 minutes (16). During the esophageal infusions, the patients sat upright in a chair and spontaneously reported pulmonary and reflux symptoms. Pulmonary function studies including spirometry and airway resistance were performed after the placement of the esophageal pH probe, after the insertion of the 8 French feeding tube, and after each esophageal infusion. Peak expiratory flow rate decreased with esophageal acid infusion in all four groups including normal controls ($p < 0.01$) (Fig. 2). Furthermore, esophageal acid clearance improved peak expiratory flow rate in all groups except in the asthma with GERD group, which had a further decrease in peak expiratory flow rate. The bronchoconstrictor response was not dependent on a positive Bernstein test or evidence of proximal reflux, a prerequisite for microaspiration. Another interesting finding is that asthmatics with GERD also had an increase in specific airway resistance with esophageal acid, which continued to increase despite acid clearance. These results agree with Wright et al.'s data, which showed a decrease in airflow independent of whether the subject had pulmonary disease (9). Since microaspiration was not required for bronchoconstriction, a vagally mediated esophago-pulmonary reflex is present in all individuals. This reflex may be a protective mechanism for the lung, in that bronchoconstriction would decrease the lung's exposure to caustic

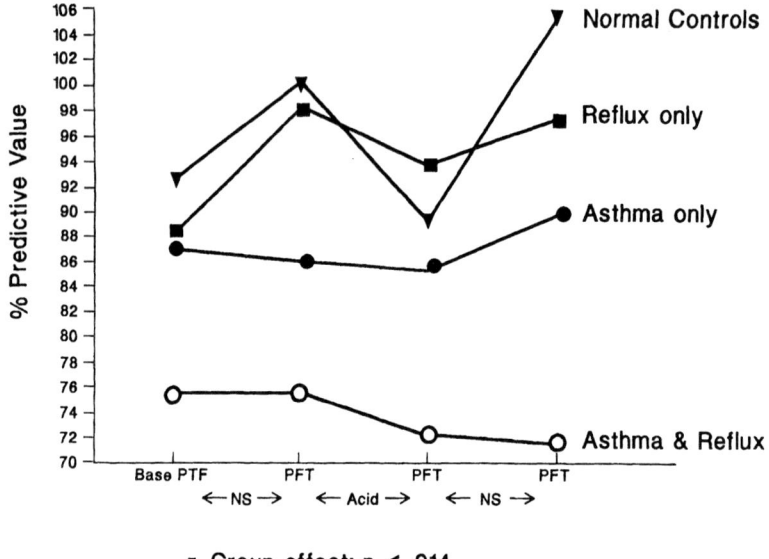

Figure 2 Peak expiratory flow rate data expressed as percent predicted during esophageal infusions of normal saline solution (NS) and acid. (From Ref. 16.)

agents. Another interesting finding is that asthmatics with GERD had no improvement in peak expiratory flow rate despite esophageal acid clearance, as documented by normalization of esophageal pH at the distal esophagus during the second saline infusion (16). The other study groups had complete recovery of peak expiratory flow rate with esophageal acid clearance. Asthmatics with GERD may have an exaggerated vagal reflex, which represents an aberration in parasympathetic tone. Another possible mechanism is that esophageal acid triggered, through a reflex, airway inflammation resulting in continued bronchoconstriction (16) (see Chap. 2).

Subsequently, we infused esophageal acid with subjects in the supine position to examine if microaspiration was a factor (17). Thirty nonsmoking adults were divided into two groups: 20 asthmatics with GERD and 10 subjects with GERD. Patients underwent dual probe esophageal pH monitoring during esophageal infusions of normal saline, 0.1 N HCl, and normal saline, each lasting 18 minutes. Since the previous study showed a decrease in peak expiratory flow rate and an increase in respiratory resistance despite esophageal acid clearance in asthmatics with GERD, two 20-minute recovery periods were added to follow airway responses. The subjects remained in a supine position throughout the study. Spirometry and specific airway resistance were measured at baseline, after each esophageal infusion, and with each recovery period. Proximal esophageal acid exposure, a prerequisite for microaspiration, was assessed by the proximal esophageal pH probe. As in our previous study, peak expiratory flow rate decreased with esophageal acid in the asthma with GERD group and did not recover immediately despite esophageal acid clearance (17). The decrease in peak expiratory flow rate was not associated with the presence of proximal esophageal acid exposure. Specific airway resistance also increased in the asthma with GERD group with esophageal acid and continued to increase despite acid clearance, especially during the second recovery phase ($p < 0.009$). The presence of proximal esophageal acid exposure was not associated with deterioration in specific airway resistance. These data show that esophageal acid infusion, given in the supine position, caused a decrease in peak expiratory flow rate and an increase in specific airway resistance, which did not improve despite esophageal acid clearance. These responses were not dependent on proximal esophageal acid exposure (17). Interestingly, specific airway resistance continued to worsen during the recovery phase in the asthma with GERD group, which may represent a prolonged bronchoconstrictor effect. These data suggested that a vagally mediated reflex was important and that microaspiration is not necessary for esophageal acid-induced bronchoconstriction. Also, in this study a positive Bernstein test was not required for the bronchoconstrictor response (17). Additionally, vagolytic doses of intravenous atropine partially ablated the bronchoconstrictor response in our model, further implicating a vagally mediated reflex (18).

To further evaluate the role of the autonomic nervous system in esophageal acid-induced bronchoconstriction, we performed autonomic function testing in 15 asthmatics with GERD, hypothesizing that asthmatics with GERD have exaggerated vagal responsiveness (19). Autonomic function testing included a passive tilt (a 3-minute 80° upward tilt on a motorized table with a comfortable foot rest, followed by 3 minutes of continous monitoring on the return of the horizontal position), a Valsalva maneuver (a sustained forced expiration through a mouthpiece connected to an aneroid manometer set at (30 mmHg lasting 15 seconds, followed by deep inspiration), heart rate variation with quiet and deep breathing (six breaths per minute), hand grip (maximum force for 15 seconds), and an echo-stress test (cortical arousal was induced by listening on earphones to an out-of-phase reproduction of a recording while reading aloud the same paragraph). Simultaneous heart rate and blood pressure readings were collected at set intervals throughout the testing period. The autonomic function test results of the asthmatics with GERD were compared to the responses of 23 age-matched normal control subjects. Results of the autonomic function tests were classified as normal, hypervagal, hyperadrenergic, or mixed (a combination of hypervagal and hyperadrenergic responses). The overall response score was determined by the results of the tilt, Valsalva maneuver, and deep breathing maneuvers. Hypervagal responses on the tilt test and Valsalva maneuver are illustrated in Figure 3. Table 1 displays the autonomic function test results in the asthmatics with GERD. In the tilt test, 60% of asthmatics with GERD had a hypervagal response, 31% had a hypervagal response during the Valsalva maneuver, and 73% of asthmatics with GERD had a hypervagal response during the deep breathing maneuver. Interestingly, each asthmatic with GERD had at least one autonomic function test display a hypervagal response. The overall response score showed that no individual had a normal or hyperadrenergic response score. Fifty-three percent of asthmatics with GERD had a hypervagal response score, and 47% had a mixed response score (19). These data suggest that asthmatics with GERD have heightened vagal responsiveness, which may be partially responsible for the airway responses to esophageal acid.

In conclusion, there appears to be a vagally mediated reflex causing bronchoconstriction when acid is infused into the esophagus, especially in asthmatics with GERD (4–11,16,17). These airway responses may be modest; however, they are present. Esophageal acid–induced bronchoconstriction is present in normal controls in some studies (9,16,17). Also, investigators have shown that the presence of esophagitis augments the bronchoconstrictor response (4,5,6,8,10,11). It appears that microaspiration, as defined by the presence of proximal esophageal acid, is not required for esophageal acid–induced bronchoconstriction (16,17). It is noteworthy that multiple investigators have shown that vagolytic doses of atropine diminish airway responses (8,9,18). Asthmatics with GERD also have evidence of autonomic dysfunction, with many individuals having a hypervagal response (19). Two studies have shown a delayed bronchoconstrictor response after esophageal acid clearance (17,18). This may reflect augmentation of airway inflammation through neurogenic stimulation.

Figure 3 Hypervagal response. Comparison of percent change in heart rate compared with baseline (x axis) and blood pressure (BP) (individual readings at time points) response to tilt test and Valsalva maneuver in control subjects and one study patient showing a hypervagal response. Note the subnormal increase in heart rate during the 80° tilt and inappropriate bradycardia during the recumbent phase. During the Valsalva maneuver, the study subject showed a subnormal increase in heart rate during the release phase and an inappropriate bradycardia during the recovery phase as compared with control subjects. (From Ref. 19.)

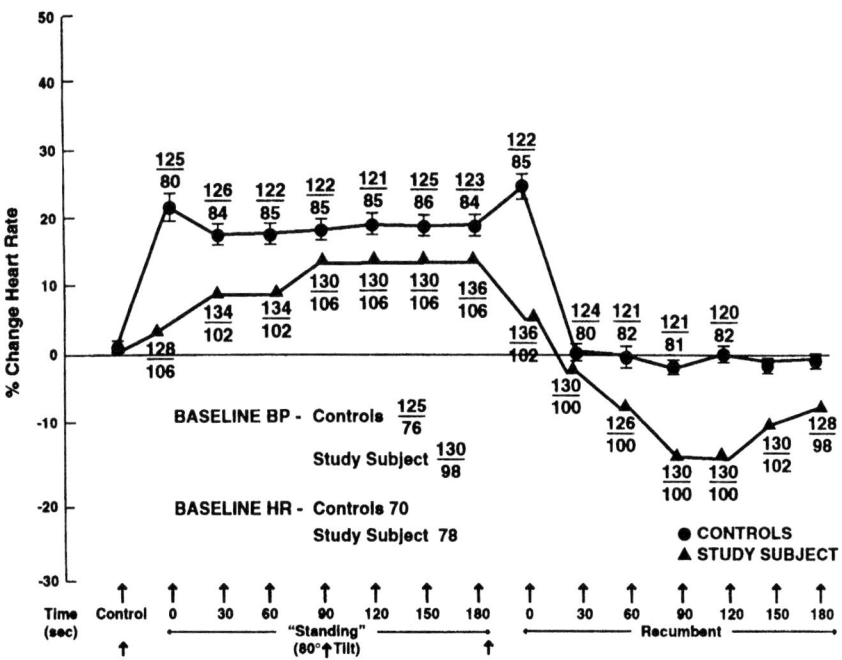

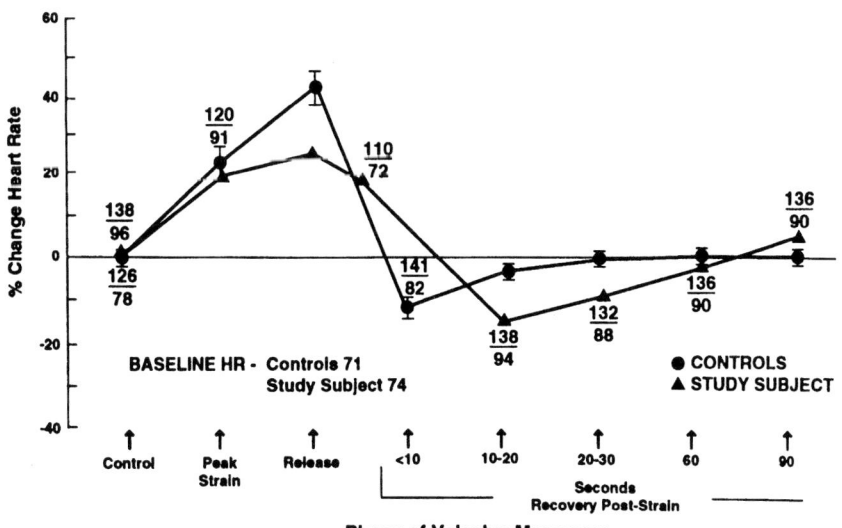

Table 1 Autonomic Function Test Results in 15 Asthmatics with GERD

	Response[a]			
Test	Normal	Hypervagal	Hyperadrenergic	Mixed
Tilt	0 (0%)	9 (60%)	1 (7%)	5 (33%)
Valsalva[b]	2 (15%)	4 (31%)	2 (15%)	5 (39%)
Deep breathing	4 (27%)	11 (73%)	0 (0%)	0 (0%)
Echo stress	12 (80%)	0 (0%)	3 (20%)	0 (0%)
Hand grip	2 (13%)	13 (87%)	0 (0%)	0 (0%)
Overall	0 (0%)	8 (53%)	0 (0%)	7 (47%)

[a]Expressed as number of individuals with each response (percentage of group).
[b]13 of 15 patients were able to hold pressure for 15 seconds.
Source: Ref. 19.

B. Heightened Bronchial Reactivity

Esophageal reflux may also cause neural enhancement of bronchial reactivity. Although the experimental observations discussed in the previous section suggest that, while individual exceptions occur, esophageal acid triggers bronchoconstriction, others have shown a poor temporal correlation between reflux episodes during esophageal pH monitoring and the onset of respiratory symptoms. Sontag et al., using esophageal pH monitoring and respiratory symptom correlation in 48 asthmatics, found that 54% of wheezing episodes had no relationship to reflux episodes (20). It is possible that there is an interactive mechanism between acid in the esophagus and other stimuli that produce bronchoconstriction and that these interactive events are larger than the primary effect of isolated acid infusion on bronchomotor tone. Esophageal reflux may worsen airflow by increasing bronchomotor responsiveness to other stimuli.

To examine this possibility, Herve et al. examined the effect of esophageal acid infusion on the bronchomotor response to two nonspecific stimuli used in bronchial provocation tests: voluntary isocapnic hyperventilation of dry air and methacholine inhalation challenge (21). Twelve adult asthmatics participated irrespective of the presence of GERD and all underwent 12 hours of overnight esophageal pH monitoring. To examine airway hyperresponsiveness, voluntary isocapnic hyperventilation of dry air and methacholine challenge tests were performed after esophageal infusion of isotonic saline and, on another day, esophageal acid. Seven control subjects also participated. Of the 12 asthmatics, seven had GERD defined by esophageal pH monitoring. Esophageal acid did not affect maximum expiratory flows or voluntary isocapnic hyperventilation response of dry air in normal subjects. However, in asthmatics, esophageal acid markedly potentiated the bronchoconstriction induced by voluntary isocapnic hyperventilation compared to normal saline infusion ($p < 0.001$). Similarly, during methacholine challenge, the dose of methacholine that produced a 20% fall in FEV_1 (PD_{20}) significantly decreased with esophageal acid infusion compared with saline ($p < 0.01$), as shown in Figure 4. Comparing the bronchial responses of asthmatics with GERD versus asthmatics without GERD, the asthmatics with GERD had a greater bronchoconstrictive response compared to asthmatics without GERD ($p < 0.01$). Three asthmatics with GERD received atropine pretreatment (2 mg intramuscular), which caused an increase in the baseline maximum expiratory flow at 50% of FVC, but prevented the decrease in maximum expiratory flow at 50% of FVC during esophageal acid infusion (21).

This study showed that esophageal acid, without additional bronchial stimulation, caused slight bronchoconstriction in asthmatics with GERD, but not in normal controls or in asthmatics without GERD. Even more impressive was the fact that esophageal acid altered the underlying bronchial reactivity to other stimuli, even in asthmatics without GERD, in whom acid perfusion alone produced

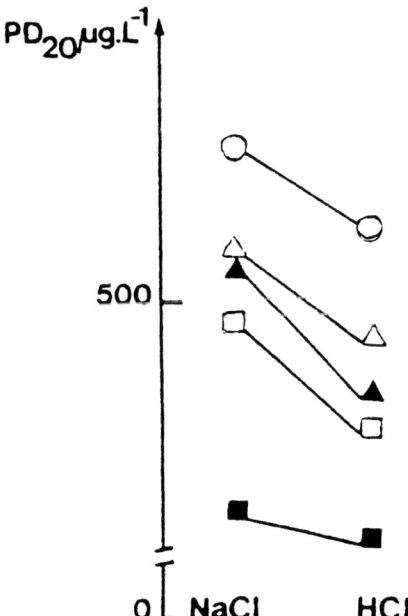

Figure 4 Provocative doses of methacholine causing a 20% decrease in FEV_1 (PD_{20}) in five asthmatics during esophageal NaCl and HCl infusion (open and closed symbols for, respectively, patients without and with GERD). The change in PD_{20} is shown for each subject. (From Ref. 21.)

no bronchoconstriction. Vagal pathways are also important since the bronchial response to esophageal acid was abolished with atropine pretreatment (21). This study supports the hypothesis that esophageal acid stimulates esophageal acid–sensitive receptors and probably interacts with cholinergic airway tone at a central nervous system level through a vagally mediated reflex.

To further support the bronchial hyperresponsiveness model, it would be optimal to show that antireflux treatment decreases airway hyperresponsiveness in provocation tests. To date, there are no studies that show that antireflux therapy decreases bronchial responsiveness. In a study performed by Teichtahl et al. omeprazole 40 mg a day for 4 weeks did not change histamine bronchial responsiveness (22). Since 17 of 20 subjects had esophagitis documented by upper endoscopy, 4 weeks of antireflux therapy might not have been adequate to heal esophagitis. The subjects did not have repeat endoscopy to document if healing of esophagitis occurred. Also, once-daily dosing of omeprazole does not suppress esophageal acid production throughout the 24-hour period, so that the therapeutic trial may not have been adequate to document a decrease in bronchial hyperreactivity (23).

The data do suggest that esophageal acid augments airway hyperreactivity in asthmatics. Asthma is a heterogeneous disease exacerbated by multiple triggers, so that when an asthmatic with GERD is exposed to an allergic trigger, such as cat dander, or a nonallergic trigger, such as cigarette smoke, they may have an exaggerated bronchoconstrictive response.

C. Microaspiration

Microaspiration of esophageal contents into the upper airway is the third mechanism of esophageal acid–induced bronchoconstriction. Microaspiration of refluxed material needs to be distinguished from macroaspiration or "flooding" of the tracheobronchial tree, which leads to clinical entities such as pneumonia, pneumonitis, lung abscess, and bronchiectasis (24,25). In the microaspiration model, gastric material refluxes to the proximal esophagus, then into the hypopharynx and possibly into the larynx and trachea. Microaspiration directly irritates the airways and causes reflex bronchoconstriction. It is well established that mechanical stimulation of the upper airway or installation of saline into the trachea causes an increase in resistance (26,27).

To examine the effect of microaspiration on airway responses, Tuchman et al. developed an animal model comparing airway responses of esophageal acid (reflex mechanism) versus tracheal acid (microaspiration mechanism) in cats (28). In a series of experiments, they showed that microaspiration of acid into the trachea causes more airway responses than esophageal acid reflux. Their experimental preparation used anesthetized adult cats breathing spontaneously through an airway cannula in the trachea. Pulmonary mechanics including pulmonary airflow, total lung resistance, and dynamic compliance were measured. A pleural catheter measured pleural pressure. Esophageal manometry located the LES and the UES, and an esophageal pH probe was placed in the upper esophagus to monitor for proximal esophageal reflux. Measurements of airway mechanics were determined before, during, and after either 0.9% saline or 0.2 N HCl infusion into the trachea or esophagus in 13 animals. To determine the mechanism of the observed response to tracheal acid, bilateral cervical vagotomy was done. To determine if the presence of esophagitis augmented airway responses after esophageal acid, 0.2 N HCl was infused into the midesophagus over a 30-minute period for 2–3 days before the study, with esophagitis documented by biopsies (28).

Figure 5 shows the lung mechanics after esophageal acid infusion of 10 ml of 0.2 N HCl over a 20-second period. In most animals, no gross change in respiratory pattern was evident from viewing the raw tracings (28). Further analysis shows that there was a 1.42-fold increase in total lung resistance compared to baseline after esophageal acid ($p < 0.05$) (28) A significant increase in total lung resistance occurred in only 60% of the animals tested. The presence of esophagitis did not enhance the airway response to esophageal acid.

In contrast, tracheal acidification with 0.05 ml of 0.2 N HCl resulted in significant alterations in lung mechanics, which was observed in all animals. Figure 6 shows that with tracheal acidification, there is interruption of tracheal airflow with large pleural pressure changes and a decrease in tidal volume. There

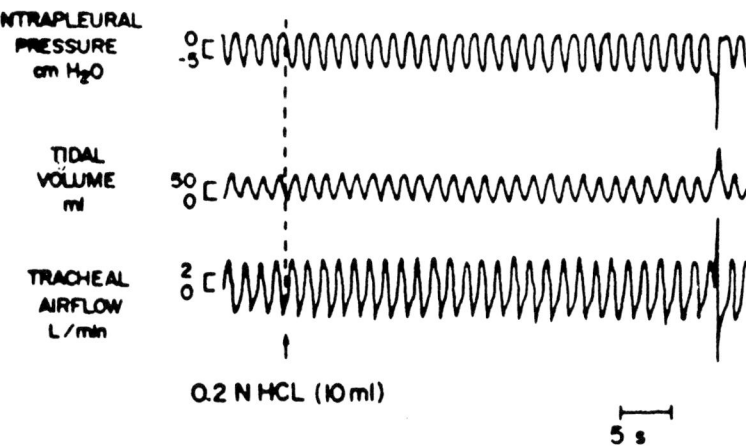

Figure 5 Lung mechanics after esophageal acid infusion. Baseline measurements are to the left of the dotted line. Ten milliliters of 0.2 N HCl into the esophagus caused minimal increase in pleural pressure and tracheal airflow. (From Ref. 28.)

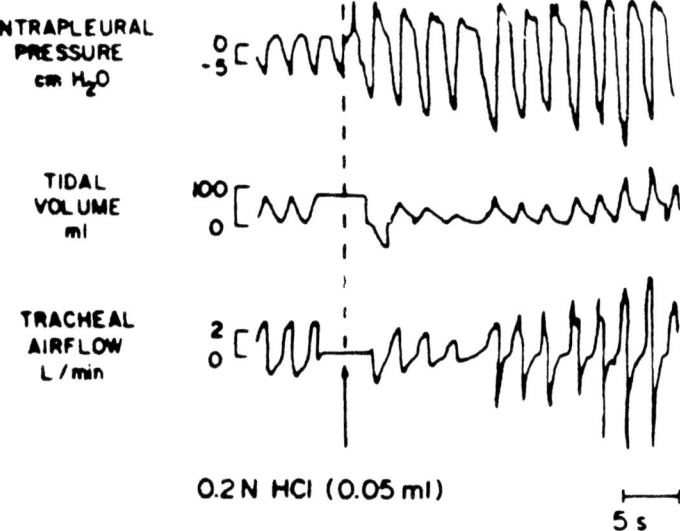

Figure 6 Lung mechanics after intratracheal acid infusion. Baseline measurements are to the left of the dotted line. Immediately after tracheal acidification of 0.05 ml of 0.2 N HCl, there is an increase in intrapleural pressure and a decrease in tidal volume and airflow. (From Ref. 28.)

was a 4.65-fold increase in total lung resistance compared to baseline ($p < 0.005$), as shown in Figure 7. Also, the bronchial response to tracheal acidification was concentration dependent, with 0.001 N HCl causing no significant change in resistance versus a 3-fold increase in resistance with 0.1 N HCl and a 4.65-fold increase with 0.2 N HCl (28).

The vagus nerve also plays a role in the microaspiration model. The increase in total lung resistance associated with tracheal acidification was abolished with bilateral cervical vagotomy, as shown in Figure 7 (28). No alteration in breathing pattern was noted after tracheal acidification in vagotomized animals (28). Scintigraphy of the chest in cats after tracheal instillation of 0.05 ml of technicium labeled 99m-sulfur colloid showed that the instilled liquid remained in the trachea and did not spread into the major bronchi or lung parenchyma (28).

It is much more difficult to monitor airway responses in humans with tracheal acidification or to monitor for microaspiration. Three methods have been used to demonstrate microaspiration of gastric contents into the lungs of humans: (a) inspection of sputum or bronchoalveolar lavage for lipid-laden alveolar macrophages, (b) radioactive labels, and (c) pH monitoring in the upper esophagus or trachea.

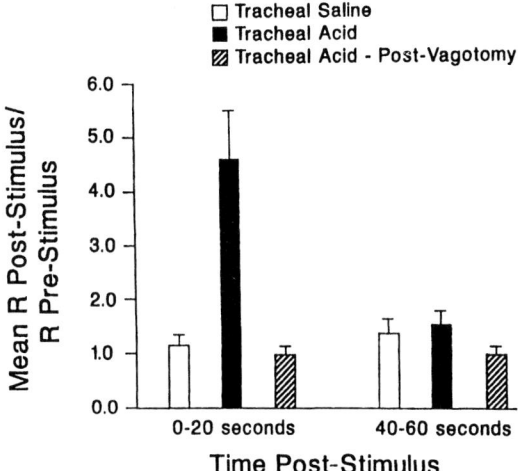

Figure 7 Total lung resistance after intratracheal infusion of 0.05 ml of 0.9% NaCl, 0.2 N HCl prevagotomy, and 0.2 N HCl postvagotomy. Intratracheal acid produced a highly significant increase in the resistance ratio compared to saline. The effect of intratracheal acid was abolished by bilateral cervical vagotomy. (From Ref. 28.)

Lipid-laden alveolar macrophages were evaluated in adults as a marker of aspiration by examining lower respiratory secretions obtained by bronchoalveolar lavage and stained for Oil-Red-O (29). Corwin and Irwin found that low numbers of intracellular Oil-Red-O–stained alveolar macrophages may be helpful in excluding aspiration as a cause of lung disease (29). Normal controls also had lipid-laden alveolar macrophages. Unfortunately, the finding of lipid-laden macrophages in children and adults has a very low specificity, making the test clinically impractical and difficult to correlate with bronchoconstriction (29,30).

Another method used to assess for microaspiration is scintigraphic monitoring using technetium 99 isotope-sulfur colloid. A radiolabeled meal or liquid is ingested and the subjects are later scanned. Increased uptake over the lungs is evidence for aspiration (31–34). In most studies, subjects went to sleep after eating (31–34). While many asthmatics had positive scans, only approximately 25–31% of those tested showed evidence of aspiration (30–35). One study showed evidence of aspiration in 38% of control subjects (35). Since the subjects were given the test meal prior to lying in the supine position and sleeping, they were predisposed to develop reflux and aspiration. Esophageal pH was monitored concurrently in five subjects with no respiratory symptoms. Two of the five subjects had abnormal scintiscans and prolonged episodes of esophageal acid (34). Despite reports of its usefulness in documenting aspiration, it has many limitations. The small amount of microaspiration required to cause bronchospasm may escape detection with currently employed scanning methods. Aspiration may be undetected if mucociliary action of the bronchial epithelium clears the technetium. Aspiration may occur only intermittently so that multiple scans are required to increase the test's sensitivity. There is also high background radioactivity in the abdomen, which may make the test difficult to interpret. In conclusion, scintigraphic monitoring is not very useful in assessing mechanisms of GERD-associated bronchoconstriction.

Monitoring pH in the proximal esophagus and upper airway allows correlation of acid events with respiratory symptoms and alterations in airway function. Most investigators used dual pH probes with the distal sensor in the esophagus 5 cm above the LES and the proximal probe near the UES in the upper esophagus. Pharyngeal probes above the UES have been unreliable because of drying artifact of the probe (34).

To evaluate the frequency of proximal esophageal reflux, a marker for microaspiration, Gastal et al. evaluated asthmatics referred to an esophageal laboratory for the possibility of GERD (37). Although, 44% of asthmatics had abnormal esophageal acid contact times in the distal esophagus, abnormal amounts of esophageal acid in the proximal probe was found in only 24% of asthmatics. They concluded that microaspiration was not as important as reflux-mediated bronchospasm (37). They did not monitor airway responses during the evaluation period.

Varkey et al. evaluated 19 consecutive asthmatics and 7 normal controls with dual esophageal pH monitoring (5 cm above the LES and 5 cm below the UES) and a probe in the pharynx 2 cm above the UES (38). Patients with moderate or severe asthma had 31% of reflux episodes associated with a full in pH at the proximal esophagus and 5% of episodes associated with acid in the pharyngeal probe, documenting that microaspiration does exist and is more prevalent in asthmatics than in normal controls (38). The investigators did not monitor airflow with reflux events.

The best human data that show the significance of microaspiration in acid-induced bronchoconstriction were reported by Donnelly et al., with follow-up data reported by Jack et al. from Liverpool (39,40). They monitored simultaneous tracheal and esophageal pH in asthmatics and measured airway responses with peak expiratory flow rates. The tracheal pH probe was placed by introducing the probe through a 13 or 14 French cannula, which was placed through the skin and the cricothyroid membrane under anesthesia. The tracheal pH probe was positioned under bronchoscopic guidance 2 cm above the carina. The cannula was removed and the probe taped to the patients' neck. The esophageal pH probe was placed 5 cm above the LES. Four patients with GERD underwent simultaneous pH monitoring and recorded peak expiratory flow rates hourly during 24 hours. Thirty-seven episodes of gastroesophageal reflux at the esophageal probe were recorded lasting more than 5 minutes. Of these, five esophageal events were closely followed by a fall in tracheal pH from a mean of 7.1 to 4.1. Figure 8 displays one such episode. When esophageal acid events occurred without a fall in tracheal pH, peak expiratory flow rates dropped an average of 8 liters per minute. When esophageal acid events were followed by a fall in tracheal pH, peak expiratory flow rates decreased 84 liters per minute (40). Unlike esophageal acid events without evidence of microaspiration, tracheal microaspiration of acid caused significant acute changes in lung function in asthmatics with GERD. This study shows that microaspiration, if present, significantly augments airway responses and plays a key role in the pathophysiology of acid-associated bronchoconstriction.

D. Conclusions on the Pathophysiology of Esophageal Acid–Induced Bronchoconstriction

Data suggest that all three mechanisms play a role in esophageal acid–induced bronchoconstriction. Animal and human studies show that there is evidence of bronchoconstriction with esophageal acid in the distal esophagus (4,11,16,17).

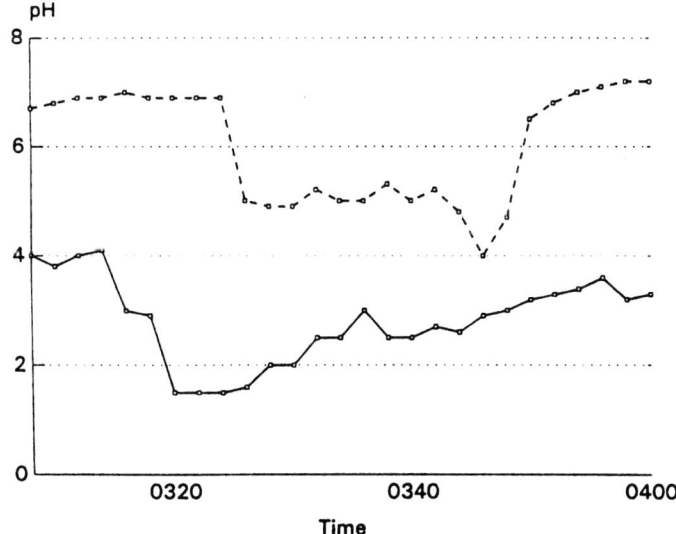

Figure 8 Segment from tracheal pH (broken line) and esophageal pH (solid line) showing an esophageal acid event followed by a prolonged drop in tracheal pH. The subject was awake and wheezing during this time and required an inhaled bronchodilator. (From Ref. 39.)

The bronchoconstriction elicited is somewhat modest, but present. There is debate as to whether this vagally mediated reflex is present in all individuals or primarily in asthmatics with GERD. Studies performed by Wright et al. and a series of studies performed by our laboratory show that even normal controls have evidence of bronchoconstriction with esophageal acid (9,16,17). The magnitude of airway change is a decrement of approximately 10 liters per minute in peak expiratory flow rate (16,17). Numerous studies have shown that airway resistance increases with esophageal acid (5–8,16,17). Most studies did not rule out the possibility of microaspiration as the cause for the airway responses. However, our laboratory, performing dual probe esophageal pH monitoring, found that proximal esophageal acid, a prerequisite of microaspiration, was not necessary to elicit bronchoconstriction (16,17).

Some investigators, however, did not find evidence of bronchoconstriction with esophageal acid (12–14). Tan et al.'s study was well done, but it failed to reveal evidence of acid-induced bronchoconstriction with spontaneous esophageal acid or esophageal acid infusion (14).

Further proof that a vagally mediated reflex is active was shown by Mansfield et al. in a dog model where bilateral vagotomy obliterated the airway responses to esophageal acid (4). Multiple investigators used atropine either intravenously or intramuscularly and showed that airway responses with esophageal acid were ablated or at least partially decreased with esophageal acid (8,9,18).

There is also conflict in the literature as to whether distal esophagitis is required to elicit airway responses. The requirement of distal esophagitis could paritally explain Tan et al.'s and Wesseling et al.'s failure to elicit airway responses with esophageal acid (13,14). Other investigators have shown, however, that distal esophagitis, as defined by a positive Bernstein test, was not required to elicit airway responses (9,16,17). Further investigation needs to be performed to clarify this. In at least two studies, there is evidence of a prolonged increase in airway resistance, despite esophageal acid clearance (16,17). This may reflect neurogenically mediated inflammation and mediator release. Currently, there are no studies evaluating molecular mechanisms of airway inflammation in esophageal acid–induced bronchoconstriction.

The second mechanism, heightened bronchial reactivity, is a subset of the vagally mediated reflex mechanism. Esophageal acid does cause an increase in airway bronchial reactivity as tested by methacholine challenge testing and voluntary isocapnic hyperventilation (21). Atropine also inhibits this heightened bronchial reactivity, so the vagus nerve also plays a role in this model (21).

Animal and human studies show that microaspiration causes significant alterations in pulmonary mechanics (28,40). The magnitude of airway responses to acid placed directly into the trachea is fivefold over baseline versus 1.5-fold with esophageal acidification in an animal model (28). In human studies, tracheal acidification caused a tenfold worsening in airflow, with peak expiratory flow rate decreasing 85 liters per minute versus an 8 liter per minute decrease with distal esophageal acid. (40).

Figure 9 shows that there is a vagally mediated response with distal esophageal acid causing bronchoconstriction through the vagus afferents projecting into the central nervous system, and the efferent limb mediating bronchoconstriction

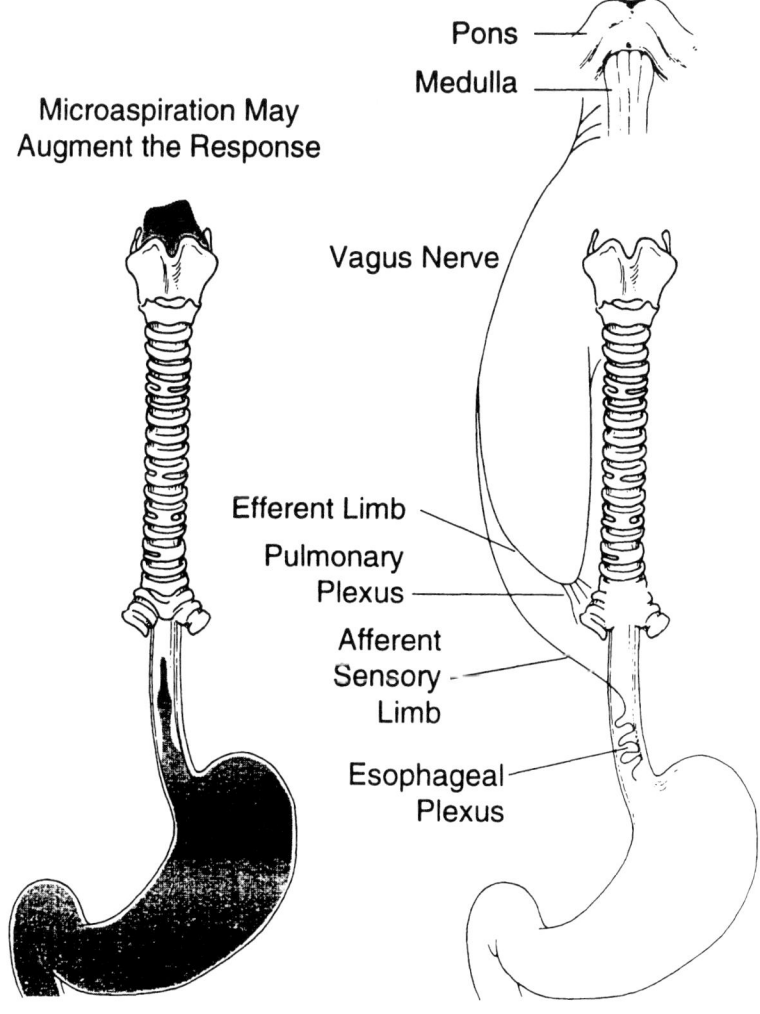

Figure 9 Esophageal acid induced bronchoconstriction where distal esophageal acid stimulates the afferent sensory limb of the vagus nerve, resulting in reflex-induced bronchoconstriction. Microaspiration augments the bronchoconstrictive response.

through cholinergic mechanisms. If microaspiration is present, there is augmentation of the bronchoconstrictive response.

There is evidence that the vagus nerve plays a prominent role in all three mechanisms. Even in the microaspiration model, bilateral vagotomy ablated the response to tracheal acidification (28). In the tracheobronchial tree, there are C fiber endings, which could mediate bronchoconstriction, and slowly adapting stretch receptors, which could also cause bronchoconstriction (2). Figure 10 shows how all three mechanisms interact through the vagus nerve leading to airway inflammation.

II. Factors That Could Promote GERD in Asthmatics

The incidence and severity of GERD in asthmatics is higher than in the normal population. In a GERD questionnaire sent to 109 asthmatics and 135 subjects in two control groups, Field et al. noted that 77% of the asthmatics experienced heartburn, 55% had regurgitation, and 24% had dysphagia versus 54, 41, and 11%, respectively, of patients from a family practice population (41). Likewise, the prevalence of abnormal esophageal acid contact times is higher in asthmatics than in normal controls. Sontag et al. evaluated 104 consecutive asthmatics and 44 normal controls with esophageal manometry and pH monitoring and found abnormal amounts of acid reflux in 82% of asthmatics (42). In addition, asthmatics, compared to controls, had decreased LES pressures, more frequent reflux episodes, and higher esophageal acid contact times (42).

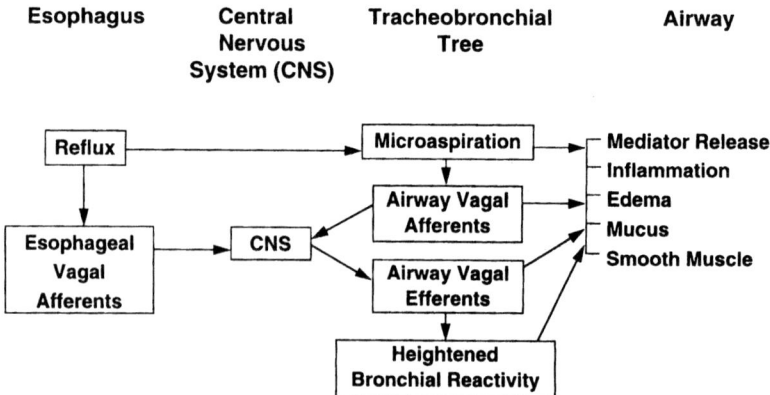

Figure 10 Esophageal acid–induced bronchoconstriction, showing the role of the vagus nerve, heightened bronchial reactivity, and microaspiration resulting in airway inflammation. (From Ref. 42a.)

There are a number of physiologic parameters that may contribute to the development of GERD. Gastric factors include delayed gastric emptying and gastric distention placing greater stress on the antireflux barrier (43). The lower esophageal sphincter (LES) plays a key role in the antireflux barrier (44). Intrinsic muscles in the high-pressure zone of the distal esophagus and the crural diaphragm contribute to LES pressure generation (44). Transient LES relaxation and a low resting LES pressure predisposes to the development of reflux (44). Another factor that contributes to GERD is the length of the esophagus, which is in the abdominal cavity. DeMeester et al. noted that the amount of esophageal acid inversely correlated with the length of the esophagus below the diaphragm (45). A hiatal hernia may also impair esophageal acid emptying (44,46).

Factors that predispose asthmatics to develop GERD include the possibility of autonomic dysfunction, since a substantial component of esophageal neurogenic tone in humans is from cholinergic innervation from the vagus nerve (44). Also, with bronchospasm there is an increase in the pressure gradient between the thorax (esophagus) and abdominal cavity (stomach) promoting reflux (47). Another factor is that asthmatics may have a higher prevalence of hiatal hernia than normal controls (48). Overinflation of the diaphragm may decrease the LES pressure because of the inability of the crural diaphragm to contribute to LES pressure generation. Also, bronchodilators, including theophylline and β_2-adrenergic agonists, may promote reflux (Table 2).

A. Autonomic Regulation

Lower esophageal sphincter tone, including relaxation of the sphincter, is mediated through the dorsal nucleus of the vagus nerve (44). Asthmatics have evidence of widespread cholinergic hyperresponsiveness. Asthmatics have increased eccrine sweat production after intradermal stimulation by methacholine (49). Also, asthmatics have increased pupillary cholinergic responsiveness compared to normal controls (50). Kallenback et al. showed evidence of enhanced parasympathetic neural drive to the sinoatrial node in asthmatics, as manifested by a greater

Table 2 Predisposing Factors in Asthmatics That Could Predispose to the Development of GERD

1. Autonomic dysregulation
2. Increased pressure differential between the thorax and the abdomen
3. High incidence of hiatal hernia
4. Crural diaphragm alterations
5. Bronchodilators may decrease LES pressure and increase gastric acid secretion (theophylline and oral β_2-adrenergic agonists)

magnitude of respiratory sinus arrhythmia induced by deep breathing, than in normal controls (51). Our laboratory performed autonomic function tests on 15 asthmatics with GERD, and there was evidence of autonomic dysfunction (19). In 73 autonomic function tests performed, a normal response was found in 20 (27%), a hypervagal response in 37 (51%), a hyperadrenergic response in 6 (8%), and a mixed response in 10 (14%) (Table 1) (19). These data suggest that there may be heightened vagal responsiveness in asthmatics with GERD. Autonomic dysregulation could result in decreased LES pressure and transient relaxation of the LES, the principal mechanisms of reflux (44). Further research into autonomic regulation needs to be performed before further conclusions can be reached.

B. Pressure Differential Between the Thorax and the Abdomen

At the end of expiration, the pressure gradient between the stomach (abdominal cavity) and esophagus (thorax) is 4–6 mmHg. Therefore, a normal LES pressure of 10–35 mmHg at end-expiration is sufficient to counteract this pressure gradient (44). Contraction of inspiratory muscles causes more negative pleural pressures (esophageal), and contraction of abdominal muscles causes increases in gastric pressure, thus increasing the pressure gradient, favoring gastroesophageal reflux (44). With an acute asthma exacerbation, there are wide pressure swings with a much more negative intrathoracic pressure with inspiration and a more positive abdominal pressure, exaggerating the pressure gradient (47). Also, this effect is coupled with active expiratory efforts generated primarily by contraction of the abdominal muscles, resulting in higher gastric pressures. Coughing is also associated with contraction of the abdominal muscles increasing abdominal pressure and promoting GERD (52).

Moote et al. showed that methacholine-induced airflow obstruction was associated with longer periods of reflux than during baseline studies (53). However, Ekström and Tibbling could not reproduce these data using histamine-induced bronchoconstriction in 10 asthmatics with GERD (54).

Another clinical entity associated with large pleural (esophageal) pressure changes is obstructive sleep apnea. During an apneic event, there is upper airway collapse with upper airway obstruction with increased respiratory efforts (55). There is increased work of breathing shown by increased intercostal EMG activity and increased esophageal pressure. Kerr et al. noted that reflux events were prominent during apneic events (56). Nasal continuous positive airway pressure (CPAP) decreased the frequency of GERD (56). Although the exact mechanism is not known, CPAP raises thoracic (pleural) pressure and probably esophageal pressure. Also, treatment of obstructive sleep apnea with CPAP decreased the wide pleural pressure swings. Kerr et al. also showed that nasal CPAP decreased esophageal acid events in patients with GERD without obstructive sleep apnea (57).

A small randomized double-blind crossover study was performed on five nocturnal asthmatics with GERD. Singh et al. observed daily asthma and gastric symptoms on and off ephedrine 15 mg for one week (58). Asthma treatment reduced asthma symptoms from six to one days per week, with a reduction of gastric symptoms from 4.8 to 1.6 days per week (58). Although definitive conclusions cannot be made, reflux may have improved because of the reduction in the abdominal-thoracic pressure gradient.

C. Asthmatics Have a High Incidence of Hiatal Hernia

Although reflux occurs without the presence of a hiatal hernia, many GERD patients have a hiatal hernia, which can serve as a reservoir for gastric contents (59). Mittal et al. observed that transient relaxation of the LES is more likely to be followed by an episode of reflux if there is a hiatal hernia with retained acid than in the absence of a hiatal hernia (60). Asthmatics may have a higher incidence of hiatal hernia. Mays examined 28 asthmatics with severe asthma with upper gastrointestinal (UGI) series and compared them with a control group of 468 subjects that had a UGI series to establish the baseline incidence of hiatal hernia (48). Eighteen (64%) of the asthmatics had a hiatal hernia compared to 92 (19%) of normal control subjects ($p < 0.001$) (48). In a more recent study, Sontag et al. performed endoscopy on 186 consecutive, unselected asthmatics (61). A hiatal hernia was present during endoscopy if gastric folds were seen extending at least 2 cm above the diaphragmatic hiatus during quiet respirations (61). Fifty-eight percent of asthmatics had a hiatal hernia (61).

D. The Role of the Diaphragmatic Crura in LES Pressure Formation

The sphincter mechanisms at the boundary between the esophagus and stomach protect against acid reflux and consists of smooth muscle of the distal esophagus forming the LES and the skeletal muscle of the crural diaphragm (Fig. 11) (44). The crural part of the diaphragm originates embryologically from the esophageal mesentary, unlike the costal part of the diaphragm, which originates from the pleuroperitoneal membrane (62). The crural part of the diaphragm, especially the right crus, forms the esophageal hiatus (63). Multiple investigators have shown that transient relaxation of the LES and the crural diaphragm are responsible for GERD. There is relaxation of the LES associated with an inhibition of the diaphragmatic EMG associated with an increase in esophageal pressure leading to a reflux episode (64,65). Transient relaxation of the LES may last as long as 60 seconds (64,65). Transient relaxation of the LES is mediated through the brainstem, with the efferent pathway being the vagus nerve (44).

Asthmatics may have alterations of their crural diaphragm. Hyperinflation associated with bronchospasm places the diaphragm at a functional disadvantage

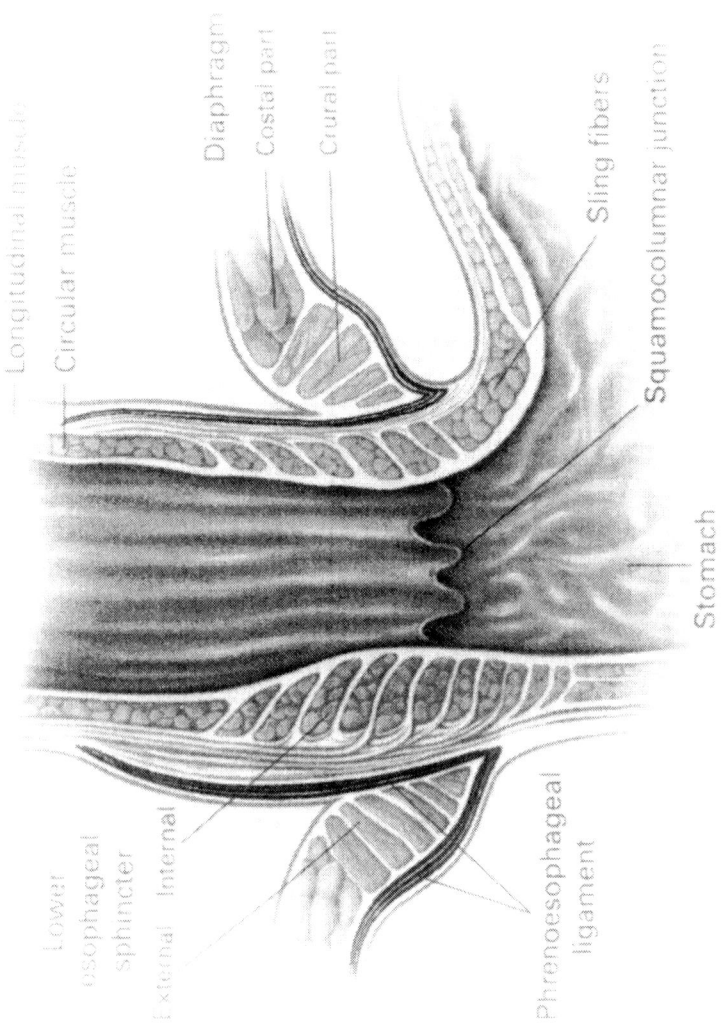

Figure 11 Anatomy of the esophagogastric junction. The lower esophageal sphincter and the crural diaphragm constitute the intrinsic and extrinsic sphincters. The two sphincters are anatomically superimposed and are anchored to each other by the phrenoesophageal ligament. (From Ref. 44.)

because of geometric flattening (66). Flattening and stretching of the diaphragmatic crura may occur with chronic hyperinflation and air trapping.

E. Bronchodilator Medications May Alter GERD

There are data showing that bronchodilators may worsen GERD; however, there is debate about the clinical importance of this. Theophylline and oral β_2-adrenergic agonists have significant effects on LES pressure.

Theophylline Effects on GERD

Theophylline is a methylxanthine that alters gastric acid secretion and LES pressure. Foster et al. evaluated gastric acid secretion and gastrin release in nine patients with chronic obstructive pulmonary disease (67). Patients received intravenous aminophylline 6 mg/kg over a 20-minute period. Intravenous aminophylline caused a significant increase in gastric acid secretion from 0.66 to 2.19 mEq/min ($p < 0.01$) (67). Oral aminophylline (400 mg) also caused a significant increase in gastric acid secretion from 2.43 to 4.06 mEq/min ($p < 0.05$) (67). The effect of theophylline on acid secretion was also shown by Johannesson et al. (68). Theophylline 5.0 mg/kg given intravenously by an infusion pump over 20 minutes resulted in serum theophylline levels of 10.0 mg/liter and an increase in gastric acid secretion and gastric volume compared to placebo in healthy male volunteers ($p < 0.01$). There was no effect of theophylline on serum gastrin (68). Stein et al. monitored the effect of theophylline on LES pressure in four normal controls and six asthmatics with GERD (69). Intravenous theophylline 6.6 mg/kg was given over 10 minutes (69). Theophylline levels were monitored at 30, 60, and 90 minutes after the start of the aminophylline infusion with all subjects maintaining therapeutic theophylline levels (10–20 mg/liter 60 minutes after the start of the infusion. Lower esophageal sphincter pressures were measured at baseline and at 60 minutes after the start of the aminophylline infusion. Figure 12 shows individual responses of the LES pressure in asthmatics with GERD given theophylline. All but one subject had a decrease in mean LES pressure ($p < 0.02$) (69).

Berquist et al. evaluated the effect of a single oral 10 mg/kg dose of theophylline versus placebo in 24 normal subjects and monitored LES pressure and esophageal pH while instilling 150 ml 0.1 N HCl into their stomachs (70). Four hours after theophylline dosing, there was a mean 25% decrease in LES pressure. Forty-seven percent of the theophylline-treated individuals complained of heartburn versus 11% of the placebo group. This shows that theophylline decreases LES pressure and increases the incidence of a positive acid reflux test and symptoms of heartburn compared with adults given placebo (70).

Further studies evaluating the impact of theophylline on reflux in asthmatics with GERD were performed by Ekström et al. (71). They evaluated 25 adult

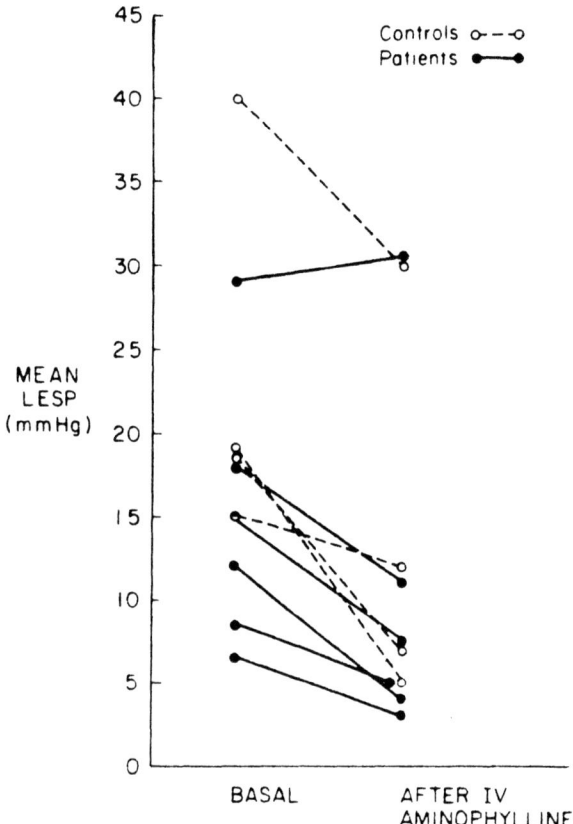

Figure 12 Mean lower esophageal sphincter pressure (LESP) at baseline and at 60 minutes after the start of a 20-minute intravenous aminophylline infusion in four normal controls and six asthmatics with GERD symptoms. Intravenous aminophylline caused a significant drop in LESP. (From Ref. 69.)

asthmatics with moderate-to-severe asthma and a history of GERD in a single-blind placebo-controlled trial. Patients underwent two consecutive esophageal pH tests, one with and one without their ordinary dose of slow-release theophylline. Patients also recorded respiratory and GERD symptoms. Peak expiratory flow rate and FEV_1 were recorded. Daytime reflux increased by 24% on theophylline. Symptoms of heartburn and regurgitation increased by 170%, while respiratory symptoms and pulmonary function studies improved on the day in which theophylline was given. The increase in GERD during theophylline treatment was more pronounced in patients with a therapeutic serum theophylline level (71).

There are, however, conflicting results. Hubert et al. performed a double-blind crossover study in 16 asthmatics, not selected for GERD, who were given a week of slow-release theophylline or placebo (72). Patients monitored peak expiratory flow rate three times daily, with spirometry weekly and theophylline levels at 2 and 7 hours after p.m. dosing. Esophageal pH testing was performed at the end of therapy with either theophylline or placebo. FEV_1 and FVC improved during the theophylline period versus placebo. Similarly, there was no significant difference in the number of reflux episodes, total duration of reflux, number of reflux episodes lasting more than 5 minutes, or the percent of time the pH was less than 4 (72). They concluded that conventional treatment with slow-release theophylline did not significantly increase GERD. Two letters to the editor questioned their results (73,74). Mansfield questioned the statistical analysis performed (74). However, statistical analysis using Wilcoxon signed-rank test failed to reveal a significant change in reflux parameters with placebo versus theophylline (74). Stein pointed out that the study population used by Hubert et al. were asthmatics who may not have had GERD (73).

In conclusion, theophylline increases gastric acid secretion and decreases LES pressure. This makes asthmatics more prone to develop GERD. Investigators have found that higher levels of theophylline resulted in higher esophageal acid contact times. There are conflicting data in the literature. Most placebo-controlled trials were done on small patient populations. Some populations were not pure and included asthmatics with or without GERD. Since theophylline could worsen GERD, it should be used cautiously, especially at high doses.

Effects of β_2-Adrenergic Agonists on GERD

Foster et al. examined basal gastric acid secretion in nine patients with chronic obstructive pulmonary disease after using inhaled epinephrine hydrochloride, isoproterenol hydrochloride, and metaproterenol sulfate, finding that the agents did not cause significant changes in basal gastric acid output (67). They concluded that β_2-adrenergic agonist therapy, in general, does not significantly alter gastric acid secretion (67). Interestingly, Christensen found that there was relaxation of the LES with β_2-adrenergic agonists (75). However, adrenergic agents used in asthma did not significantly effect esophageal motility (75). DiMarino et al. found that oral or intravenous β_2-adrenergic agonists decreased LES pressure (76). However, since most β_2-adrenergic agonists are given by the inhaled route, these findings may not be clinically relevant in most patients (76).

Other investigators have shown that inhaled β_2-adrenergic agonists caused no significant change in GERD parameters or esophageal motility. Schindlbeck et al. examined the effect of albuterol 1.25 mg per nebulizer on 24-hour esophageal pH testing and esophageal manometry in 10 healthy volunteers in a double-blind placebo-controlled trial (77). LES pressure, esophageal peristaltic amplitudes, and esophageal acid contact times were unchanged during placebo treatment versus nebulized albuterol (77). They concluded that inhaled albuterol does not significantly alter reflux parameters (77). Michoud et al. studied the effect of an oral β_2-adrenergic agonist, salbutamol, on GERD in 10 healthy volunteers and 8 asthmatics (78). Patients were given salbutamol 4 mg or placebo with the order of administration randomized in a double-blinded fashion. There was no significant difference in LES pressure, peak esophageal contraction pressure, number or duration of reflux episodes between asthmatics and normal controls on placebo versus oral salbutamol (78). Although multiple studies have shown no significant alteration in GERD with inhaled β_2-adrenergic agonists, Bittinger et al. studied seven patients with chronic obstructive pulmonary disease and noted higher total reflux times after inhalation of 400 mg of fenoterol (79). Although this was a small study, they concluded that obstructive pulmonary disease should be treated with the lowest possible doses of inhaled β_2-adrenergic agonists (79).

It appears that the β_2-adrenergic agonists have less effect on esophageal function than theophylline. Ruzkowski et al. studied nine male patients with chronic obstructive pulmonary disease and GERD with nebulized albuterol 0.5 mg four times a day versus theophylline and monitored 24-hour esophageal pH testing and pulmonary function (80). Pulmonary function results were similar with the two treatments. Theophylline caused higher esophageal acid contact times than albuterol. Patients on albuterol also had fewer reflux episodes lasting longer than 5 minutes than while on theophylline (80).

Inhaled β_2-adrenergic agonists are important therapeutic agents for the treatment of asthma, especially during an acute exacerbation. Most studies show that inhaled β_2-adrenergic agonists do not cause significant alterations in esophageal manonmetry, LES pressure, gastric acid secretion, or esophageal acid contact times. There is some controversy concerning whether inhaled β_2-adrenergic agonists can predispose patients to develop GERD.

Studies Evaluating Multiple Bronchodilators

Sontag et al. examined the frequency of esophagitis in 186 consecutive asthmatics on versus off bronchodilators (61). One hundred and forty asthmatics underwent endoscopy while taking their usually prescribed bronchodilators, including theophylline, terbutaline, inhalers, and prednisone, and 46 were studied without bronchodilators. Thirty-eight percent of asthmatics had esophagitis on bronchodilators versus 39% of asthmatics not on bronchodilators (p = nonsignificant) (61). Although the study did not analyze the effects of individual medications, their results show that asthmatics on chronic bronchodilator therapy have the same prevalence of esophagitis compared to asthmatics not on bronchodilators (61). They concluded that bronchodilators did not adversely affect the esophageal mucosa (61).

Sontag et al. also evaluated 104 consecutive asthmatics with esophageal manometry and 24-hour esophageal pH testing (42). Seventy-four asthmatics were studied while taking their usual bronchodilators, including theophylline, oral terbutaline, inhalants (adrenergic, anticholinergic, corticosteroid) and prednisone, while others were not on routine bronchodilators (42). There was no significant difference in LES pressure (13.0 ± 1.0 on medications vs. 12.6 ± 1.8 off medications), percent time where distal esophageal pH < 4 (10.8 ± 1.2 on medications vs. 12.9 ± 2.6 off medications), or number of episodes where pH < 4 (3.4 ± 0.3 on medications vs. 3.7 ± 0.5 off medications) (42). Chronic bronchodilator therapy did not adversely affect LES pressure or esophageal acid contact time (42).

Field et al. examined GERD symptoms in 109 consecutive asthmatics (41). Ninety-three percent of asthmatics used β_2-adrenergic agonists, 84% used inhaled corticosteroids, and approximately 33% used oral corticosteroids or theophylline (41). None of the asthma medications were associated with an increased likelihood of having heartburn or regurgitation (41).

Although these studies show that patients on bronchodilators have no increase in GERD symptoms, esophagitis or esophageal acid contact times compared to asthmatics not on routine bronchodilators, they cannot conclude that bronchodilators do not influence an individual patient's GERD, since individuals were not studied on and off bronchodilators.

F. Conclusions

In conclusion, there are many physiologic alterations associated with asthma that may promote GERD. Factors controlling the competence of the gastroesophageal junction may be altered during an asthma attack. Normally, gastric pressure is positive in relation to pleural and esophageal pressure because the latter structures are in the chest (44). With increased airflow obstruction during an asthma attack, very negative pleural pressures can increase the pressure gradient between the thorax and abdominal cavity, predisposing the patient to develop reflux (47).ced The diaphragmatic crura contributes to pressure generation of the LES and may be altered in asthmatics (44). Overinflation and air trapping may also lead to flattening of the diaphragm, further impairing the antireflux barrier (66). Asthmatics with GERD have autonomic dysfunction, which may predispose asthmatics to develop GERD since the vagus nerve innervates the esophagus and vagal input influences LES pressure and esophageal motility (19). Bronchodilator medications may be detrimental to the competency of the gastroesophageal junction, especially theophylline and other methylxanthines, which increase gastric acid secretion and decrease LES pressure (67–69). There is continued debate about the influence of bronchodilator medications on the severity of GERD. Theophylline has the highest potential to produce GERD in asthmatics. Inhaled β_2-adrenergic agonists probably have minimal effect on esophageal parameters (77). Airway disease in asthmatics with GERD should be treated aggressively with antiinflammatory agents and bronchodilators. If possible, theophylline and oral β_2-adrenergic agonists should be avoided. Data also support that bronchodilators do not alter reflux symptoms or esophageal parameters (41,42,61).

III. Lessons from Clinical Experience with Acid Suppression

Many clinical investigations have examined whether antireflux therapy improves asthma outcome. Many studies have looked at predictors of asthma response. These predictors shed light on the pathophysiologic mechanisms of acid-induced bronchoconstriction (Table 3).

One possible predictor of asthma response in asthmatics with GERD is endoscopic healing of esophagitis with antireflux therapy. This point was brought out by Meier et al., who performed a prospective double-blind crossover study examining 15 asthmatics with GERD (81). Using omeprazole 20 mg twice a day for 6 weeks, with an endpoint of a greater than a 20% net change in FEV_1, they found that 4 of 15 patients had omeprazole-responsive asthma. They noted that only patients with complete endoscopic healing of esophagitis had omeprazole-responsive asthma ($p < 0.01$) (81). That healing of esophagitis is necessary for asthma improvement points out that esophagitis may play a significant role in reflux-associated bronchoconstriction. Acid reflux into the distal esophagus where esophagitis is present could stimulate acid-sensitive receptors inducing a vagally mediated reflex.

One of the most respected studies in the literature examining asthma response was performed by Larrain et al. (82). They performed a prospective placebo-controlled trial where 90 nonallergic adult-onset asthmatics with less than Grade 1 esophagitis were randomized to receive cimetidine 300 mg four times a day, placebo, or a modified posterior gastropexy. After 6 months, more than 75% of the patients in the two therapy groups had a significant decrease in pulmo-

Table 3 Predictors of Asthma Response

1. Healing of esophagitis with antireflux therapy (81,82)
2. Difficult-to-control asthma (83)
3. History of reflux-associated respiratory symptoms (84,86)
4. Intrinsic asthma (85)
5. Onset of reflux symptoms before respiratory symptoms (85)
6. Normal esophageal motility (86)
7. Abnormal amounts of proximal esophageal acid (87,88)
8. Presence of regurgitation (88)

nary symptoms and medication usage scores (82). This study shows that nonallergic asthmatics without endoscopic evidence of esophagitis or grade 1 esophagitis had asthma improvement with aggressive antireflux therapy. Again, the role of healing of esophagitis is implicated.

Irwin et al. prospectively examined difficult-to-control asthmatics requiring prednisone and implemented a systematic management protocol (83). They found that GERD was a possible contributing factor in 25 of 31 (81%) patients and 64% had a favorable asthma response with antireflux therapy (83). Also, GERD was clinically "silent" in 24% of patients. They concluded that difficult-to-control asthmatics need to be investigated for GERD, since therapy of reflux may improve asthma outcome (83).

Ekström et al. performed a prospective double-blind crossover study on 48 moderate to severe asthmatics with GERD and treated them with ranitidine 150 mg twice a day for 4 weeks (84). They found that a history of reflux-associated respiratory symptoms predicted asthma improvement resulting in a significant decrease in nighttime asthma symptom score and a decrease in the number of metered dose inhaler puffs used per day (84). This implicated the importance of GERD and pulmonary symptom correlation in predicting a favorable asthma response.

Perrin-Fayolle et al. reported a retrospective study examining asthma improvement in 44 asthmatics with GERD who were more than 5 years status post-Nissen transabdominal gastropexy (85). Subjects who were younger in age had nocturnal asthma attacks, and those with intrinsic asthma had improved asthma outcome (85). The onset of reflux symptoms before respiratory symptoms, severe GERD, and medical therapy response also predicted asthma improvement (85).

DeMeester et al. performed a prospective study in 17 patients with pulmonary symptoms unresponsive to medical antireflux therapy who underwent fundoplication (86). Of 17 patients, 9 were free of respiratory symptoms in the postoperative state. Asthma success rate was higher in subjects who had normal esophageal motility. Seven of nine (78%) patients with normal esophageal motility preoperatively denied respiratory symptoms postoperatively, while only 2 of 8 (25%) patients with reflux with abnormal esophageal motility denied respiratory symptoms postoperatively (86). There was also a correlation between pulmonary symptoms and esophageal reflux events. Patients with pulmonary symptoms during or within 3 minutes of a reflux event had higher success rates than other patients (86). This was the first study that showed that 24-hour esophageal pH monitoring may predict which patients have improvement in asthma symptoms with aggressive antireflux therapy (86).

The role of 24-hour esophageal pH monitoring in predicting asthma outcome was also noted in a study performed by Schnatz et al. who retrospectively examined 54 patients with cough or asthma triggered by gastroesophageal reflux (87). Patients received H_2 blockers, omeprazole, surgery, or lifestyle therapy only for therapy of GERD. They found that 71% of subjects had good pulmonary symptom response with antireflux therapy (87). Nine of 11 (82%) with distal only esophageal reflux had a favorable response. Likewise, 4 out of 4 (100%) with proximal only reflux had a favorable response. Of patients with both distal and proximal reflux, 11 of 19 (58%) had improvement in pulmonary symptoms (87). None of the five patients who had normal esophageal acid contact times had pulmonary improvement. This study indicates that the presence of distal and proximal reflux may predict a favorable asthma outcome with antireflux therapy and that normal esophageal acid contact times may indicate that asthma symptoms will not respond to antireflux therapy (87).

Our laboratory performed a prospective study examining predictors of asthma response in 30 asthmatics with GERD measuring asthma symptoms—peak expiratory flow rates before and after 3 months of documented acid suppression therapy with omeprazole (88). Asthma response was defined by a priori definition with an asthma symptom score reduction of greater than 20%. Twenty of 30 (67%) subjects were asthma symptom responders (88). Predictors of asthma response were identified by comparing demographic and esophageal variables in the asthma symptom responders and the nonresponders. Higher amounts of total proximal reflux, higher baseline asthma symptom score, higher baseline reflux symptom score, the presence of regurgitation, asthma exacerbated by upper respiratory tract infection, and asthma exacerbated by allergy showed a trend toward asthma improvement (88). In a forward stepwise logistic regression analysis examining models to predict asthma outcome, the presence of regurgitation more than once a week or excessive proximal reflux (defined as a greater than 1.1 percentage of time where esophageal pH was less than 4) predicted a greater than 20% improvement in asthma symptoms (88). The presence of regurgitation or excessive proximal reflux identified all responders with a 100% sensitivity. These findings were absent in all nonresponders, giving a 100% negative predictive value, a specificity of 44%, and a positive predictive value of 79% (88). Proximal esophageal reflux and regurgitation may be associated with microaspiration.

In conclusion, there are many possible predictors of asthma response (Table 3). These include the presence of regurgitation as documented by Harding et al. and the presence of proximal esophageal acid in 24-hour pH monitoring documented by Harding et al. and Schnatz et al. (87,88). Nonallergic asthma also seems to be a possible predictor of asthma response as documented by Larrain et al. and Perrin-Fayolle et al. (82,85). Complete healing of esophagitis was important in Meier et al.'s study, as well as less than Grade 1 esophagitis in Larrain et al.'s study (81,82). Irwin et al. found that reflux may play a significant role in difficult-to-control asthmatics (83). Ekström et al. showed that reflux-associated respiratory symptoms may predict asthma response (84). Nocturnal asthma may also be a predictor, as is the onset of GERD symptoms before respiratory symptoms, as documented by Perrin-Fayolle et al. (85). These predictors show that multiple pathogenic mechanisms may be responsible for airway responses to esophageal acid. Regurgitation and proximal esophageal acid may signify the role of microaspiration, and healing of esophagitis and reflux-associated respiratory symptoms may implicate a vagally mediated reflex. Further research will illustrate how GERD and airway disease interact.

Acknowledgments

The author wishes to acknowledge Mr. Martin M. Robbins for his invaluable assistance in editing this manuscript, Dr. Joel Richter for his insight, and Drs. K. Randall Young and Jeffrey Hawkins for their support. Dr. Harding is supported by a Sleep Academic Award through the National Heart, Lung, and Blood Institute.

References

1. Osler WB. Bronchial Asthma. In: Osler WB, ed. The Principles and Practice of Medicine. 8th ed. New York: D. Appleton and Company, 1912:627–631.
2. Karlsson JA, Sant'Ambrogio G, Widdicombe J. Afferent neural pathways in cough and reflex bronchoconstriction. J Appl Physiol 1988; 65:1007–1023.
3. Cunningham ET Jr, Ravich WJ, Jones B, Donner MW. Vagal reflexes referred from the upper aerodigestive tract: an infrequently recognized cause of common cardio respiratory responses. Ann Intern Med 1992; 116:575–582.
4. Mansfield LE, Hameister HH, Spaulding HS, Smith NJ, Glab N. The role of the vagus nerve in airway narrowing caused by intraesophageal hydrochloric acid provocative and esophageal distention. Ann Allergy 1981; 47:431–434.
5. Mansfield LE, Stein MR. Gastroesophageal reflux and asthma: a possible reflex mechanism. Ann Allergy 1978; 41:224–226.
6. Spaulding HS Jr, Mansfield LE, Stein MR, Sellner JC, Gremillion DE. Further investigation of the association between gastroesophageal reflux and bronchoconstriction. J Allergy Clin Immunol 1982; 69:516–521.
7. Ducoloné A, Vandevenne A, Jovin H, Grob J-C, Coumaros D, Meyer C, Burghard G, Methlin G, Hollender L. Gastroesophageal reflux in patients with asthma and chronic bronchitis. Am Rev Respir Dis 1987; 135:327–332.
8. Andersen LI, Schmidt A, Bundgaard A. Pulmonary function and acid application in the esophagus. Chest 1986; 90:358–363.
9. Wright RA, Miller SA, Corsello BF. Acid-induced esophagobronchial-cardiac reflexes in humans. Gastroenterology 1990; 99:71–73.
10. Kjellen G, Tibbling L, Wranne B. Bronchial obstruction after oesophageal acid perfusion in asthmatics. Clin Physiol 1981; 1:285–292.
11. Davis RS, Larsen GL, Grunstein MM. Respiratory response to intraesophageal acid

infusion in asthmatic children during sleep. J Allergy Clin Immunol 1983; 72:393–398.
12. Ekström T, Tibbling L. Esophageal acid perfusion, airway function, and symptoms in asthmatic patients with marked bronchial hyperreactivity. Chest 1989; 96:995–998.
13. Wesseling G, Brummer R-J, Wouters EFM, ten Velde GPM. Gastric asthma? No change in respiratory impedance during intraesophageal acidification in adult asthmatics. Chest 1993; 104:1733–1736.
14. Tan WC, Martin RJ, Pandey R, Ballard RD. Effects of spontaneous and simulated gastroesophageal reflux on sleeping asthmatics. Am Rev Respir Dis 1990; 141:1394–1399.
15. Pack Al. Acid: a nocturnal bronchoconstrictor? Am Rev Respir Dis 1990; 141:1391–1392.
16. Schan CA, Harding SM, Haile JM, Bradley LA, Richter JE. Gastroesophageal reflux-induced bronchoconstriction. An intraesophageal acid infusion study using state-of-the-art technology. Chest 1994; 106:731–737.
17. Harding SM, Schan CA, Guzzo MR, Alexander RW, Bradley LA, Richter JE. Gastroesophageal reflux-induced bronchoconstriction. Is microaspiration a factor? Chest 1995; 108:1220–1227.
18. Harding SM, Guzzo MR, Maples RV, Alexander RW, Richter JE. Gastroesophageal reflux induced bronchoconstriction: vagolytic doses of atropine diminish airway responses to esophageal acid infusion (abstr). Am J Respir Crit Care Med 1995; 151:A589.
19. Lodi U, Harding SM, Coghlan HC, Guzzo MR, Walker LH. Autonomic regulation in asthmatics with gastroesophageal reflux. Chest 1997; 111:65–70.
20. Sontag S, O'Connell S, Khandelwal S. Does wheezing occur in association with an episode of gastroesophageal reflux? (abstr). Gastroenterology 1989; 96:A482.
21. Herve P, Denjean A, Jian R, Simonneau G, Duroux P. Intraesophageal perfusion of acid increases the bronchomotor response to methacholine and to isocapnic hyperventilation in asthmatic subjects. Am Rev Respir Dis 1986; 134:986–989.
22. Teichtahl H, Kronborg IJ, Yeomans ND, Robinson P. Adult asthma and gastroesophageal reflux: the effects of omeprazole therapy on asthma. Aust NZ J Med 1996; 26:671–676.
23. Kuo B, Castell DO. Optimal dosing of omeprazole 40 mg daily: effects on gastric and esophageal pH and serum gastrin in healthy controls. Am J Gastroenterol 1996; 91:1532–1538.
24. Overholt RH, Ashraf MM. Esophageal reflux as a trigger in asthma. NY State J Med 1966; 66:3030–3032.
25. Bannister WK, Sattilaro AJ, Otis RD. Therapeutic aspects of aspiration pneumonitis in experimental animals. Anesthesiology 1961; 22:440–443.
26. Tomori Z, Widdicombe JG. Muscular, bronchomotor and cardiovascular reflexes elicited by mechanical stimulation of the respiratory tract. J Physiol 1969; 200:25–49.
27. Colebatch HJH, Halmagyi DFJ. Reflex airway reaction to fluid aspiration. J Appl Physiol 1962; 17:787–794.

28. Tuchman DN, Boyle JT, Pack Al, Scwartz J, Kokonos M, Spitzer AR, Cohen S. Comparison of airway responses following tracheal or esophageal acidification in the cat. Gastroenterology 1984; 87:872–881.
29. Corwin RW, Irwin RS. The lipid-laden alveolar macrophage as a marker of aspiration in parenchymal lung disease. Am Rev Respir Dis 1985; 132:576–581.
30. Nussbaum E, Maggi JC, Mathis R, Gallant SP. Association of lipid-laden alveolar macrophages and gastroesophageal reflux in children. J Pediatr 1987; 110:190–194.
31. Ghaed N, Stein MR. Assessment of a technique for scintigraphic monitoring of pulmonary aspiration of gastric contents in asthmatics with gastroesophageal reflux. Ann Allergy 1979; 42:306–308.
32. Crausaz FM, Favez G. Aspiration of solid food particles into lungs of patients with gastroesophageal reflux and chronic bronchial disease. Chest 1988; 93:376–378.
33. Greyson ND, Reid RH, Liu YC, Thomas P. Radionuclide assessment in nocturnal asthma. Clin Nucl Med 1982; 7:318–319.
34. Chernow B, Johnson LF, Janowitz WR, Castell DO. Pulmonary aspiration as a consequence of gastroesophageal reflux. A diagnostic approach. Dig Dis Sci 1979; 24:839–844.
35. Ruth M, Carlsson S, Mansson I, Bengtsson U, Sandberg N. Scintigraphic detection of gastro-pulmonary aspiration in patients with respiratory disorders. Clin Physiol 1993; 13:19–33.
36. Weiner GJ, Koufman JA, Wu WC, Cooper JB, Richter JE, Castell DO. The pharyngoesophageal dual ambulatory pH probe for evaluation of atypical manifestations of gastroesophageal reflux (GERD) (abstr). Gastroenterology 1987; 92:1694.
37. Gastal OL, Castell JA, Castell DO. Frequency and site of gastroesophageal reflux in patients with chest symptoms. Studies using proximal and distal pH monitoring. Chest 1994; 106:1793–1796.
38. Varkey B, Pathial K, Shaker R, Dodds WJ, Hogan WJ. Pharyngoesophageal reflux index in asthmatics (abstr). Chest 1992; 102:152s.
39. Donnelly RJ, Berrisford RG, Jack CIA, Tran JA, Evans CC. Simultaneous tracheal and esophageal pH monitoring: investigating reflux-associated asthma. Ann Thorac Surg 1993; 56:1029–1034.
40. Jack CIA, Calverley PMA, Donnelly RJ, Tran J, Russell G, Hind CRK, Evans CC. Simultaneous tracheal and esophageal pH measurements in asthmatic patients with gastro-esophageal reflux. Thorax 1995; 50:201–204.
41. Field SK, Underwood M, Brant R, Cowie RL. Prevalence of gastroesophageal reflux symptoms in asthma. Chest 1996; 109:316–322.
42. Sontag SJ, O'Connell S, Khandelwal S, Miller T, Nemchausky B, Schnell TG, Serlovsky R. Most asthmatics have gastroesophageal reflux with or without bronchodilator therapy. Gastroenterology 1990; 99:613–620.
42a. Harding SM. Pulmonary abnormalities in gastroesophageal reflux disease. In: Richter JE, ed. Ambulatory Esophageal pH Monitoring. Practical Approach and Clinical Applications. Baltimore: Williams and Wilkins, 1997:149–164.
43. Altorki NK, Skinner DB. Pathophysiology of gastroesophageal reflux. Am J Med 1989; 86:685–689.

44. Mittal RK, Balaban DH. The esophagogastric junction. N Engl J Med 1997; 336: 924–932.
45. DeMeester TR, Wernly JA, Bryant GH, Little AG, Skinner DB. Clinical and in vitro analysis of determinants of gastroesophageal competence: a study of the principles of antireflux surgery. Am J Surgery 1979; 137:39–45.
46. Sloan S, Kahrilas PJ. Impairment of esophageal emptying with hiatal hernia. Gastroenterology 1991; 100:596–605.
47. Holmes PW, Campbell AM, Barter CE. Changes of lung volumes and lung mechanics in asthma and normal subjects. Thorax 1978; 33:394–400.
48. Mays EE. Intrinsic asthma in adults: association with gastroesophageal reflux. JAMA 1976; 236:2626–2628.
49. Kaliner M. The cholinergic nervous system and immediate hypersensitivity. J Allergy Clin Immunol 1978; 58:308–314.
50. Kaliner M, Shelhamer JH, Davis PB, Smith LJ, Venter JC. Autonomic nervous system abnormalities and allergies. Ann Intern Med 1982; 96:349–357.
51. Kallenback JM, Webster T, Dowdeswell R, Reinach SG, Millar NSC, Zwi S. Reflex heart rate control in asthma: evidence of parasympathetic overactivity. Chest 1985; 87:644–648.
52. Pellegrini CA, DeMeester TR, Johnson LF, Skinner DB. Gastroesophageal reflux and pulmonary aspiration: incidence, functional abnormality, and results of surgical therapy. Surgery 1979; 86:110–119.
53. Moote DW, Lloyd DA, McCourtie DR, Wells GA. Increase in gastroesophageal reflux during methacholine-induced bronchospasm. J Allergy Clin Immunol 1986; 78:619–623.
54. Ekström TKA, Tibbling LIE. Can mild bronchospasm reduce gastroesophageal reflux? Am Rev Respir Dis 1989; 139:52–55.
55. Culebras A. Sleep apnea syndromes. In: Culebras A, ed. Clinical Handbook of Sleep Disorders. Boston: Butterworth-Heinemann, 1996:181–231.
56. Kerr P, Shoenut JP, Millar T, Buckle P, Kryger MH. Nasal CPAP reduces gastroesophageal reflex in obstructive sleep apnea syndrome. Chest 1992; 101:1539–1544.
57. Kerr P, Shoenut JP, Steens RD, Millar T, Micflikier AB, Kryger MH. Nasal continuous positive airway pressure. A new treatment for nocturnal gastroesophageal reflux? J Clin Gastroenterol 1993; 17:276–280.
58. Singh V, Jain NK. Asthma as a cause for, rather than a result of, gastroesophageal reflux. J Asthma 1983; 20:241–243.
59. Pope CE II. Acid-reflux disorders. N Engl J Med 1994; 331:656–660.
60. Mittal RK, Lange RC, McCallum RW. Identification and mechanism of delayed esophageal acid clearance in subjects with hiatus hernia. Gastroenterology 1987; 92: 130–135.
61. Sontag SJ, Schnell TG, Miller TQ, Khandelwal S, O'Connell S, Chejfec G, Greenlee H, Seidel UJ, Brand L. Prevalence of oesophagitis in asthmatics. Gut 1992; 33:872–876.
62. Langman J. Medical Embryology. Baltimore: Williams and Wilkins, 1978.
63. Delattre JF, Palot JP, Ducasse A, Flament JB, Hureau J. The crura of the diaphragm and diaphragmatic passage. Anat Clin 1985; 4:271–283.

64. Mittal RK, Holloway RH, Penagini R, Blackshaw LA, Dent J. Transient lower esophageal sphincter relaxation. Gastroenterology 1995; 109:601–610.
65. Mittal RK, Rochester DF, McCallum RW. Electrical and mechanical activity in the human lower esophageal sphincter during diaphragmatic contraction. J Clin Invest 1988; 81:1182–1189.
66. Roussos C, Macklem PT. The respiratory muscles. N Engl J Med 1982; 307:786–797.
67. Foster LJ, Trudeau WL, Goldman AL. Bronchodilator effects on gastric acid secretion. JAMA 1979; 241:2613–2615.
68. Johannesson N, Andersson KE, Joelsson B, Persson CGA. Relaxation of lower esophageal sphincter and stimulation of gastric secretion and diuresis by antiasthmatic xanthines. Am Rev Respir Dis 1985; 131:26–31.
69. Stein MR, Towner TG, Weber RW, Mansfield LE, Jacobson KW, McDonnell JT, Nelson HS. The effect of theophylline on the lower esophageal sphincter pressure. Ann Allergy 1980; 45:238–241.
70. Berquist WE, Rachelefsky GS, Kadden M, Siegel SC, Katz RM, Mickey MR, Ament ME. Effect of theophylline on gastroesophageal reflux in normal adults. J Allergy Clin Immunol 1981; 67:407–411.
71. Ekström T, Tibbling L. Influence of theophylline on gastro-esophageal reflux and asthma. Eur J Clin Pharmacol 1988; 35:353–356.
72. Hubert D, Gaudric M, Guerre J, Lockhart A, Marsac J. Effect of theophylline on gastroesophageal reflux in patients with asthma. J Allergy Clin Immunol 1988; 81:1168–1174.
73. Stein MR. Effect of theophylline on gastroesophageal reflux (letter). J Allergy Clin Immunol 1990; 85:140–141.
74. Mansfield LE. Effects of theophylline in gastroesophageal reflux (letter). J Allergy Clin Immunol 1989; 84:407–408.
75. Christensen J. Effects of drugs on esophageal motility. Arch Intern Med 1976; 136:532–537.
76. DiMarino AJ, Cohen S. Effect of an oral beta-2 adrenergic agonist on lower esophageal sphincter pressure in normals and in patients with achalasia. Dig Dis Sci 1982; 27:1063–1066.
77. Schindlbeck NE, Heinrich C, Huber RM, Muller-Lissner SA. Effects of albuterol (salbutamol) on esophageal motility and gastroesophageal reflux in healthy volunteers. JAMA 1988; 260:3156–3158.
78. Michoud MC, Leduc T, Proulx F, Perreault S, DuSouich P, Duranceau A, Amyot R. Effect of salbutamol on gastroesophageal reflux in healthy volunteers and patients with asthma. J Allergy Clin Immunol 1991; 87:762–767.
79. Bittinger M, Barnert J, Weinbech M. Dose-dependant relationship between gastroesophageal reflux (GER) and inhalative therapy with fenoterol in chronic obstructive lung disease (COLD)-a preliminary report. Dis Esophagus 1994; 7:276–279.
80. Ruzkowski CJ, Sanowski RA, Austin J, Rohwedder JJ, Waring JP. The effects of inhaled albuterol and oral theophylline on gastroesophageal reflux in patients with gastroesophageal reflux disease and obstructive lung disease. Arch Intern Med 1992; 152:783–785.
81. Meier JH, McNally PR, Punja M, Freeman SR, Sudduth RH, Stocker N, Perry M,

Spaulding HS. Does omeprazole (Prilosec) improve respiratory function in asthmatics with gastroesophageal reflux? A double-blind, placebo-controlled crossover study. Dig Dis Sci 1994; 39:2127–2133.
82. Larrain A, Carrasco E, Galleguillos F, Sepulveda R, Pope CE, II. Medical and surgical therapy of nonallergic asthma associated with gastroesophageal reflux. Chest 1991; 99:1330–1335.
83. Irwin RS, Curley FJ, French CL. Difficult-to-control asthma: contributing factors and outcome of a systematic management protocol. Chest 1993; 103:1662–1669.
84. Ekström T, Lindgren BR, Tibbling L. Effects of ranitidine therapy on patients with asthma and a history of gastroesophageal reflux: a double blind crossover study. Thorax 1989; 44:19–23.
85. Perrin-Fayolle M, Gormand F, Braillon G, Lombard-Platet R, Vignal J, Azzar D, Forichon J, Adeleine P. Long-term results of surgical therapy for gastroesophageal reflux in asthmatic patients. Chest 1989; 96:40–45.
86. DeMeester TR, Bonavina L, Iascone C, Courtney JV, Skinner DB. Chronic respiratory symptoms and occult gastroesophageal reflux: a prospective clinical study and results of surgical therapy. Ann Surg 1990; 211:337–345.
87. Schnatz PF, Castell JA, Castell DO. Pulmonary symptoms associated with gastroesophageal reflux: use of ambulatory pH monitoring to diagnose and to direct therapy. Am J Gastroenterol 1996; 91:1715–1718.
88. Harding SM, Richter JE, Guzzo MR, Schan CA, Alexander RW, Bradley LA. Asthma and gastroesophageal reflux: acid suppressive therapy improves asthma outcome. Am J Med 1996; 100:395–405.

8

Medical Treatment of Gastroesophageal Reflux Disease and Airway Disease

MANI S. KAVURU and JOEL E. RICHTER

The Cleveland Clinic Foundation
Cleveland, Ohio

I. Introduction

There is a substantial literature that suggests a relationship between gastroesophageal reflux disease (GERD) and bronchial asthma (1). The possible associations between these two conditions are several (2):

1. These are two very common diseases that coexist independently in some patients.
2. Gastroesophageal reflux either exacerbates or is causally related to the pathogenesis of asthma in a subset of patients.
3. Bronchial asthma and/or antiasthma medications exacerbate or induce gastroesophageal reflux disease.

It is likely that all three of these possibilities occur in subsets of patients with bronchial asthma. The magnitude of the association between GERD and asthma and its clinical significance remains unclear from the literature. Gastroesophageal reflux, with its primary symptoms of heartburn and acid regurgitation, is very common in the general population. A recent random sample of 2200 Olmstead County, Minnesota, residents aged 25–74 years found that 20% of the respondents had reflux symptoms at least weekly and nearly 60% had experienced either heartburn or acid regurgitation within the past year (3). The prevalence of GERD in asthmatics is reported to range from 34 to 89% (4–8). Reasons for this wide variability include the use of self-reported questionnaire data (9), comorbid confounding factors (alcohol, cigarette smoking, gender) (8,10), and the variability of definition and choice of diagnostic techniques to establish GERD (11). This chapter will assume that a relationship exists between GERD and asthma and will review various medical treatments for GERD and their effects on asthma symptoms, pulmonary function studies, and the need for asthma medications.

An explosion of information has recently implicated airway inflammation in the pathogenesis of airway hyperreactivity in asthma (12). However, even though our understanding of the pathogenesis of asthma has increased in the past decade, so has asthma morbidity and mortality. Although several possible reasons have been offered for these trends, there appears to be a general consensus that suboptimal use of conventional asthma therapy by both patients and physicians plays an important role. The most recent asthma practice guidelines (National Asthma Education and Prevention Program, Expert Panel Report II) stressed the importance of chronic maintenance anti-inflammatory therapy in all patients with persistent asthma, along with educational and avoidance measures (13). Literature suggests that a subset of asthmatics have suboptimal asthma control, based on symptoms and need for acute health care services, despite maximal conventional therapy (12). It is likely that GERD plays a role in a subset of these asthmatics as well (14).

A number of relevant issues exist regarding therapy for GERD associated with asthma. What are the clinical data showing the effectiveness of each type of medical therapy? Which group of asthmatics should receive therapy for GERD? Is empiric medical therapy for GERD-related asthma adequate, or are specific diagnostic tests followed by therapy more appropriate? For long-term maintenance therapy, what are the goals and what are the key outcome parameters? What is the optimal dose, duration, and agent for therapy? What are the long-term costs of no therapy versus the costs of medical therapy? With suboptimal asthma control, is it better to increase chronic asthma maintenance therapy and/or add therapy for GERD?

II. Methodology Issues

A number of methodologic limitations exist in the published literature relating GERD and asthma (Table 1). The major limitation in all the published studies is the lack of attempt to optimize conventional, "standard" therapy for the underlying asthma. Today this means the use of daily inhaled corticosteroids (15). Inadequate use of inhaled corticosteroids is a major treatment shortcoming for

Table 1 Methodologic Limitations of Studies Relating GERD and Asthma

---
Lack of attempt to optimize conventional asthma therapy
Lack of objective assessment or documentation of acid suppression
Absence of a control group
Small number of patients
Outcome parameters for asthma control are not consistent
Studies only involve patients with symptomatic GERD

---

many patients with poorly controlled asthma. The study of a "novel" intervention for GERD-related asthma without instituting conventional asthma therapy is an important source of variability in the published studies. A second major limitation in most studies is the lack of objective assessment of acid suppression while asthmatic patients are being treated for GERD. In the absence of documented control of acid reflux, one cannot conclude that therapy for GERD did not improve the associated asthma. A third limitation is the absence of a control group in some studies. Based on data from a variety of experimental antiinflammatory therapies for chronic "steroid-dependent" asthma, it is known that the placebo arm of these asthma studies could improve 20–40% simply by participating in a clinical trial, i.e., the "Hawthorne effect" (12). A fourth limitation is that the total number of asthmatics subjected to GERD therapy is quite small (77 patients in five reports for omeprazole and 125 patients in five reports for H_2-receptor antagonists). Any beneficial effects of antireflux therapy associated with a small improvement in asthma control might not have been detected because of small sample size (β-error). A fifth limitation is that the choice of outcome parameters for asthma improvement are not consistent in the published studies. The beneficial effect on symptom scores has been much greater than other objective parameters, such as peak expiratory flow or forced expiratory volume in one second (FEV_1). Finally, it is important to note that all published trials on therapy for GERD-associated asthma involve asthmatics with symptoms of heartburn or acid regurgitation. Therefore, findings cannot be extended to asthmatics with so-called "silent GERD," where the reflux disease is diagnosed by a positive pH probe or endoscopic evidence of esophagitis in the absence of GERD symptoms.

This chapter will assume that a relationship exists between GERD and asthma and that there is a need for aggressive treatment of the reflux disease to better control the asthma. We will limit our discussion to studies of adults with bronchial asthma and not include atypical presentations of GERD such as cough. Interventions to be considered will include lifestyle changes, antacids, alginic acid, H_2-receptor antagonists, pro-kinetic agents, and acid proton pump inhibitors.

III. Medical Treatment

The primary goal of managing GERD with or without associated extraesophageal disease is complete symptom resolution (16–19). Additional therapeutic endpoints include healing of esophagitis when present, prevention of complications such as peptic stricture or Barrett's esophagus, and the maintenance of symptom control in patients with chronic disease. The overall management strategies can be classified as lifestyle changes, pharmacologic manipulations of gastric acid and motility, or surgery. See Table 2 for a summary of antireflux medications.

A. Lifestyle Modifications

Lifestyle changes include eating smaller meals and avoiding the supine position soon after meals, dietary modification to avoid certain types of foods as well as alcohol, weight reduction, smoking cessation, and elevation of the head of the bed for sleep. The lifestyle changes are intuitively appealing to physicians since they do not have side effects. These changes have other obvious medical benefits; they are within the "patient's control," and these changes are "simply the right thing to do." Although all patients could be counseled about these lifestyle changes, the reality is that probably only a small subset of patients experiences significant relief with these interventions alone (20). Data to support each of these recommendations are, in fact, fairly limited.

Table 2 Antireflux Medications for the Treatment of GERD

Antacids
Alginic acid (Gaviscon)
H_2-receptor antagonists
   Cimetidine (Tagamet)
   Famotidine (Pepcid)
   Nizatidine (Axid)
   Ranitidine (Zantac)
Prokinetic agents
   Metoclopramide (Reglan)
   Bethanechol (Urecholine)
   Domperidone[a]
   Cisapride (Propulsid)
H^+/K^+-ATPase (proton pump) inhibitors
   Omeprazole (Prilosec)
   Lansoprazole (Prevacid)
   Pantoprazole[a]

[a]Currently not available in the United States.

Nocturnal acid reflux can be particularly damaging, as the normal acid-clearance mechanisms are impaired. Gravity is not effective, as we usually sleep in the supine or prone position. During sleep esophageal peristalsis is minimal and saliva (pH 6.8–7.4) is not made—the reason we awaken with a "cotton mouth or dry mouth" in the morning. Limited data suggest that elevating the head of the bed 6–8 inches protects the esophagus from acid reflux during sleep (21,22). Placing pillows under the head is usually not enough; the head and upper body elevation typically requires placement of a foam wedge underneath the mattress or blocks underneath the headboard to elevate the entire bed. The impact of this maneuver reduced the time of esophageal pH < 4 from 22 to 14% in one study (21). This recommendation should target patients with nocturnal reflux symptoms and/or nocturnal asthma symptoms such as wheezing, chest tightness, and coughing.

Cigarette smoking through the pharmacologic effect of nicotine contributes to GERD by decreasing lower esophageal sphincter (LES) pressure, increasing the frequency of reflux episodes, and decreasing acid clearance (23–25). Smoking cessation alone can significantly improve respiratory symptoms in patients with asthma. In the only study to investigate the impact of cessation of cigarette smoking on GERD, it was found that the immediate discontinuation of smoking decreased the number of daily reflux episodes but did not affect the total esophageal acid exposure in patients without esophagitis (26). Therefore, the contribution of cigarette smoking to GERD may only be modest; nevertheless, it should be recommended vigorously to all patients for the other overwhelming medical benefits.

Patients who give a history of worsening reflux symptoms with certain foods should be counseled about avoiding these products. Foods can aggravate reflux symptoms by a number of mechanisms, including increased gastric volume producing gastric distention and transient LES relaxation, food contents directly lowering LES pressure, and direct irritant effects of food, possibly due to hyperosmolarity on inflamed esophageal mucosa (27). Fatty foods, alcohol, and chocolates are generally best avoided, especially prior to assuming the supine position (28,29). Also, a variety of medications, both prescribed and over-the-counter, can lower esophageal sphincter pressure and have direct effects by producing gastric and esophageal mucosal damage. Drugs in the former group include progesterone, theophylline (30–32), several prostaglandins, anticholinergic drugs, oral β-adrenergic agonists (33), α-adrenergic agonists, dopamine, diazepam, meperidine, morphine, and calcium channel blockers. Medications commonly causing direct injury to the esophagus include doxycycline, slow-release potassium, ascorbic acid, ferrous sulfate, aspirin, nonsteroidal anti-inflammatory drugs, quinidine, and alendronates. It appears that inhaled β-agonists such as salbutamol do not affect esophageal function (33,34). Whether obesity actually contributes to GERD and whether weight loss has beneficial effects is unknown.

Kjellen et al. studied the effect of conservative treatment of GERD in a group of 62 patients with asthma and symptomatic GERD (35). The intervention included lifestyle changes (avoid eating for 3 hours before bedtime, avoid aspirin-type medications, elevate head of bed, finish meals with a glass of warm water) and Gaviscon. Study design was randomized allocation to an intervention group and a control group, but patients were not blinded to the treatment. All patients had esophageal dysfunction by a variety of studies (this study antedated esophageal pH testing). The esophageal symptoms improved in 87% of treatment group and 11% of control group. Baseline asthma, which was characterized as exogenous or endogenous, was treated with inhaled steroids in only 18 of 62 patients (29%). Improvement in asthma was statistically significant for the treatment group based on symptoms and need for β-agonists. However, there was no description of the validity of the questionnaire or how symptoms were scored. Also, the reduction in β-agonist use was from 4.4 to 3.8 puffs/day ($p < 0.05$) for the treatment group and 3.9 to 3.6 puffs/day for the control group. Less than one puff reduction is probably not clinically significant, especially in patients who were not treated with inhaled steroids. Also, there was no significant improvement in objective pulmonary function studies.

B. Antacids/Alginic Acid

Used on an as-needed basis, antacids and alginic acid are the mainstay of rapid, safe, effective relief of heartburn symptoms. Antacids primarily work by neutralizing acid, albeit for relatively short periods of time. Therefore, patients need to take antacids frequently, usually 20–30 minutes after meals and bedtime, depending on the severity of symptoms. Liquid forms are preferable to tablets, although the latter are the most popular preparation of this medication. Containing antacids and alginic acid, Gaviscon is a popular over-the-counter treatment for GERD. The active component of this medication, alginic acid, interacts with saliva to form a highly viscous solution that floats on the surface of the gastric pool, acting as a mechanical barrier. The barrier reduces the number of reflux episodes and diminishes esophageal acid exposure during the day but not at night (36). Antacids and alginic acid are effective for relieving mild to moderate intermittent reflux symptoms (37,38). They are particularly useful in patients with situational heartburn brought on by lifestyle changes or pregnancy. Even in high doses, these agents are not effective in healing esophagitis.

Excessive use of antacids may be associated with side effects. Magnesium-containing antacids produce diarrhea, while aluminum-containing products are constipating. The potential for magnesium or aluminum toxicity further limits their use in patients with significant renal disease. Low-sodium antacids (e.g., magaldrate-Riopan) are preferable for individuals on salt-restricted diets. Antacids and alginic acid are the initial agents of choice for treating reflux symptoms in pregnant women since they are nontoxic. In this special situation, adverse effects are rare but include interference with iron absorption, with ingestion of sodium bicarbonate, metabolic alkalosis and fluid overload in both the fetus and mother.

C. H_2-Receptor Antagonists

The four currently available H_2-receptor antagonists (H_2-RAs), cimetidine, ranitidine, famotidine, and nizatidine, act competitively and reversibly to inhibit stimulation of the parietal cell by histamine (39). The plasma concentration of the drug correlates approximately with the degree of inhibition. These agents block nocturnal acid secretion more effectively, having minimal effect on meal-stimulated acid secretion. H_2-receptor antagonists have no significant effect on gastric emptying, LES pressure, or pancreatic secretion.

Overall, H_2-RAs decrease acid reflux by 30–50%. Standard doses of H_2-RAs given twice a day (morning and before supper) alleviate symptoms of GERD and heal mild to moderate erosive esophagitis. A recent summary of studies evaluating the treatment of GERD by H_2-RAs suggests an aggregate symptomatic response in 1132 of 1887 patients (60%) and a healing rate for 506 of 1003 (50%) patients, compared to placebo rates of 27% and 24%, respectively (40,41). The typical duration for these studies ranges from 6 to 12 weeks. Some patients, failing a course of standard dose of H_2-RAs, may be hypersecretors of acid; they may require higher and more frequent doses of the H_2-RAs. Ranitidine is the only H_2-RA approved for the maintenance healing of erosive esophagitis. The recommended dose is 150 mg twice daily, with placebo-controlled trials having been carried out for one year.

All the H_2-RAs are now available over the counter, usually at 50% the prescription dose. Their use is similar to that of antacids for the treatment of intermittent heartburn, although the rapidity of relief is not as good as with antacids. The over-the-counter H_2-RAs are superior to antacids in preventing reflux episodes after large meals, exercise, or other provocative situations when given 30 minutes before the refluxogenic activity.

The H_2-RAs have an excellent side-effect profile and a low incidence of the following adverse reactions: central nervous system disturbances (especially cimetidine in high concentrations), headaches, diarrhea, gynecomastia, and impotence. Drug interactions (cimetidine binds to the cytochrome P-450 system with greater affinity than does ranitidine) include those with theophylline, warfarin, phenytoin, and benzodiazepines. Neither famotidine nor nizatidine interacts with the cytochrome P-450 system. The H_2-RAs cross the placental blood barrier and are excreted in breast milk. A recent large case-control study in Canada, however, found no adverse side effects in pregnant women taking this class of drugs at any stage of pregnancy (42). Therefore, the H_2-RAs can be used in pregnant women with very severe reflux symptoms not responding to lifestyle changes or antacids.

Table 3 summarizes the adult studies with H_2-RAs for asthma and GERD. These studies include four placebo-controlled crossover trials (43–46) and one case series (47) using either cimetidine or ranitidine.

Goodall et al. conducted a placebo crossover trial of 20 adult asthmatics with GERD recruited from a pulmonary outpatient clinic (43). Cimetidine 200 mg 4 times a day or placebo was given over 6 weeks with a 1-week washout period. At baseline, 18 of 20 patients had abnormal acid reflux, by manometry and pH monitoring, reflux of barium, or endoscopy. On cimetidine, reflux symptoms improved significantly in 14 of 20 patients compared with placebo (a drop in GERD symptom score from 2.8 to 1.1, $p < 0.02$). Baseline asthma severity was probably mild to moderate. All patients had nocturnal asthma symptoms, but the baseline asthma therapy was not described. Despite effective treatment of the gastroesophageal reflux, there were only minimal changes in a variety of asthma outcome parameters. The daytime symptom score did not change, and the night score decreased slightly from 1.1 to 0.7, reaching statistical significance ($p < 0.05$), but of uncertain clinical significance. Four peak flow readings were obtained per day, but only the night peak flow increased from 310 to 335 ($p < 0.05$). There was no significant change in the FEV_1, and no change in the use of rescue albuterol. Overall, this is essentially a negative trial, but the study limitations include the lack of documented control of GERD, a less than standard dose of cimetidine, and a relatively short duration of treatment.

Harper et al. reported on 15 adult nonsmokers with symptomatic GERD, all of whom had pH testing (10 of 15 with erosive esophagitis, total reflux time of 22.5% with pH <4) (47). Therapy was ranitidine 150 mg twice a day for 8 weeks. These were nonallergic asthmatics, only 4 of which had nocturnal asthma symptoms. Interestingly, some patients were pretreated at baseline with prednisone for the various procedures in this study. This could have artifactually increased the baseline FEV_1, thereby lessening the degree of possible improvement. Within one week of beginning ranitidine therapy, there was significant reduction in heartburn and regurgitation scores, but significant improvement in pulmonary symptom scores took 7 weeks of therapy. Pulmonary function tests (PFTs), including FEV_1, FVC, and percent of FEV_1, were improved significantly after 8 weeks of therapy. Although not a placebo-controlled study, this study suggests that improvement of asthma may not immediately parallel improvement of esophageal symptoms but may take much longer.

In a placebo crossover trial, Nagel et al. studied 44 adult asthmatics with esophageal pH testing (44). Twenty-one of the 44 patients had nocturnal asthma symptoms along with a drop in early morning peak flows ("morning dipping"). Fifteen of 44 patients (34%) also had GERD and were the subjects participating in this trial. Of the patients with GERD by pH testing (mean 20% of the time pH < 4), only seven had symptoms of heartburn or regurgitation. Ranitidine 450 mg a day or placebo was used only for 7 days with a 3-day washout. Asthma symptom scores improved in only 3 of 15 patients; there was no objective change in the peak flows or the need for rescue medications. This was a reasonable population of asthmatic patients to study, although the glaring study limitation is the very short duration of antireflux therapy and the absence of documented control of GERD.

Ekstrom et al. recruited 48 asthmatics, all of whom had symptomatic GERD, from the outpatient medical clinic for a 4-week intervention with placebo or ranitidine 150 mg bid with a 2-week washout period (45). The severity of acid reflux was modest by pH testing (4.4% time pH <4); 27 of 48 subjects had a positive acid perfusion test. The subjects had moderate-to-severe asthma that was well characterized, and 32 of 48 patients were documented to be on inhaled corticosteroids. Importantly, 20 of 48 patients were on oral prednisone therapy with a dose of about 6.5 mg per day. These authors showed symptomatic improvement in GERD but did not objectively assess reflux control. Overall, there was only a slight improvement in the nighttime asthma score, which was statistically significant at $p = 0.02$. There was no change in the morning or day symptom scores, nor objective changes in FEV_1, peak flow, or histamine challenge studies. There was only a trivial reduction in inhaled β-agonist use.

D. Promotility Agents

The newer promotility agents, cisapride and domperidone, are effective in the treatment of mild to moderate heartburn and healing mild erosive esophagitis. This class of drugs improves GERD by augmenting lower esophageal sphincter pressure, increasing the amplitude of esophageal peristalsis and thereby improving acid clearance, and accelerating gastric emptying or modifying duodenogastric reflux, if abnormal.

The older agents, including metoclopramide and bethanechol, were not particularly effective and were frequently associated with central nervous system side effects. Recent data shows that cisapride at 10 mg four times a day (30 minutes before meals and bedtime) provides symptomatic relief and healing of esophagitis with results comparable to cimetidine 400 mg four times a day or ranitidine 150 mg twice a day and superior to placebo. Some data suggest there may be benefit combining the promotility agents with the H_2-RAs (41). Additional data suggest that cisapride may be effective as maintenance therapy for mild GERD (48). Side effects are infrequent with cisapride and usually consist of abdominal pain, diarrhea, or headaches. Metoclopramide has been used safely as an antiemetic agent during pregnancy for about 30 years. A recent case-control study found no adverse effects on mother or child in pregnant women taking cisapride (49). This study included 129 pregnant women, 88 of whom took cisapride during the period of fetal organogenesis.

Table 3 H$_2$-Receptor Antagonists for Asthma and Gastroesophageal Reflux: Summary of Adult Studies

Author, year (Ref.)	Design	N	Age (M/F)	Recruitment source	Duration of intervention (weeks)	Dose	Baseline GERD Dx	Baseline GERD Severity
Goodall, 1981 (43)	Placebo crossover	20	54 (13/7)	Pulmonary outpatient clinic	6 weeks	Cim 200 mg 4x/day	GERD Sx 19/20 18/20 had abnormal studies	?
Harper, 1987 (47)	Case series, pre-, post- comparison	15	48 (6/9)	N/S	8 weeks	Ran 150 mg bid	GERD Sx 15/15 10/15 erosive esophagitis	Total reflux scores 22.5% ± 9.9%
Nagel, 1988 (44)	Placebo crossover	15	42 (11/4)	Pulmonary clinic	1 week, 3 days washout	Ran 450 mg/d	7/15 GERD Sx	pH < 4 20% time
Ekstrom, 1988 (45)	Placebo crossover	48	58 (30/18)	Outpatient medical clinic	4 weeks, 2 week run-in & washout	Ran 150 mg bid	48/48 GERD Sx	GERD > 1×/wk pH < 4 4.4% time 27/48 ⊕ acid-perf
Larrain, 1991 (46)	Placebo controlled 3-arm randomized trial	28 = plac 27 = exp	P: 42 (9/19) Exp: 43 (2/25)	Pulmonary clinic	6 months	Cim 300 mg 4x/d	P: 19/28 GERD Sx Exp. 19/27	N/S

Abbreviations: cim = cimetidine; ran = ranitidine; β-MDI = β-agonist metered dose inhaler; ICs = inhaled corticosteroids; N/S = not specified; FEV$_1$ = forced expiratory volume in one second; PEF = peak expiratory flow; PC$_{20}$ = provocative concentration of methacholine for 20% drop in FEV$_1$; EGD = endoscopy; P: placebo; exp = experimental.

There are no published studies of promotility agents being used to treat adult asthmatics with GERD. An initial study in the pediatric literature assessed 29 infants (2–4 months old) with GERD by 24-hour pH monitoring (50). These babies were randomized to therapy with body positional treatment in addition to either placebo or cisapride. After 16 days of therapy, there was no significant

	Baseline asthma		Documentation of acid control		Asthma outcome measures			
Dx	Severity	Rx	Sx	pH	Sx	PEF or FEV1	βMDI/ pred use	Comment
Nocturnal asthma 20/20	Mild-mod? baseline FEV_1 ~ 2.0; 17 years	N/A	Sx scope improved in 14/20 c/w plac From 2.8 to 1.8 (p < 0.02)	—	Night score ↓ed 1.1 →0.7 (p < 0.05) Day: NO Δ	x4/day FEV_1 no Δ	No Δ in β-MDI	
Non-allergic asthma Nocturnal asthma Sx in 4/15	Baseline FEV_1 72%, ratio 0.95	N/S	Improved Sx scores	Clear-cut improvement in EGD 10/10 Resolved in 8/10	Increase in Sx for 4 weeks, then sig. decrease	Increase in FEV_1 to 82% (p < .001)	Meds increased in 6/15, decreased 3/15, unchanged in 4/15	No good correlation between changes in FEV_1 & esoph Sx Some patients were pretreated with pred before procedures— FEV_1 may have ↑ed
Well established 21/44 had nocturnal asthma	N/S	N/S	No	No	Scores improved 3/15 deteriorated 5/15 6/15 → no Δ	No Δ AM, PM PEF	No Δ	44 adult asthmatics underwent pH test 21/44 → "morning dipping" with noct Sx, ↓ PEF 15/44 → GERD → participated in study (34%) No difference in GERD in patients with noct Sx c/w others
Well established	Mod-severe; 14 years	ICs = 32/48 Theo ~ 26/48 Pred = 20/48 (dose ~ 6.5/ d) p.o β-MDI ~ 33/48	GERD score improved from 0.69 → 053 (p.0002)	No	Sight improvement in night asthma score 0.61 → 0.53 (p.02) No Δ in AM or day score	No Δ in PEF, FEV_1, PC_{20}	β-MDI puffs/ day 5.6 → 5.0	350 asthma pts N = w/asthma & GERD Sx > 1×/wk Most rep Sx improvement occurred in pts with hx reflux assoc. resp Sx (N = 27) 21 (No hx of reflux-assoc. Sx) → no response
N/S	Duration: 10 years	P: 14/28 pred Exp: 13/27 NO ICs	N/A	N/A	N/S	N/S	N/S	

change in the total number of reflux episodes or the number of reflux episodes per hour; however, there was a significant improvement in the number of reflux episodes lasting longer than 5 minutes (0.30 vs. 0.59, $p < 0.01$), suggesting that cisapride improves acid clearance. A second study evaluated the effect of cisapride on esophageal pH monitoring in children with reflux-associated cough (51). Over one month, there was a significant reduction in the cough episodes at night as well as GERD (time pH < 4 decreased from 18 to 4.9%). A third uncontrolled, open-label study included 36 children with poorly controlled asthma and no GERD symptoms (52). By pH test, 27 of 36 patients (75%) were documented to have GERD. All patients were treated with cisapride (0.2 mg/kg qid) for 3 months. A second pH test was performed on 11 of 27 patients, 9 of whom showed improvement in time pH < 4. Follow-up was conducted for 19 patients, 16 (84%) of whom had improvement in asthma symptoms.

E. H^+/K^+-ATPase (Acid Proton Pump) Inhibitors

Acid-forming parietal cells are located in the oxyntic glands of the gastric fundus and body (53). Parietal cell membrane consists of three classes of receptors: histamine, paracrine receptors; gastrin, endocrine receptors; and acetylcholine, neurocrine (muscarinic) receptors. All of these receptors mediate the final step in the secretion of hydrochloric acid through the activation of the H^+/K^+-ATPase acid pump (Fig. 1).

Antacids have no direct influence on gastric acid secretion. These agents work by neutralizing the gastric acid secreted by parietal cells, thereby increasing the intragastric pH. Both the H_2-RAs and the acid proton pump inhibitors block acid secretion. The H_2-RAs only block histamine receptors on the parietal cell surface, while the gastrin and acetylcholine receptors are still active and can augment acid secretion. On activation of the parietal cell, the enzyme H^+/K^+-ATPase moves from the cytoplasm of the gastric parietal cell to the permeable membrane of the secretory canaliculi (53). The enzyme can subsequently move hydrogen ions across the parietal cell membrane in exchange for potassium ions, thereby secreting acid with a pH of about 1.0. Both of the currently available substituted benzimidazoles, more commonly called proton pump inhibitors (omeprazole and lansoprazole), bind to the H^+/K^+-ATPase enzyme, thus blocking acid secretion. Since both nocturnal and meal-stimulated acid is inhibited, a single morning dose maintains gastric pH at 5 or more for almost 24 hours, decreases gastric volume by over 60%, and normalizes acid reflux parameters in over 80% of patients (53–55). Proton pump inhibitors have no effect on LES pressure.

In general, the proton pump inhibitors are well tolerated and easy to use with dosing either once or twice a day. Rare side effects include diarrhea, nausea, dry mouth, dizziness, weakness, headaches, and numbness. However, these side effects are no more common than with placebo in the published studies. Omeprazole inhibits selective isoenzymes of the cytochrome P-450 system, including those that metabolize phenytoin, warfarin sodium, and benzodiazepines (but not theophylline or propranolol). On the other hand, lansoprazole minimally inhibits this system and does not appear to significantly interfere with other drugs metabolized by cytochrome P-450 (56). The major long-term concern with using the proton pump inhibitors is their ability to produce a profound decrease in gastric acid secretion. This causes a secondary increase in gastrin production from the

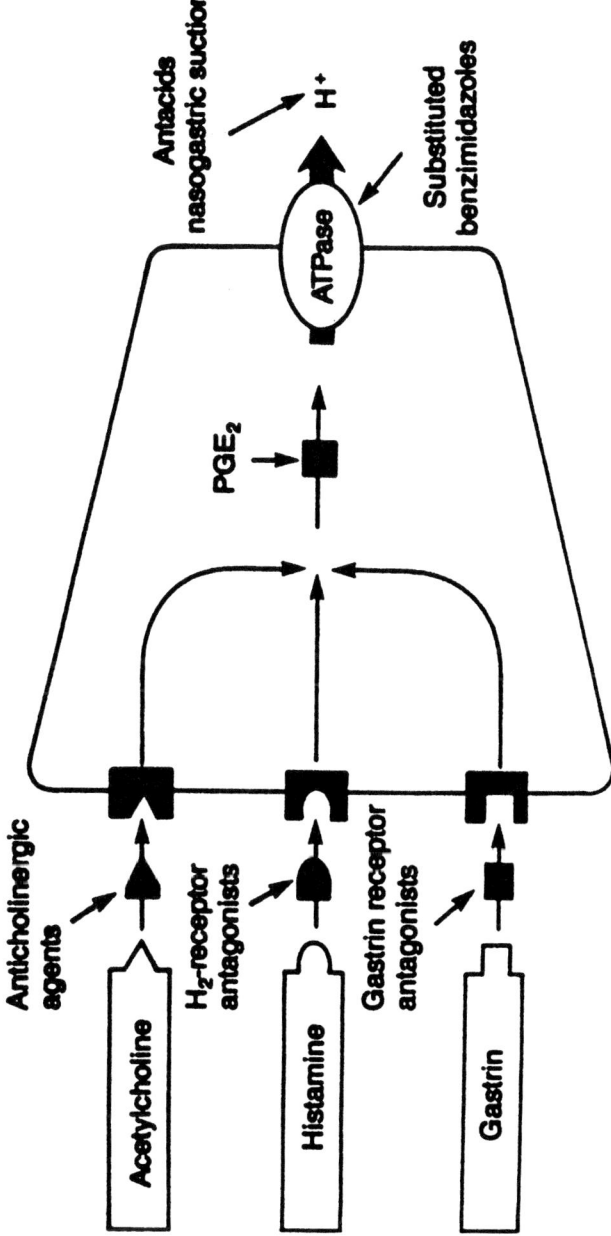

Figure 1 Schematic diagram of a parietal cell: therapeutic modalities to affect gastric acid. Parietal cell membrane consists of three classes of receptors: acetylcholine, histamine, and gastrin. The final step in the secretion of hydrochloric acid is through the activation of ATPase acid pump. PGE_2 = prostaglandin E_2. Substituted benzimidazoles are proton pump inhibitors. See text for details.

antral G cells resulting in serum gastrin levels usually elevated two to four times above basal values. Theoretically, the prolonged gastrin stimulation of enterochromaffin-like (ECL) cells could produce tropic changes in the gastric mucosa and was associated with increased stomach tumors in rats treated for a lifetime. However, the human experience with the use of proton pump inhibition is over a decade, with a number of patients with severe reflux esophagitis taking the drug continuously for up to 10 years. There have not been any reported cases of gastric carcinoid-type tumors in patients receiving either omeprazole or lansoprazole, with the rare exception of subjects with the multiple endocrine adenomatosis syndrome where carcinoid tumors are commonly seen. The consensus from published studies and close FDA surveillance of the proton pump inhibitors is that these drugs at therapeutic doses are unlikely to result in clinically significant gastric mucosal change (54–58).

Several recent review articles have summarized the results of randomized trials with proton pump inhibition in the treatment of GERD (40,53). Controlled studies show that omeprazole 20 mg q AM or lansoprazole 30 mg q AM completely abolishes reflux symptoms in most patients with GERD, regardless of severity, usually within 5 weeks. Complete healing of esophagitis occurs after 8 weeks in more than 80% of patients (54,59,60). In those not healing after this time, prolonged therapy with the same dose or increasing the dose usually results in nearly 100% healing (58), although rare patients are resistant to doses of omeprazole up to 180 mg/day (61). Head-to-head comparison found no efficacy difference in either symptom relief or esophagitis healing between omeprazole or lansoprazole (60). Both proton pump inhibitors also are effective for maintaining the healing of esophagitis, regardless of severity, for up to 1 year in controlled studies and up to 5 years in case series (55,58). The maintenance dose of omeprazole is usually 20 mg/day, while lansoprazole 15 mg/day is as effective as 30 mg for long-term therapy. Proton pump inhibitors are the most effective medical therapy for treating GERD, with long-term results similar to antireflux surgery.

Table 4 summarizes the available published adult studies of omeprazole therapy for asthma and associated GERD. Studies with lansoprazole have not been published. Available data include one case report (62), three placebo-controlled crossover trials (63–65), and one prospective case series with a pretest and posttest comparison (66).

A case report by Depla et al. describes a 25-year-old man with well-established severe bronchial asthma with nocturnal symptoms (62). This patient's maintenance asthma therapy included inhaled albuterol, ipratropium, beclomethasone (dose not specified), as well as oral terbutaline. Esophageal pH monitoring found severe GERD with pH < 4 for 27% of the time. The upper endoscopy was normal. The patient previously failed reflux therapy with ranitidine 750 mg per day. Omeprazole 20 mg a day was used for 12 weeks. There was dramatic improvement in GERD based on symptoms as well as a follow-up pH study showing the acid-exposure time decreasing to normal value (4%). From an asthma standpoint, there was definite improvement in symptoms, FEV_1 (before-therapy range was 2.85–3.81 liters; after-therapy value was 3.88 liters), and a reduction in the need for nocturnal rescue inhaler therapy. This single-case report well documents improvement in both GERD and asthma with the institution of omeprazole therapy.

Ford et al. conducted a placebo-controlled crossover trial of 11 asthmatics, with a mean age of 63 years, recruited from an outpatient pulmonary clinic, with a history of asthma predating GERD (3.4 years vs. 6.4 months) (63). All patients had moderately severe bronchial asthma with nocturnal symptoms despite treatment with inhaled corticosteroids in 8 of 11 patients (dose not specified). All patients also had symptoms of GERD, an abnormal upper endoscopy, and a positive pH test in 9 of 11 patients. Patients were randomly assigned to initial therapy with omeprazole 20 mg per day or placebo, and after a one-week washout, they were crossed over to the other agent. Although reflux symptoms resolved in 5 of 10 patients on omeprazole therapy, there was no objective documentation of acid control by follow-up pH testing. Compliance with therapy was noted to be 96%. One patient was excluded secondary to uncontrolled asthma. There was no improvement in asthma control based on day or nighttime symptom scores, a.m. and p.m. peak expiratory flows, or any changes in the need for inhaled rescue bronchodilators. The strength of this study included well-characterized asthmatics, and most patients had continued respiratory symptoms despite being on maintenance therapy with inhaled corticosteroids. The obvious limitations included the short treatment duration, lack of documented reflux control, and perhaps an inadequate dose of omeprazole.

Meier et al. conducted a 6-week placebo-controlled crossover study of 15 adult asthmatics with symptomatic GERD with a 2-week wash-in period and a 2-week run-in period (64). Omeprazole 20 mg twice a day was used. Patients were recruited from an allergy clinic from a database of 3000 asthmatics. Thirty of these patients had both asthma and weekly heartburn, of which 15 were selected for the study. All patients had well-established asthma, but there was no mention of nocturnal asthmatic symptoms nor a description of baseline asthma therapy. All subjects had moderately severe GERD with endoscopic esophagitis and an average distal acid exposure over 24 hours of 22%. Asthma outcome was described as omeprazole-responsive asthma based on a 20% improvement in FEV_1 (4 of 15 or 27%) or non–omeprazole-responsive asthma (11 of 15 or 73%). Data regarding symptoms or medication use were not given. Follow-up endoscopy showed that all responders had endoscopic healing of esophagitis, whereas only 6 of 11 nonresponders showed esophagitis healing. Overall, this study suggests that a subset of asthmatics with GERD will respond to aggressive antireflux therapy. This subset may have been larger if there was titration of omeprazole dose to documented control of GER and/or a longer duration of therapy with

Table 4 Omeprazole for Asthma and Gastroesophageal Reflux: Summary of Adult Studies

Author, year (Ref.)	Design	N	Age (M/F)	Recruitment source	Smoking hx	Duration of intervention (weeks)	Dose	Baseline GERD Dx	Baseline GERD Severity
Depla, 1988 (62)	Case report	1	25 (M)	N/S	N/S	12 weeks	20 mg qd	Normal EGD ⊕ pH test	pH < 4 27% time Severe
Ford, 1994 (63)	Placebo crossover	11	63 (6/5)	Pulmonary OPD	2/11	4 weeks, with 1 week run-in, washout	20 mg qd	11/11 EGD 9/11 pH test 11/11 Sx	N/S
Meier, 1994 (64)	Placebo crossover	15	49 (9/6)	Allergy clinic Database of 3000 asthma 30 = asthma & weekly pyrosis 15 = met criteria	None	6 weeks, 2 weeks run-in, washout	20 mg bid	N/S	EGD esophageal and/or distal pH < 4 22% time
Harding, 1996 (65)	Prospective case series, pretest & posttest comparison	30	46 (12/18)	Outpatient pulmonary medical clinics	None	4 weeks pre-therapy phase; 4–12 weeks acid titration phase; 3 mos acid suppressive doses	20–60 mg/d	29/30 (97%) had increased distal acid reflux; 1 only abn proximal reflux	Sx ≥ 2x/mo pH < 4 12.1% time
Teichtahl, 1996 (66)	Placebo crossover	20	46 (12/8)	Outpatient pulmonary/ gastroenterology clinics	None	4 weeks, with 2 weeks run-in, washout	40 mg/d	19/20 had GERD Sx	pH < 4 12% time

FEV$_1$ = Forced expiratory volume in one second; EGD = endoscopy; Sx = symptoms; PEF = peak expiratory flow; ORA = omeprazole responsive asthma; terb = terbutaline; beclo = beclomethasone; ICs = inhaled corticosteroids; β-MDI = β-agonist metered dose inhaler; N/S = not specified.

complete esophagitis healing in the additional 5 patients. This is particularly relevant in this study as the nonresponders had two to three times the amount of distal or proximal GER compared to the responders. However, this study also confirms that some patients with asthma and symptomatic GERD may not improve their asthma despite good control of reflux symptoms and healing of esophagitis.

The largest study to date, as well as the most compelling data for treating GERD in asthma, was published by Harding et al. involving 30 adult asthmatics with GERD (65). This study included 18 women and 12 men (mean age 46 years), who were recruited from the outpatient pulmonary and medical clinics for this prospective, open-label case series with pretest and posttest comparisons of the effects of therapy. All patients had control of acid reflux documented by serial pH testing using doses of omeprazole ranging between 20 and 60 mg/day. There was a 4-week run-in period, followed by a period of 4–12 weeks for acid titration,

	Baseline asthma		Documentation of acid control		Asthma outcome measures			
Dx	Severity	Rx	Sx	pH	Sx	PEF or FEV$_1$	β-MDI pred use	Comment
Well established Nocturnal Sx	Severe	Albuterol Ipratropium P.O. terb Beclo (? dose)	Yes	Yes (4% pH <)	Improved	FEV$_1$ 2.85– 3.81 before; 3.88 after	↓ Nocturnal β-MDI	
Well established ⊕ nocturnal Sx	Moderate	ICs = 8 PRN β-MDI	No GER Sx in 5/10 on omep	No	Night: 0: 1 ± 0.6 P: 1 ± 0.7 day 0: 1 ± 0.7 P: 0.9 ± 0.7	AM PEF: O = 262 ± 86 P = 255 ± 86 PM PEF: O: 280 ± 81 P: 277 ± 78		1 pt excluded 2° to uncontrolled asthma Asthma: 3.4 mos; GERD 6 mos.
Well established No mention of nocturnal Sx	N/S	N/S	0	All 4/15 om-resp. had complications esop. head 6/11 non-ORA showed complete history	N/S	4/15 = ORA FEV$_1$ ↑ed 20%	N/S	10/15 had complete healing; all ORA were complete healers Overall 27% pts ORA
Well established No mention of nocturnal Sx	Moderately severe (77%) FEV$_1$ 72%	ICs = 16/30 Pred = 15/30 Mean = 3 meds	Yes Sx score (0–84) decreased from 21.4 → 3.7	Yes (titration omep for acid supp)	Sx score (0–105) decreased from 32.2 to 19.0 20/30 were Sx responders	6/30 (20%) were PEF responders (PEF increase of 20%)	5/30 (17%) were med usage responders; 4/15 (27%) were able to reduce dose of pred > 40%	Spiro Sensormedics Morris/Polgar ? what is size of screened population, time. 30/38 completed
Well established ⊕ nocturnal Sx	FEV$_1$ 70 ±7%	Stable Rx for 1 mo. before ICs: 21/25 Pred: 3 Theo: 9	Improved in omep group c/w placebo (p < .05)	No	No change in Sx	AM PEF 76 ± 4 vs. 76 ± 4% PM PEF 82±	No change	Asthma: 275 mos; GERD: 83 mos

followed by 3 months of therapy with acid-suppressive dosages. All patients had reflux symptoms at least weekly, with 97% of the patients having increased distal acid reflux, mean total acid reflux 12.1% (normal < 5.8%). With acid suppression, the GERD symptom score dramatically improved from 21.5 to 3.7. The underlying asthma in these nonsmokers was fairly well characterized as being moderately severe; however, there was no mention of the frequency of nocturnal symptoms. At baseline, patients used a mean of three asthma medications, including inhaled corticosteroids in 16 of 30 patients and oral prednisone in 15 of 30 patients. Follow-up evaluation also showed that proton pump inhibitor therapy was effective in improving asthma control. The asthma symptom score (a range of 0 to 105) improved from 32 to 19, and 20 of 30 patients (66%) were found to have at least a 20% improvement in asthma symptoms. Lung function responders were defined as having a peak flow increase of 20% from baseline; this was seen in 6 of 30 patients (20%). The use of asthma medication decreased in 5 of 30 patients (17%), and 4 of 15 (27%) asthmatics were able to reduce their dose of prednisone by greater than 40%. Further analysis showed that the presence of regurgitation (>1 per week) or excessive proximal esophageal reflux predicted asthma response to omeprazole therapy at 100% sensitivity and a positive predictive value of 79%. The strength of this study lies in the fact that control of acid reflux was accomplished in all patients with omeprazole therapy. Also, the duration of therapy for GERD and asthma was the longest to date. The authors noted that 27% of the patients required more than 20 mg per day of omeprazole to accomplish acid suppression, 6 patients needed 40 mg, and 2 patients required 60 mg per day. Although the mean symptom score improved significantly in the group as a whole, some asthmatics improved much more dramatically (5 of 30 patients had a symptom score improve by greater than 50 points). On the other hand, the objective improvement in lung function was disappointing and clinically modest (only 6 of 30 patients had a peak flow increase of greater than 20%). This study needs to be repeated using a control group of subjects.

Teichtahl et al. conducted a placebo-controlled crossover trial for an intervention period of 4 weeks (omeprazole 40 mg) with a 2-week run-in and a 2-week washout (66). Twenty adults with asthma and GERD were recruited from outpatient pulmonary and gastroenterology clinics. Actually, 30 patients entered the run-in, 25 were randomized, and 20 finally completed the study. All patients had GERD symptoms, and a baseline pH test showed an average acid exposure time with pH <4 of 12%. Baseline asthma was well characterized as moderate disease, and all patients had nocturnal symptoms. The disease was stable for one month before the study and inhaled corticosteroids were appropriately administered in 21 of 25 patients, an additional 9 patients took theophylline and 3 patients were taking oral prednisone. The mean duration for asthma was much longer than GERD (275 months vs. 83 months). Compliance was greater than 75%. GERD symptoms were improved in the omeprazole group compared to the placebo group (p <0.05). However, there was no other documentation of acid control to assess the adequacy of dose or duration. As far as the effect on asthma is concerned, this is a negative trial as there was no change in any of the asthma-outcome measures, including symptoms, peak flows, FEV_1, airway reactivity, or the use of medications. Again, one wonders whether there was adequate control of acid reflux and whether the duration of therapy was sufficient.

IV. Surgical Therapy

The published experience with antireflux surgery for GERD in adult patients with asthma is summarized in Table 5 (46,67–71). Most of the surgical trials have a variety of design flaws including lack of a control group, poor documentation of airflow obstruction both preoperatively and postoperatively, poor documentation of baseline asthma severity and baseline asthma medical therapy, and lack of objective documentation of GERD control in the postoperative state.

Although proton pump inhibitors can relieve GERD symptoms and heal esophagitis in the vast majority of patients, this has not eliminated the need to consider surgery in a subset of patients (72). In fact, a good response to medical therapy may help to identify the subset of patients who will do well after surgery (73). Antireflux surgery should be reserved for patients with complicated GERD who will require lifetime medical therapy (74). Some indications for surgery include: (1) patient requires lifelong therapy with high-dose H_2-RAs or proton pump inhibitors, (2) refractory reflux disease with intolerable symptoms or esophagitis that has proved difficult to treat, (3) recurrent esophageal strictures, (4) esophagotracheal aspiration resulting in recurrent pneumonia, asthma, or laryngitis, or (5) bleeding from Barrett's ulcers or as a result of a hiatal hernia causing linear gastric erosions (72). Several preoperative factors influence whether and what kind of surgery is beneficial: (1) functional status of the lower esophageal sphincter and esophageal pump as assessed by the adequacy of peristalsis, (2) esophageal length, (3) presence of acid hypersecretion, (4) degree of delayed gastric emptying, and (5) relative surgical risk based on age and co-morbid diseases. Further discussion about the specific surgical procedures will be considered elsewhere (see Chap. 9).

Two studies attempted to compare medical and surgical therapy for GERD in patients with both asthma and GERD (46,70). Unfortunately, neither study used proton pump inhibitors or documented control of acid reflux by 24-hour esophageal pH testing. Also, one of these studies was published only in abstract form making critical evaluation difficult.

Larrain et al. conducted a three-arm open-label prospective long-term randomized controlled trial of medical vs. surgical treatment of GERD in 81 nonallergic asthmatics (46). The minimum follow-up period was 6 months. Patients were randomized to placebo, cimetidine 300 mg four times a day, or the Hill antireflux surgical repair for GERD. Eighty-one patients completed this study, including 28 in the placebo group, 27 in the cimetidine group, and 26 in the surgery group. Baseline GERD symptoms were present in 60 of 81 (75%) patients, and the presence of GER was documented by either barium studies or pH testing. There was no description of the underlying asthma severity, medical therapy, or the comparability of asthma disease severity in each of the three groups. It is notable that 32 of the 81 patients had a history of cigarette smoking. Asthma symptoms improved in all three groups, with the greatest improvement occurring in the surgery (77%) and cimetidine groups (74%). It is noteworthy that the placebo group also had a 36% improvement in their mean asthma score. It is important to note that despite symptom improvement, there was no statistically

Table 5 Antireflux Surgery for Adults with Asthma and GERD

Author, year (Ref.)	Design	N	Baseline GERD	Baseline asthma	Type of surgery	Medical therapy	Follow-up	Comments
Sontag (67)	Case series	13	GERD symptoms in all By pH test or endoscopy	11/13 daily BDs 7/13 steroid-dependent	N/S	N/S	1–5 yr	4/11 = stopped BDs 6/11 = reduced BDs by >50% 2/7 weaned off steroids 3/13 died after surgery
Perrin-Fayolle (68)	Case series	44	GERD symptoms in all No objective documentation	Severe $FEV_1\%$: 68% No baseline inhaled steroids	Nissen fundoplication	18/44 had a 3-month trial of medical therapy	>5 yr	Cure: 1 (2.5%) Improvement: 18 (41%) No improvement: 15 (34%)
Tardif (69)	Case series	10	GERD symptoms in all Positive pH test	Severe asthma 5/10 prednisone-dependent	N/S	N/S	21 months	GERD was cured in 8/10 Only 5/10 asthma improved, no cures Reduce prednisone 3/10

Study	Design	N	Inclusion	Comparison	Medical Rx	Duration	Results
Sontag, 1990 (70)	3-arm open-label, prospective, randomized	Total: 73 AA: 26 Ran: 24 Surg: 33	Positive pH test and esophagitis All had GERD symptoms No details	All groups were comparable No details on severity or baseline Rx	Nissen fundoplication	GERD: Ran 150 mg tid > 1 yr.	1–5 yr	Asthma improved or "cured" in 75% in surg group (c/w 9.1%, 4.3%) (? what criteria) D/C prednisone in 33% surg group (c/w 11%, 0%) Published only as an abstract
Larrain, 1991 (46)	3-arm open-label, prospective, randomized	Total: 81 Plac: 28 Cim: 27 Surg: 26	By Ba⁻ or pH test GERD symptoms in 60/81	No description of asthma severity in each group ? baseline RX 32/81 hx of smoking	Hill antireflux surgical repair	Cim 300 mg qid	6 months	Asthma symptoms improved in all 3 groups, with surg > CIM > placebo Placebo improved >40% No significant objective improvement in FEV₁
Johnson, 1996 (71)	Case series	118	GERD in all	Respiratory Sx in 63/118 ? asthma in 14/63	Fundoplication	N/S	3 yr	Relieved resp Sx 38/50 (76%) GERD improved in 43/50 (86%) Motility abnormality 17/50 (34%)

AA = antacid; Ran = ranitidine; Cim = cimetidine; BDs = bronchodilators; N/S = not specified; Ba⁺ = barium studies; Rx = therapy.

significant improvement in objective measures of airflow obstruction including FEV_1. This study did not capture ambulatory peak flow measures or peak flow variability.

Sontag et al. performed a three-arm open-label, prospective, randomized, placebo-controlled study comparing ranitidine 150 mg three times a day, surgery with the Nissen fundoplication, and placebo in asthmatics with GERD (70). A total of 73 patients completed the study—26 in the control group (who used as-needed antacids), 24 in the ranitidine group, and 33 in the surgery group. All patients had symptoms of GERD with baseline documentation of reflux by pH testing and/or endoscopy. Details were not given regarding the severity of the GERD. There was no information given regarding the baseline asthma severity, the baseline medications required to control asthma, or whether the severity and type of asthma were accounted for and matched across the three groups. The total duration of follow-up was 1–5 years. The authors concluded that asthma improved or was cured in 75% of the patients in the surgery group, compared with 9.1% in the ranitidine group and 4.3% in the placebo group. However, details were not given as to how the improvement was defined. It was also noted that 33% of the patients in the surgery group were able to discontinue oral prednisone therapy compared with 11% in the ranitidine group and none in the placebo group. Due to the overall lack of detail in this abstract, it is difficult to make further conclusions about this study.

Both the Larrain and Sontag studies are ambitious attempts to compare medical versus surgical therapies in a randomized fashion. However, they do not adequately answer the question, which subset of patients should undergo surgery for GERD in the setting of suboptimal asthma control.

V. Proposed Approach to GERD-Associated Asthma

Our approach to GERD in asthmatics is summarized in Figure 2. We favor an aggressive empiric therapy for both GERD and asthma, with judicious use of diagnostic studies. For patients with suboptimal control of asthma, based on frequent symptoms, daily use of bronchodilators, need for prednisone bursts, and emergency visits, we carefully optimize conventional asthma therapy. Based on consensus guidelines, this would include patient education, trigger-avoidance measures, appropriate use of peak flow monitoring, and daily inhaled corticosteroids in appropriate doses. For patients who continue to have poor asthma control, a careful investigation is pursued to exclude asthma mimics and search for co-morbid disease or exacerbating factors, including environmental allergies, chronic nasal and sinus disease (rhinitis, polyposis, sinusitis), pulmonary infiltrates, and gastroesophageal reflux. For patients who have symptomatic GERD and, perhaps, prominent nocturnal symptoms, we recommend specific lifestyle

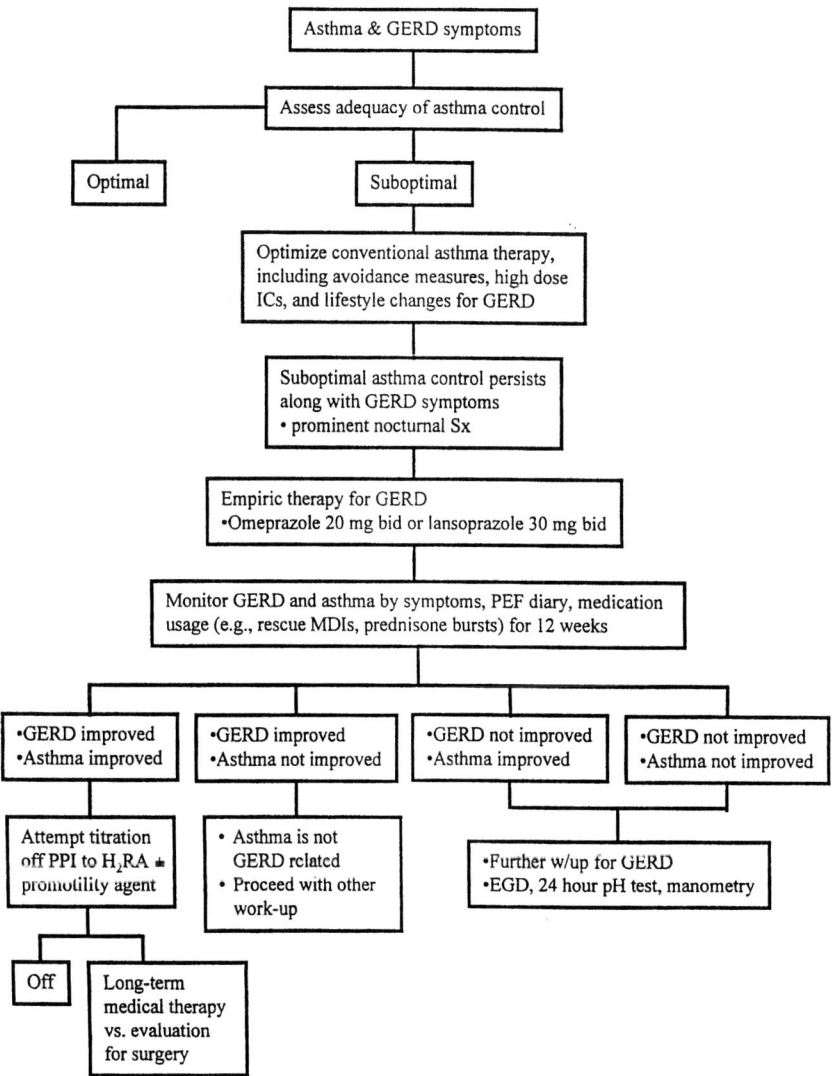

Figure 2 Proposed approach to GERD-associated asthma. For patients with suboptimal asthma control, optimize conventional asthma therapy according to guidelines including inhaled steroids. For persistent asthma, investigate comorbid disease and exclude asthma mimics. For GERD symptoms, trial of proton pump inhibitor for 12 weeks. If both asthma and GERD are improved, GERD is a significant factor that requires long-term management. See text for details. MDI: β-agonist metered dose inhaler; IC: inhaled corticosteroid; PPI: proton pump inhibitor; EGD: endoscopy; PEF: peak expiratory flow.

changes and empiric therapy with proton pump inhibitors, 12-week trial at a dose of 20 mg bid for omeprazole or 30 mg bid with lansoprazole. We subsequently monitor both GERD and asthma by symptoms, peak flow diary, and rescue medication use.

The outcome of this intervention could fall into one of four groups. Both GERD and asthma may be improved, which would suggest that GERD is an important trigger. In this subset, the next challenge is long-term management including gradual titration off proton pump inhibition to H_2-RA and/or promotility drugs, long-term proton pump inhibitor therapy, or evaluation for surgery. GERD may be improved, but asthma may remain unchanged, suggesting that GERD is not an important trigger. If GERD is not improved with an empiric trial of proton pump inhibitor, further workup should include specific diagnostic studies such as pH testing with manometry and endoscopy to ensure that acid reflux has been adequately controlled.

VI. Future Directions

Many questions remain regarding the relationship and proper therapy for GERD-associated asthma. Certainly, a large multi-institutional placebo-controlled study is needed to adequately address the efficacy of aggressive acid suppression in improving acid-related asthma symptoms. We would suggest a very high dose of proton pump inhibitor (omeprazole 40 mg bid or lansoprazole 60 mg bid) to best assure control of acid reflux, short of individual pH titration (an impossible task in a large study). The duration of the study should be at least 3–4 months, though others would argue one year since asthma exacerbation may have seasonal variations. Additionally, the therapy for asthma should be clearly defined and should include therapy as outlined by the consensus guidelines. The group to study is problematic, since many asthmatics may be ''silent'' refluxers. Therefore, a large study of all difficult to treat asthmatics, regardless of reflux symptoms, may best address the practical issue of whom to treat. By including detailed demographic analysis as well as comprehensive pulmonary and reflux evaluations (endoscopy, manometry, 24-hour pH test) and not stratifying for the symptomatic or physiologic presence of abnormal GERD, a study with adequate sample size (probably 150–200 patients per group) could help to validate or refine suggested predictors for a therapeutic response to acid suppression. If predictors are not identified but asthmatics do well with aggressive acid suppression, then an empiric trial will be the best diagnostic and therapeutic approach to these patients. If acid reflux can be defined as a common trigger for asthma, later studies can address the role of less aggressive therapy for GERD using H_2-RAs and promotility agents. Finally, cost analysis and quality-of-life studies will be necessary to assess the cost trade-offs (i.e., expensive antireflux medications vs. possibly less antiasthma medications) improvement in quality of life, and health care utilization in these patients.

We hope this review has clarified some of the problems with current medical studies assessing the treatment of GERD-associated asthma. Future directions and studies are outlined that should help to resolve this issue over the next 10 years, improving the care of our patients with asthma.

References

1. Harding SM, Richter JE. Gastroesophageal reflux disease and asthma. Sem Gastro Dis 1992; 3(3):139–150.
2. Ayres JG, Miles JF. Oesophageal reflux and asthma. Eur Respir J 1996; 9:1073–1078.
3. Locke GR, Talley NJ, Fett SL, Zinsmeister AR, Melton LJ. Prevalence and clinical spectrum of gastroesophageal reflux: a population based study in Olmstead County, Minnesota. Gastroenterology 1997; 112:1448–1456.
4. Mays EE. Intrinsic asthma in adults: association with gastroesophageal reflux. JAMA 1976; 236:2626–2628.
5. Perpina M, Ponce J, Marco V, Benlloch E, Miralbes M, Berenguer J. The prevalence of asymptomatic gastroesophageal reflux in bronchial asthma and in non-asthmatic individuals. Eur J Respir Dis 1983; 64:582–587.
6. Ducolone A, Vandevenne A, Jovin H, Grob JC, Coumaros D, Meyer C, Burghard G, Methlin G, Hollender L. Gastroesophageal reflux in patients with asthma and chronic bronchitis. Am Rev Respir Dis 1987; 135:327–332.
7. Sontag SJ, Schnell TG, Miller TQ, Khandelwal S, O'Connell S, Chejfec G, Greenlee H, Seidel WJ, Brand L. Prevalence of oesophagitis in asthmatics. Gut 1992; 33:872–876.
8. Sontag SJ, O'Connell S, Khandelwal S, Miller T, Nemchausky B, Schnell TG, Serlovsky R. Most asthmatics have gastroesophageal reflux with or without bronchodilator therapy. Gastroenterology 1990; 99:613–620.
9. Field SK, Underwood M, Brant R, Cowie RL. Prevalence of gastroesophageal reflux symptoms in asthma. Chest 1996; 109:316–322.
10. Sontag SJ, O'Connell S, Khandelwal S, Miller T, Nemchausky B, Schnell TG, Serlovsky R. Effect of positions, eating, and bronchodilators on gastroesophageal reflux in asthmatics. Dig Dis Sci 1990; 35:849–856.
11. Goldman JM, Bennett JR. Gastroesophageal reflux and asthma; a common association, but of what clinical importance? Gut 1990; 31:1–3.
12. Kavuru MS, Pien L, Litwin D, Erzurum SC, Ahmad M. Asthma: current controversies and emerging therapies. Clev Clin J Med 1995; 62:293–304.
13. National Heart, Lung, and Blood Institute. National Asthma Education and Prevention Program. Expert Panel Report 2. Guidelines for the diagnosis and management of asthma. Bethesda, MD: National Institutes of Health, 1997. Publication no. 97-4051.

14. Irwin RS, Curley FJ, French CL. Difficult-to-control asthma. Chest 1993; 103:1662–1669.
15. Kamada AK, Szefler SJ, Martin RJ, Boushey HA, Chinchilli VM, Drazen JM, Fish JE, Israel E, Lazarus SC, Lemanske RF. Issues in the use of inhaled glucocorticoids. Am J Respir Crit Care Med 1996; 153:1739–1748.
16. DeVault KR, Castell DO. Guidelines for the diagnosis and treatment of gastroesophageal reflux disease. Arch Intern Med 1995; 155:2165–2173.
17. Pope CE. Acid-reflux disorders. N Engl J Med 1994; 331:654–660.
18. Simpson WG. Gastroesophageal reflux disease and asthma. Arch Intern Med 1995; 155:798–804.
19. Howden CW, Castell DO, Cohen S, Freston JW, Orlando RC, Robinson M. The rationale for continuous maintenance treatment of reflux disease. Arch Intern Med 1995; 155:1465–1471.
20. Kitchin LI, Castell DO. Rationale and efficacy of conservative therapy for gastroesophageal reflux disease. Arch Intern Med 1991; 151:448–454.
21. Hamilton JW, Boisen RJ, Yamamoto DT, Wagner JL. Sleeping on a wedge diminishes exposure of the esophagus to refluxed acid. Dig Dis Sci 1988; 33:518–522.
22. Johnson LF, DeMeester TR. Evaluation of elevation of the head of the bed, bethanechol, and antacid form tablets on gastroesophageal reflux. Dig Dis Sci 1981; 26:673–680.
23. Dennish GW, Castell DO. Inhibiting effect of smoking on the lower esophageal sphincter. N Engl J Med 1971; 284:1136–1137.
24. Kahrilas PJ, Gupta RR. Mechanisms of acid reflux associated with cigarette smoking. Gut 1990; 31:4–10.
25. Kadakia SC, Kikendall JW, Maydonovitch C, Johnson LF. Effect of cigarette smoking on gastroesophageal reflux measured by 24-hour ambulatory esophageal pH monitoring. Am J Gastroenterol 1995; 90:1785–1790.
26. Waring JP, Eastwood TF, Austin JM, Sanowski RA. The immediate effects of cessation of cigarette smoking on gastroesophageal reflux. Am J Gastroenterol 1989; 9:1076–1078.
27. Holloway RH, Hongo M, Berger K, McCallum RW. Gastric distension: a mechanism for postprandial gastroesophageal reflux. Gastroenterology 1985; 89:779–784.
28. Becker DJ, Sinclair J, Castell DO, Wu WC. A comparison of high and low fat meals on postprandial esophageal acid exposure. Am J Gastroenterol 1989; 84(7):782–786.
29. Vitale GC, Cheadle WG, Patel B, Sadek SA, Michel ME, Cuschieri A. The effect of alcohol on nocturnal gastroesophageal reflux. JAMA 1987; 258:2077–2079.
30. Berquist WE, Rachelefsky GS, Kadden M. Effect of theophylline on gastroesophageal reflux in normal adults. J Allergy Clin Immunol 1981; 67:407–411.
31. Hubert D, Gaudric M, Guerre J, Lockhart A, Marsac J. Effect of theophylline on gastroesophageal reflux in patients with asthma. J Allergy Clin Immunol 1988; 81:1168–1174.
32. Ruzkowski CJ, Sanowski RA, Austin J, Rohwedder JJ, Waring JP. The effects of inhaled albuterol and oral theophylline on gastroesophageal reflux disease and obstructive lung disease. Arch Intern Med 1992; 152:783–785.

33. Schindlbeck NE, Heinrich C, Huber RM, Muller-Lissner SA. Effects of albuterol (salbutamol) on esophageal motility and gastroesophageal reflux in healthy volunteers. JAMA 1988; 260:3156–3158.
34. Michoud MC, Leduc T, Proulx F, Perreault S, DuSouich P, Duranceau A, Amyot R. Effect of salbutamol on gastroesophageal reflux in healthy volunteers and patients with asthma. J Allergy Clin Immunol 1991; 87:762–767.
35. Kjellen G, Tibbling L, Wranne B. Effect of conservative treatment of oesophageal dysfunction or bronchial asthma. Eur J Respir Dis 1981; 62:190–197.
36. Castell DO, Dalton CB, Becker D, Sinclair J, Castell JA. Alginic acid decreases postprandial upright gastroesophageal reflux. Dig Dis Sci 1992; 37:589–593.
37. Buts JP, Barudi C, Otte JB. Double-blind controlled study on the efficacy of sodium alginate (Gaviscon) in reducing gastroesophageal reflux assessed by 24 h continuous pH monitoring in infants and children. Eur J Pediatr 1987; 146:156–158.
38. Stanciu C, Bennett JR. Alginate-antacid in the reduction of gastro-oesophageal reflux esophagitis. Lancet 1974; 1:109–111.
39. Richter JE, Castell DO. Gastroesophageal reflux: pathogenesis, diagnosis, and therapy. Ann Intern Med 1982; 97:93–103.
40. DeVault KR, Castell DO. Current diagnosis and treatment of gastroesophageal reflux disease. Mayo Clin Proc 1994; 69:867–876.
41. Vigneri S, Termini R, Leandro G, Badalamenti S, Pantalena M, Savarino V, DiMario F, Bettaglia G, Mela GS, Pilotto A, Plebani M, Davi G. A comparison of five maintenance therapies for reflux esophagitis. N Engl J Med 1995; 333:1106–1110.
42. Magee LA, Inocencion G, Kamboj L, Rosetti F, Koren G. Safety of first trimester exposure to histamine H_2 blockers. A prospective cohort study. Dig Dis Sci 1996; 4:1145–1149.
43. Goodall RJ, Earis JE, Cooper DN, Bernstein A. Relationship between asthma and gastro-oesophageal reflux. Thorax 1981; 36:116–121.
44. Nagel RA, Brown P, Perks WH, Wilson RS, Kerr GD. Ambulatory pH monitoring of gastro-oesophageal reflux in ''morning dipper'' asthmatics. Br Med J 1988; 297: 1371–1373.
45. Ekstrom T, Lindgren BR, Tibbling L. Effects of ranitidine treatment on patients with asthma and a history of gastro-oesophageal reflux: a double blind cross over study. Thorax 1989; 44:19–23.
46. Larrain A, Carrasco E, Galleguillos F, Sepulveda R, Pope CE 2d. Medical and surgical treatment of nonallergic asthma associated with gastroesophageal reflux. Chest 1991; 99:1330–1335.
47. Harper PC, Bergren A, Kaye MD. Anti-reflux treatment in asthma: improvement in patients with associated gastroesophageal reflux. Arch Intern Med 1987; 147:56–60.
48. Blum AL, Adami B, Bouzo MH, Brandstatter G, Fumagalli J, Galmiche JP, Hebbeln H, Hentschel E, Huttemann W, Schutz E, et al. Effect of cisapride on relapse of esophagitis. A multinational, placebo-controlled trial in patients healed with an antisecretory drug. The Italian Eurocis Trialists. Dig Dis Sci 1993; 38:551–560.
49. Bailey B, Addis A, Lee A, et al. Cisapride use during human pregnancy. A prospective, controlled multicenter study. Dig Dis Sci 1997; 42:1248–1252.
50. Vandenplas Y, deRoy C, Sacre L. Cisapride decreases prolonged episodes of reflux in infants. J Pediatr Gastroenterol Nutr 1991; 12:44–47.

51. Saye Z, Forget PP. Effects of cisapride on esophageal pH monitoring in children with reflux-associated bronchopulmonary disease. J Pediatr Gastroenterol Nutr 1989; 8:327–332.
52. Tucci F, Resti M, Fontana R, Novembre E, Lami CA, Vierucci A. Gastroesophageal reflux and bronchial asthma: prevalence and effect of cisapride therapy. J Pediatr Gastroenterol Nutr 1993; 17:265–270.
53. Maton PN. Omeprazole. N Engl J Med 1991; 324:965–975.
54. Sontag SJ, Hirschowitz BI, Holt S, Robinson MG, Behar J, Berenson NN, et al. Two doses of omeprazole versus placebo in symptomatic erosive esophagitis: the US Multicenter Study. Gastroenterology 1992; 102:109–118.
55. Robinson M, Lanza F, Avner D, Haber M. Effective maintenance treatment of reflux esophagitis with low-dose lansoprazole. Ann Intern Med 1996; 124:859–867.
56. Barradell LB, Faulds D, McTavish D. Lansoprazole. A review of its pharmacodynamic and pharmacokinetic properties and its therapeutic efficacy in acid-related disorders. Drugs 1992; 44:225–250.
57. Jansen JB, Klinkenberg-Knol EC, Meuwisesen SG, DeBruijne JW, Festen HP, Snel P, et al. Effect of long-term treatment with omeprazole on serum gastrin and serum group A and C pepsinogens in patients with reflux esophagitis. Gastroenterology 1990; 99:621–628.
58. Klinkenberg-Knol EC, Festen HP, Jansen JB, Lamers CB, Nelis F, Snel P, Luckers A, Dekkers CP, Havu N, Meuwissen SG. Long-term treatment with omeprazole for refractory reflux esophagitis: efficacy and safety. Ann Intern Med 1994; 121:161–167.
59. Hatlebakk JG, Berstad A, Carling L, Svedberg LE, Unge P, Ekstrom P, et al. Lansoprazole versus omeprazole in short-term treatment of reflux oesophagitis. Results of a Scandinavian multicentre trial. Scand J Gastroenterol 1993; 28:224–228.
60. Castell DO, Richter JE, Robinson M, Sontag SJ, Haber MM. Efficacy and safety of lansoprazole in the treatment of erosive esophagitis. The Lanzoprazole Group. Am J Gastroenterol 1996; 91:1749–1757.
61. Just R, Katzka DA, Castell DO. Omeprazole failure in a patient with gastroesophageal reflux disease. Ann Intern Med 1994; 121:899.
62. Depla AC, Bartelsman JF, Roos CM, Tytgat GN, Jansen HM. Beneficial effect of omeprazole in a patient with severe bronchial asthma and gastro-oesophageal reflux. Eur Respir J 1988; 1:966–968.
63. Ford GA, Oliver PS, Prior JS, Butland RJ, Wilkinson SP. Omeprazole in the treatment of asthmatics with nocturnal symptoms and gastro-oesophageal reflux: a placebo-controlled cross-over study. Postgrad Med J 1994; 70:350–354.
64. Meier JH, McNally PR, Punja M, Freeman SR, Sudduth RH, Stocker N, Perry M, Spaulding HS. Does omeprazole (Prilosec) improve respiratory function in asthmatics with gastroesophageal reflux? A double-blind, placebo-controlled crossover study. Dig Dis Sci 1994; 39:2127–2133.
65. Harding SM, Richter JE. The role of gastroesophageal reflux in chronic cough and asthma. Chest 1997; 111:1389–1402.
66. Teichtahl H, Kronborg IJ, Yeomans ND, Robinson P. Adult asthma and gastro-oesophageal reflux: the effects of omeprazole therapy on asthma. Aust NZ J Med 1996; 26:671–676.

67. Sontag S, O'Connell S, Greenlee H, Schnell T, Chintam R, Nemchausky B, Chejfec G, Van Drunen M, Wanner J. Is gastroesophageal reflux a factor in some asthmatics? Am J Gastroenterol 1987; 82:119–126.
68. Perrin-Fayolle M, Gormand F, Braillon G, Lombard-Platet R, Vignal J, Azzar D, Forichon J, Adeleine P. Long-term results of surgical treatment for gastroesophageal reflux in asthmatic patients. Chest 1989; 96:40–45.
69. Tardif C, Nouvet TG, Denis P, Tombelaine R, Pasquis P. Surgical treatment of gastroesophageal reflux in ten patients with severe asthma. Respiration 1989; 56:115–116.
70. Sontag S, O'Connell S, Khandelwal S, Greenlee G, Chejfec B, Nemchausky T, Schnell T, Miller T, Brand L. Anti-reflux surgery in asthmatics with reflux (GER) improves pulmonary symptoms and function [abstract]. Gastroenterology 1990; 98: A128.
71. Johnson WE, Hagen JA, DeMeester TR, Kauer WKH, Ritter MP, Peters JH, Bremner CG. Outcome of respiratory symptoms after anti-reflux surgery on patients with gastroesophageal reflux disease. Arch Surg 1996; 131:489–492.
72. Peters JH, DeMeester TR. Gastroesophageal reflux. Surg Clin North Am 1993; 73: 1119–1143.
73. DeMeester TR, Bonavina L, Iascone C, Courtney JV, Skinner DB. Chronic respiratory symptoms and occult gastroesophageal reflux: a prospective clinical study and results of surgical therapy. Ann Surg 1990; 211:337–345.
74. Richter JE. Surgery for reflux disease—reflections of a gastroenterologist (editorial). N Engl J Med 1992; 326:825–827.

9

Surgical Treatment of Gastroesophageal Reflux Disease with Emphasis on Respiratory Symptoms

STEVEN R. DeMEESTER and TOM R. DeMEESTER

University of Southern California School of Medicine
Los Angeles, California

I. Introduction

Gastroesophageal reflux disease (GERD) can be defined as an increased exposure of the esophageal body to refluxed gastric contents. The etiology of this increased exposure to gastric juice is largely biomechanical, and as a consequence it is uniquely suited to surgical therapy. The three main biomechanical causes for GERD are a defective lower esophageal sphincter (LES), ineffective esophageal clearance of refluxed material, and abnormalities of the gastric reservoir that augment physiologic reflux. Of these, a structurally defective LES is the most common cause of abnormal reflux. In 60–70% of patients with GERD, the LES can manometrically be demonstrated to be defective on the basis of one or a combination of three factors: an inadequate pressure, a short overall length, or a decreased length of esophagus exposed to the positive-pressure environment of the abdomen. Many of the remaining 30–40% of patients have early disease, and in these patients the LES is intermittently defective, usually during the postprandial period, due to gastric distension. Surgical therapy is ideal in patients with a defective LES since a fundoplication augments and restores competency to the LES and prevents intermittent unfolding of the sphincter during episodes of gastric distension.

Inefficient clearance can result in abnormal esophageal exposure to refluxed gastric juice in individuals with normal LES and gastric function because of the failure to clear physiologic reflux episodes. Important factors in esophageal clearance include gravity, esophageal motor activity, salivation, and anchoring of the distal esophagus in the abdomen. Surgical correction of a hiatal hernia reanchors the esophagus in the abdomen and can improve esophageal clearance.

Finally, gastric abnormalities that contribute to GERD include acid hypersecretion, gastric dilation such as can occur with chronic aerophagia or overeating, and delayed gastric emptying. In most patients a surgical antireflux procedure will improve gastric emptying. Thus, the combination of a fundoplication and repair of hiatal hernia in patients with GERD can improve or correct each of the three main factors responsible for abnormal gastroesophageal reflux. It is important to fully evaluate the potential causes for reflux prior to consideration of surgery, since each will influence the decision for surgery as well as the selection of an antireflux repair.

II. Considerations for Surgical Therapy

In the pre–proton pump inhibitor era, the major indication for surgery was the failure of medical therapy to control a patient's symptoms. However, symptoms of heartburn are now alleviated in nearly all patients by proton pump inhibitors, albeit frequently at very large doses. Pulmonary symptoms, on the other hand, are more difficult to treat medically. Richter reported that respiratory symptoms are improved in only about 75% of patients treated with 20 mg of omeprazole twice a day, and therapy is often required for 2–3 months before any change in symptoms is noted (1).

It is important to remember that despite symptom control with pharmacologic therapy, the underlying defect remains uncorrected in these patients and reflux continues unabated. In patients with reflux-induced respiratory symptoms, pharmacologic therapy may decrease the quantity of gastric secretions and raise the pH of the refluxate. Nonetheless, reflux, pulmonary symptoms, and pulmonary injury may continue. Furthermore, any beneficial effects of pharmacologic therapy only occur if the medication is taken. Failure to take prescribed medication regularly and failure to follow the dietary and lifestyle modifications that help control reflux often causes prompt return or worsening of symptoms. On the other hand, an antireflux operation abolishes reflux and allows return to a normal diet and lifestyle, off all medication. Currently, surgical intervention is recommended for select subsets of patients with GERD, including those with risk factors for progressive or difficult-to-manage disease, those with advanced or complicated disease, those with drug dependency, and those with extraesophageal—in particular pulmonary—manifestations of reflux disease.

A. Risk Factors for Progressive or Difficult-to-Manage GERD

Mechanically Defective LES

Careful follow-up of patients with GERD has allowed the identification of several risk factors, or markers, for patients with reflux disease who are likely to have progressive or difficult-to-manage disease. The first of these risk factors is the presence of a mechanically defective LES. An incompetent sphincter allows unrestricted reflux of gastric juice into the esophagus and overwhelms the normal clearance mechanisms. This leads to progressive esophageal injury and favors the development of complications of repetitive reflux including severe esophagitis, stricture, and Barrett's metaplasia. The severity of these complications is directly related to the prevalence of a mechanically defective sphincter (2). There is a similar tendency in the occurrence of pulmonary complications. Sontag and colleagues studied the LES characteristics in patients with asthma. They reported that, compared to controls, asthmatics had significantly lower LES pressures, greater frequency of reflux episodes, and greater acid-exposure time. These findings were independent of bronchodilator medication (3).

Composition of the Refluxate

The composition of the refluxed material is another risk factor for progressive disease. Patients who reflux both gastric and duodenal juice have been found to have a higher prevalence of esophagitis and Barrett's esophagus than do patients who reflux gastric juice alone (4). Analysis of the composition of reflux in 100 patients with gastroesophageal reflux disease demonstrated that the patients with the greatest degree of mucosal injury (complicated Barrett's esophagus) were more likely to have gastroduodenal as opposed to pure gastric reflux (Fig. 1) (5). Patients with Barrett's have been shown to have both a significantly higher prevalence and duration of abnormal esophageal bilirubin exposure (a tag for duodenal juice) compared with patients who have only esophagitis (4). Furthermore, among patients with Barrett's, significantly greater esophageal bilirubin exposure has been demonstrated in those with complications of Barrett's, including stricture and dysplasia (6). Evidence is accumulating that bile salts are the noxious component in refluxed duodenal juice and that their ability to cause cellular injury is pH dependent. For bile salts to injure mucosal cells, they must be soluble and nonionized. At a pH of 7, greater than 90% of bile salts are in solution and completely ionized. However, at a pH between 2 and 7, a mixture of ionized salt and the lipophilic, nonionized acid is present. Acidification of bile to below pH 2 results in an irreversible bile acid precipitation. Thus, under normal physiologic gastric conditions, bile acids precipitate and are of minimal significance. In a more alkaline gastric environment, however, bile salts are partially dissociated and nonionized, and this nonpolar form is able to rapidly cross cell mem-

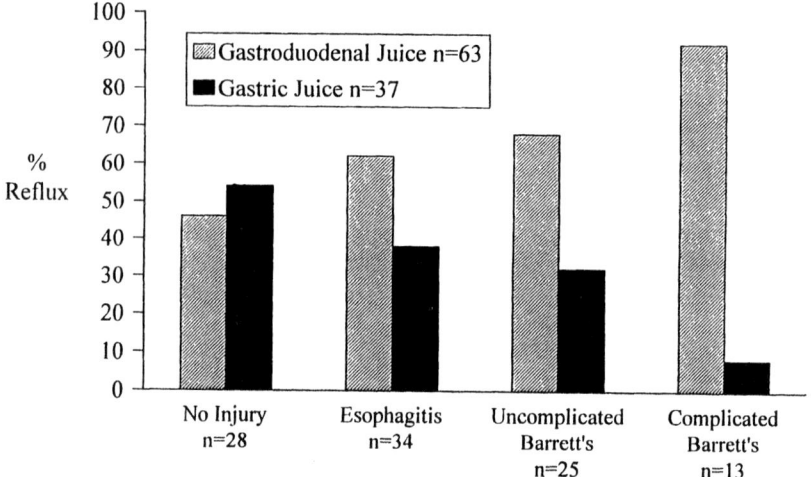

Figure 1 Prevalence of gastric and gastroduodenal reflux in patients with either no mucosal injury, esophagitis, Barrett's esophagus, or complicated Barrett's esophagus.

branes and accumulate within mucosal cells where it is toxic to the mitochondria (Fig. 2). For bile acids to remain completely ionized and innocuous in a patient with reflux disease taking acid-suppression medication, the gastric pH must be maintained above 7 for 24 hours a day, 7 days a week for the patient's lifetime. Not only is this impractical, but it is likely impossible unless very high doses of medication are used. The use of lesser doses may allow esophageal mucosal damage to occur while the patient remains relatively asymptomatic (4).

Pattern of Reflux and Extent of Esophagitis

Studies of numerous patients with reflux disease have demonstrated that those patients with supine and bipositional reflux, as opposed to upright reflux, tend to have more severe LES dysfunction and reflux disease (7). Current studies suggest that initially reflux occurs in the upright position during the postprandial period. Repetitive injury of the mucosa within the sphincter leads to the loss of sphincter function and supine reflux occurs. Esophageal body function initially compensates for reflux episodes occurring during the upright and awake periods by rapidly clearing the refluxed material. However, with bipositional reflux, esophageal body function begins to fail and severe esophagitis ensues (Fig. 3). Consequently, those patients found to have severe esophagitis at initial endoscopy are apt to be bipositional refluxers and to have a structurally defective sphincter

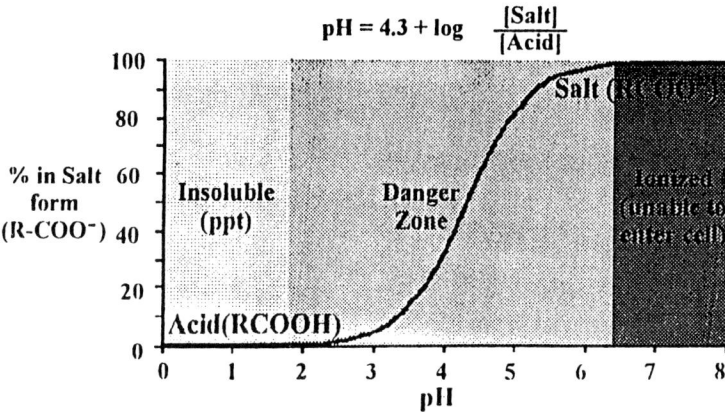

Figure 2 Dissociation curve for bile acids. Only the soluble, nonionized form of bile acids are able to cross cell membranes, accumulate, and become toxic to the mitochondria. At pH < 2 essentially all the bile acids are in an insoluble, precipitated state, while at pH > 7 the bile acids are fully ionized. Thus, the conditions necessary to produce the injurious form of bile acids exist in the partially alkaline environment of the incompletely acid-suppressed stomach.

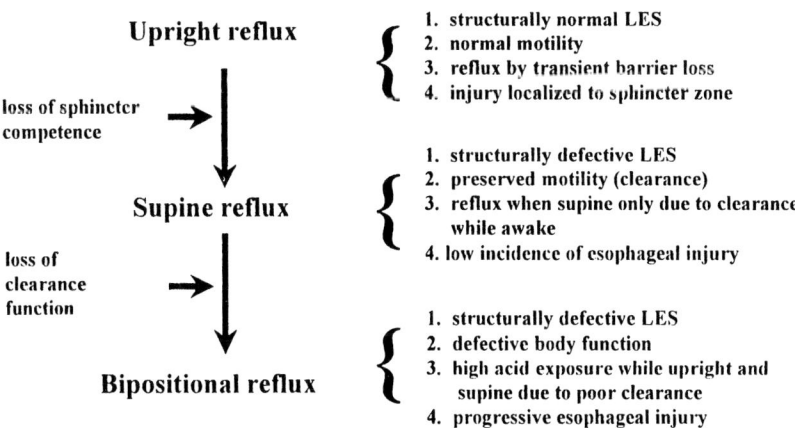

Figure 3 Postulated mechanism for the progression of reflux disease from disease confined to the lower esophageal sphincter to disease that has exploded into the esophagus.

and poor esophageal clearance. They are thus at increased risk for progressive or difficult-to-manage disease and should be considered for surgical therapy.

Genetic Factors

Males with reflux disease are more prone to develop Barrett's metaplasia than are women, and young men have many years ahead in which to develop a complication of their reflux disease. In addition, patients with increased esophageal exposure to gastric juice and a family history of Barrett's or esophageal adenocarcinoma may have a genetic predisposition toward the development of intestinal metaplasia, dysplasia, and cancer.

B. Advanced or Complicated GERD

A strong indication for surgical correction of reflux disease is the presence of advanced disease. This includes patients with complications of reflux such as stricture or Barrett's metaplasia. Appropriate management of a reflux stricture requires control of the reflux with an antireflux procedure in combination with dilatation of the stricture. Similarly, the proper therapy for a patient with Barrett's esophagus is an antireflux procedure. Evidence suggests that surgery reduces the risk for progression of metaplasia, formation of a Barrett's ulcer, and the development of dysplasia or adenocarcinoma (8,9).

C. Drug-Dependent GERD

While proton pump inhibitors are extremely effective in healing esophagitis and relieving symptoms of reflux, they only work if they are taken. Hetzel et al. found that within 6 months of stopping proton pump inhibitor medication, >80% of patients had recurrence of symptoms and esophagitis (10). Furthermore, patients who respond to a course of medical therapy but have recurrence of symptoms within 4 weeks after cessation of therapy are prone to drug dependency (2). This usually means life-long maintenance therapy with proton pump inhibitors, often with the need for dose escalation to stop breakthrough symptoms or persistent mucosal injury. Thus, a relative surgical indication is the patient who is drug dependent and unwilling to accept the inconvenience, expense, or side effects of life-long medication, as well as the dietary and lifestyle modifications imposed by their reflux disease.

D. Respiratory Manifestations of GERD

An increasingly more important group of patients who benefit from antireflux surgery are those with atypical and extraesophageal manifestations of reflux disease. These patients suffer from chest pain, chronic cough or throat clearing, wheezing, episodes of nocturnal choking and/or waking up with gastric contents in the mouth, apnic spells, hoarseness, laryngitis, or recurrent pneumonia. The end stage of repetitive pulmonary injury from reflux is bronchiectasis or pulmonary fibrosis. At the University of Southern California at least one patient has undergone bilateral lung transplantation for pulmonary fibrosis ultimately found to be secondary to chronic reflux and aspiration. Any patient with respiratory symptoms secondary to reflux should be considered for antireflux surgery, as these patients respond poorly to medical therapy compared to patients with heartburn symptoms. Despite the decrease in gastric acid secretion and neutralization of gastric pH with proton pump inhibitors, reflux, aspiration, and respiratory symptoms often persist.

Respiratory symptoms can occur with overt as well as occult gastroesophageal reflux. In patients with overt symptoms of reflux, such as regurgitation and heartburn, it is typically not difficult to recognize that reflux may be a contributing factor to the respiratory problem. However, in patients who seek medical attention for respiratory symptoms with occult reflux, a high index of suspicion will be necessary to make the diagnosis. Even with direct questioning few of these patients have typical heartburn or regurgitation symptoms (Fig. 4). Compared to patients who present with symptoms of heartburn, endoscopic esophagitis appears to be less common in patients with laryngeal or respiratory symptoms (11).

In patients with respiratory complaints consideration must be given to the possibility that gastroesophageal reflux is responsible, even in the absence of symptoms or endoscopic findings suggesting reflux. Evaluation of these patients requires 24-hour esophageal pH monitoring, often with two probes. Donnelly et

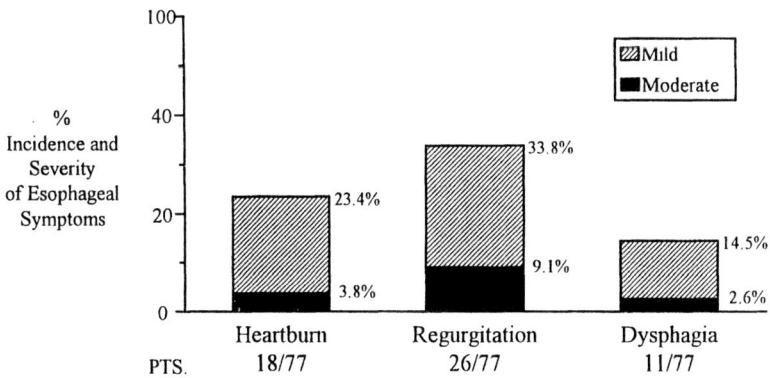

Figure 4 The incidence and severity of esophageal symptoms in 77 patients with chronic respiratory complaints resistant to medical therapy. Ultimately 54 of the 77 patients (70%) were demonstrated to have increased esophageal acid exposure on 24-hour pH monitoring.

al. (12) as well as Jack and colleagues (13) have reported using simultaneous tracheal and esophageal pH monitoring to diagnose patients with respiratory symptoms caused by reflux. Tracheal pH should stay consistently above 6, and any dip below pH 6 is definitive evidence for reflux and aspiration. Katz monitored 10 nonsmoking patients who complained of hoarseness with dual pH probes (14). The proximal probe was placed 2 cm above the upper sphincter in the hypopharynx, and a drop to or below pH 4 in the proximal probe was found in 7 of the 10 patients. Three of these 7 patients had normal 24-hour acid exposure at the lower probe and would have been classified as not having reflux. Of importance, these patients were upright refluxers with high-frequency, short-duration reflux episodes. Dobhan and Castell, also using dual probes but with the upper probe located in the proximal esophagus, have shown that acid exposure below pH 4 occurs at the proximal probe in less than 1% of the total time and 0% of the supine time in normal volunteers (15). Subsequently, in a retrospective analysis of 54 patients with pulmonary symptoms suspected to be related to reflux who underwent 24-hour pH monitoring with dual probes, Schnatz and Castell found that 33% of patients had reflux only into the distal esophagus, 55% had a combination of distal and proximal reflux, and 12% had reflux only in the proximal esophagus (16). Without using a proximal pH probe, those patients with normal distal esophageal acid exposure but abnormal proximal exposure would have been missed. This study also pointed out the importance of documenting abnormal esophageal reflux in patients with respiratory symptoms prior to treatment. In the group of 54 patients, all with respiratory symptoms believed to be secondary to gastroesophageal reflux, 24-hour pH monitoring was normal in 22% of patients. While 71% of the patients with abnormal esophageal acid exposure documented on 24-hour pH monitoring reported an improvement in their respiratory symptoms with medical treatment, none of the patients with normal esophageal acid exposure on 24-hour pH monitoring had relief of respiratory symptoms with medical therapy.

One must exercise caution, however, when excluding gastroesophageal reflux as a cause or contributing factor in patients with respiratory symptoms on the basis of one normal 24-hour pH monitoring study. Tracheal irritation and respiratory symptoms can persist for up to one week following a significant aspiration episode (17). Consequently, respiratory symptoms during a 24-hour pH test that do not correlate with a reflux episode do not exclude the possibility that intermittent episodes of reflux-induced aspiration are the cause. It is possible that intermittent aspiration episodes too infrequent to document on one 24-hour pH monitoring may produce chronic respiratory symptoms.

On the other hand, just documenting abnormal esophageal acid exposure 5 cm above the lower esophageal sphincter on 24-hour pH monitoring in patients with respiratory symptoms alone is inadequate to conclude that reflux is the cause of the respiratory symptoms (18). It is important to correlate the timing of respiratory symptoms with a reflux episode, since we now know that while reflux can stimulate the onset of respiratory symptoms, it is also true that respiratory symptoms can precede and initiate an episode of reflux. Simultaneous ambulatory esophageal manometry and pH monitoring is one technique whereby the chronology and occurrence of reflux and respiratory symptoms can be evaluated, and the primary or secondary nature of the reflux determined (Fig. 5). This distinction is critical in evaluating patients with only respiratory symptoms for antireflux surgery, since patients whose reflux episodes are induced by respiratory symptoms such as cough or wheezing will not be helped by a fundoplication (18). Furthermore, treatment of the primary respiratory disorder in these patients often not only improves their respiratory symptoms, but also decreases reflux episodes (19). The best results following fundoplication have been in patients with respiratory symptoms that developed during or within 3 minutes after a reflux episode (18).

Another important factor in patients with respiratory symptoms secondary to reflux is the function of the esophageal body. Studies have shown that in patients with reflux disease there is a direct correlation between the number of respiratory symptoms and the prevalence of a motility abnormality (Fig. 6). Overall, 45% of patients with reflux-induced respiratory disorders were found to have abnormalities in esophageal contractility or wave progression (18). The dysmotility in these patients interferes with the ability of the esophagus to clear refluxed acid, particularly in the supine position, and nonperistaltic contractions facilitate the propulsion of esophageal contents retrograde up into the pharynx. As a consequence of this intermittent aspiration of swallowed saliva and food, patients with motility disorders of the esophageal body tend to have respiratory symptoms that persist after antireflux surgery.

Sontag and colleagues have speculated that aspiration of refluxed acid may initially sensitize the pulmonary tree to a variety of other stimuli and that as the process progresses, reflux and aspiration of acid become more obscure. Antireflux surgery at this stage may prevent acid-induced wheezing, but a hypersensitive pulmonary tree may still be prone to bronchospasm in response to other stimuli (20). Consequently, the results of ambulatory pH monitoring are not always predictive of which patients will symptomatically benefit most from antireflux surgery. Figure 7 is the algorithm we use to make a decision for surgery in a patient with respiratory symptoms secondary to occult gastroesophageal reflux.

While there are few absolute requirements or contraindications for an antireflux operation, there are guidelines as to which patients with respiratory symptoms are most likely to receive the greatest benefit from surgery. In general, patients most likely to have a good outcome after a fundoplication will preoperatively demonstrate:

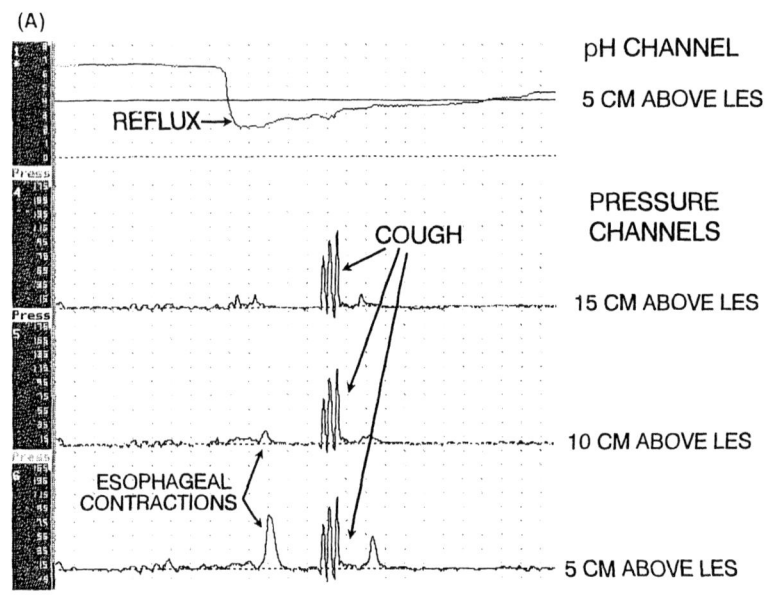
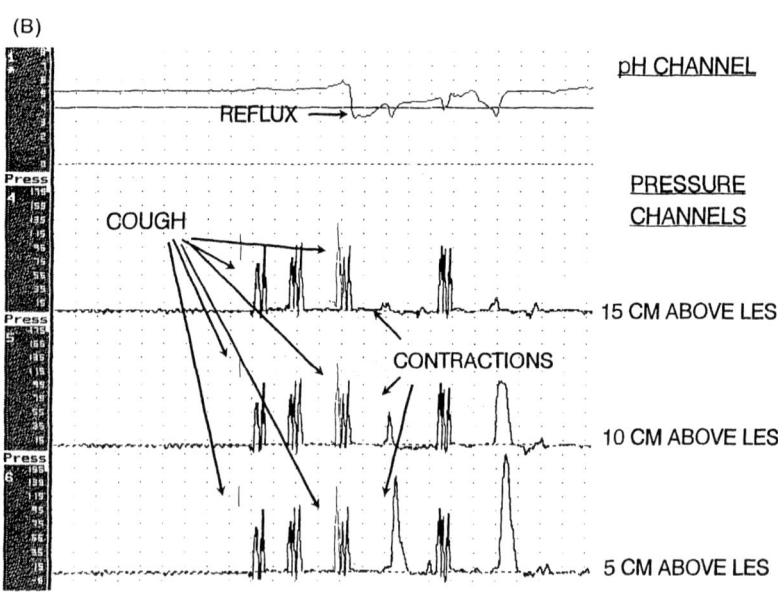

1. Increased esophageal exposure to gastric juice on 24-hour esophageal pH monitoring of the distal esophagus 5 cm above the lower esophageal sphincter
2. Increased esophageal exposure to gastric juice on 24-hour pH monitoring of the proximal esophagus 1 cm below the cricopharyngeal sphincter
3. Respiratory symptoms that occur simultaneously with or within 3 minutes after an episode of reflux documented on 24-hour pH monitoring
4. A structurally or dynamically defective LES by manometry
5. Normal gastric emptying
6. Normal esophageal body motility
7. Improvement or relief of symptoms with acid-suppression medication

III. Factors to Consider When Choosing the Proper Antireflux Procedure

After selecting patients who likely would benefit from an antireflux procedure, the approach and type of fundoplication needs to be determined. The operation should be tailored to the patient's physiology. Important factors to consider include esophageal length, esophageal body motility, the patient's age and overall health, coexistent respiratory disease or pulmonary pathology, body mass index (obesity), and a history of previous upper abdominal or gastric surgery including a prior failed antireflux procedure.

A. Esophageal Length

Perhaps the key initial determinant of the approach for an antireflux operation is the surgeon's judgment of esophageal length. This is an all-important issue, because any repair that is done under tension is likely to fail. An absolute determinant of adequate length has not been identified; however, there are several clues to suggest the potential for esophageal shortening. The first clue is the finding

---

Figure 5 (A) The technique of simultaneous ambulatory esophageal manometry and pH monitoring allows objective documentation of reflux associated with respiratory symptoms. The abrupt increase in intrathoracic pressure that occurs with coughing is recorded by the intrathoracic pressure transducers and is easily recognized by the simultaneous nature and steep slope of the pressure recording. Coughing that occurs soon after the onset of a reflux episode may be the result of occult aspiration of refluxed gastric juice or a reflex brought on by esophageal acidification. (B) On the other hand, the increase in intra-abdominal pressure that occurs with coughing may overcome the antireflux mechanism and produce a reflux episode.

of a sliding hiatal hernia that will not reduce radiographically in the upright position. A Type III, or combined sliding and paraesophageal hernia with a partial or complete intrathoracic stomach seldom reduces spontaneously, yet many of these patients have adequate esophageal length after intraoperative esophageal mobilization. Thus, nonreducibility of the hernia, like all clues, is not an absolute; rather, it is a warning sign to the surgeon that a short esophagus may be present. Similarly, the finding of more than 5 cm between the endoscopically identified gastroesophageal junction and the diaphragmatic crura suggests the potential for esophageal shortening. Lastly, both Barrett's esophagus and esophageal strictures are commonly associated with shortening of the esophagus.

When esophageal shortening is suspected, a transthoracic approach allows complete mobilization of the esophagus up to the level of the aortic arch. Careful division of vagal branches to the left and right pulmonary hilum and separation of the esophagus from the left mainstem bronchus are important aspects of esophageal mobilization and are best done transthoracically. With complete mobilization, often sufficient esophageal length is gained to allow an antireflux procedure to be accomplished without the addition of an esophageal lengthening procedure. In general, we have found that if the esophagogastric junction, marked intraoperatively with a stitch, can be reduced 2 cm below the crura, then a Nissen fundoplication can be performed with acceptable tension. Construction of a Belsey partial

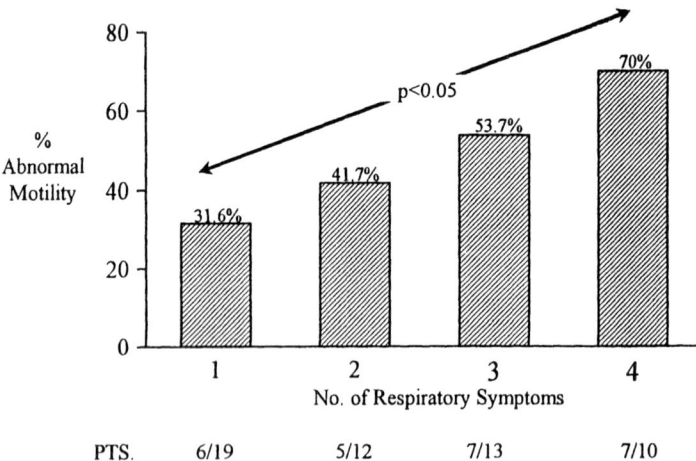

Figure 6 Prevalence of abnormal esophageal motility defined as ≥20% abnormal esophageal contractions (simultaneous or dropped waves) in 54 patients with respiratory symptoms and increased esophageal acid exposure, stratified according to the number of reported respiratory complaints.

Surgical Treatment of GERD

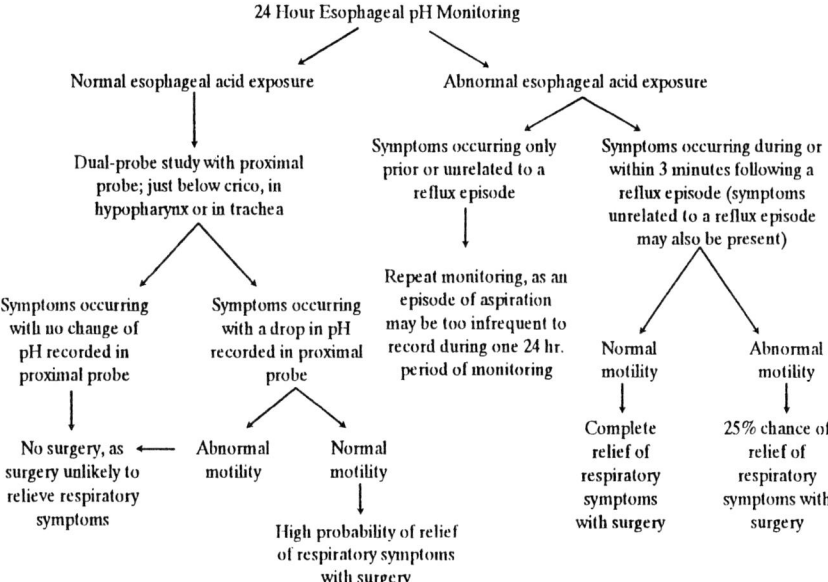

Figure 7 Proposed management algorithm to select patients with unexplained recalcitrant respiratory symptoms for antireflux surgery.

fundoplication, on the other hand, requires 4 cm of intra-abdominal esophagus, and, consequently, more often requires the addition of an esophageal lengthening procedure.

B. Esophageal Motility

Another critical factor to consider when choosing the proper antireflux operation is the status of the patient's esophageal body. Poor esophageal motility not only influences the choice of antireflux procedure, but it has a direct bearing on the anticipated outcome of the surgery as well. Patients who demonstrate peristaltic contraction amplitudes of 20 mmHg or less in the distal three-fifths of the esophagus are considered to have poor motility, as are those with a named motility disorder such as scleroderma. These patients are at risk for postoperative dysphagia since the outflow resistance of the reconstructed cardia after a complete fundoplication may exceed the peristaltic power of the body of the esophagus.

In patients with abnormal wave progression down the esophagus, such as those with nonspecific motility disorders consisting of >10% dropped waves or >20% segmental simultaneous contractions, a complete fundoplication is not associated with an increased incidence of postoperative dysphagia in our experience (21). In contrast, a patient with the manometric criteria of a named motility disorder characterized by a specific abnormal wave progression such as diffuse spasm is likely to continue to experience dysphagia after a fundoplication. For patients with reflux disease and documented poor motility, the preferred operation is a transthoracic partial fundoplication (Belsey Mark IV). A transabdominal laparoscopic option recently gaining favor is the Toupet procedure. An important observation is that esophageal shortening and poor motility often occur together, and a number of these patients will require both a gastroplasty to lengthen the esophagus and a partial fundoplication to prevent reflux (Fig. 8).

C. Factors Favoring a Transthoracic Approach

Relative indications for a transthoracic approach include obesity, prior upper abdominal operations including previous antireflux procedures, and the presence of pulmonary pathology in the left lung that requires operative evaluation or treatment. Traditionally, transthoracic antireflux operations are done through a left thoracotomy since exposure of the esophageal hiatus and diaphragmatic crura are limited from the right chest. An important indication for a transthoracic approach is evidence of a shortened esophagus by barium esophagram or endoscopy.

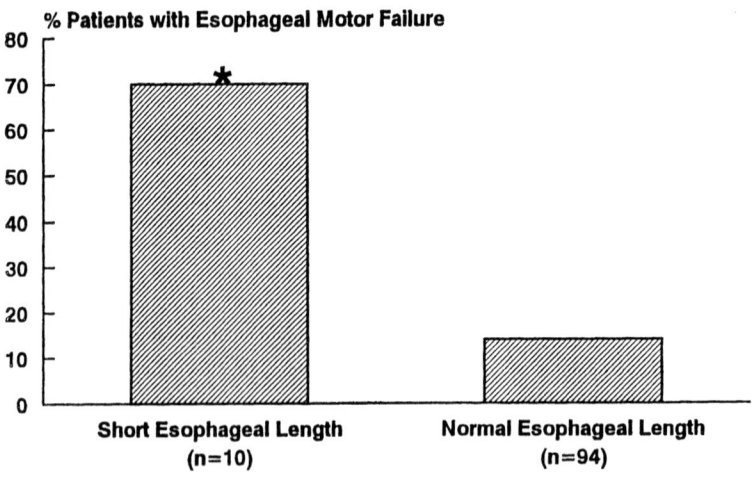

Figure 8 Prevalence of esophageal motor disorders in patients with and without short esophageal length.

D. Factors Favoring a Transabdominal Approach

Clearly, laparoscopic antireflux surgery is associated with shorter hospital stays, improved postoperative comfort, and an earlier return to normal activities compared to an open abdominal or thoracic procedure. Any patient without a specific indication for a thoracic approach should be considered for a laparoscopic fundoplication. Prior abdominal operations not directed at the stomach or esophagus have not made laparoscopic fundoplication excessively difficult and do not represent a contraindication. Extensive adhesions may necessitate innovative or additional port placement.

IV. Types of Antireflux Operations

A. Complete Fundoplication

Antireflux operations are divided into those that create a complete, or 360° fundoplication and those that create a partial fundoplication. The complete fundoplication was devised by Rudolf Nissen in 1956, and in addition to being one of the easiest to teach and learn, it continues to be the most commonly performed and the most effective antireflux procedure. The Nissen fundoplication can be done as an open transabdominal, an open transthoracic, or a laparoscopic procedure. Worldwide experience with the open Nissen procedure has demonstrated that it is an effective and durable antireflux repair associated with minimal side effects, particularly when the modifications of a very short (1–2 cm) and loose fundoplication are incorporated. Our extensive experience with the Nissen procedure has convinced us of the importance of complete fundic mobilization with division of the short gastric vessels, routine crural closure, and the creation of a loose, short fundoplication under no tension. We secure the anterior and posterior fundus to each other and the esophagus using a single pledgeted mattress suture with a 60 Fr bougie in place to size the fundoplication. Numerous reports have found that greater than 90% of adults and children continue to have relief of their reflux symptoms 10 years after a Nissen fundoplication.

Since the introduction of the laparoscopic Nissen fundoplication in 1991, many patients have benefited from the reduced hospital stay, less discomfort, and quicker return to work offered by the minimally invasive laparoscopic technique. Importantly, the technical details of performing the Nissen fundoplication are maintained in the laparoscopic approach, and thus similar excellent long-term relief of symptoms as has been demonstrated in the open procedure should be obtainable. Reports of individual and institutional experiences with several hundred laparoscopic Nissen fundoplications confirm excellent short-term results (22); however, 10-year follow-up of a large series of patients is not yet available.

In patients with a shortened esophagus on preoperative evaluation, a transthoracic approach is currently recommended. After complete esophageal mobilization is accomplished, esophageal length can be assessed, and, if necessary, an esophageal lengthening procedure can be performed. If the G-E junction can be placed 2 cm below the crura, we have found that a Nissen fundoplication can be performed with acceptable tension. In our experience, the transthoracic Nissen is associated with the best long-term relief of symptoms and lowest rate of failure of any of the available antireflux procedures or approaches (23).

B. Partial Fundoplication

The oldest and most commonly performed partial fundoplication is the Belsey Mark IV fundoplication. Described in 1952 by Ronald Belsey, it represents the fourth and final variant of the procedure. It requires a transthoracic approach and consists of a 270° anterior fundoplication. It is a more difficult procedure than the Nissen fundoplication, and Dr. Belsey noted differences in the outcome when he versus others on his staff performed the operation. Nonetheless, long-term follow up is available on large numbers of patients, and the symptomatic recurrence rate after 10 years is 14.7% (24). It is important to recognize, though, that recurrence rates increase to 45% in patients with preoperative severe esophagitis and stricture. It is now recognized that this is due to the amount of esophageal shortening commonly associated with this degree of esophageal pathology. Consequently, a Collis gastroplasty should be added to the Belsey partial fundoplication in this setting. Horbach and colleagues assessed symptoms, esophagitis on endoscopy, and the results of 24-hour pH monitoring on a group of 37 patients before and after Belsey fundoplication (25). They reported that following operation 81% of patients had relief of their reflux symptoms and endoscopic resolution of esophagitis. Normalization of total reflux time was obtained in 73% of the 37 patients. These values are somewhat less than what is reported following a complete (Nissen) fundoplication and suggest that a partial fundoplication is not as effective a barrier to reflux as a complete fundoplication.

The Toupet partial fundoplication, described in 1963 by Andre Toupet, was developed in an attempt to decrease the incidence of postoperative dysphagia and gas bloat symptoms that were seen frequently after a Nissen fundoplication at that time. The Toupet procedure and subsequent modifications consist of a posterior 180–270° partial fundoplication, as opposed to the anterior placement of the Belsey partial fundoplication. Originally done as an open transabdominal procedure, it is now also performed laparoscopically. While no long-term laparoscopic follow-up is available yet, the open Toupet procedure is reported to provide excellent relief of reflux symptoms in 90% of patients with up to 10 years of follow-up (26). In a series of laparoscopic Toupet procedures reported by Mosnier et al., early postoperative dysphagia was reported to be as high as 45%, but no patient continued to complain of dysphagia beyond 2 months (27). In our opinion, the major advantage of the Toupet procedure is that it offers a laparoscopic alternative to the traditional transthoracic Belsey fundoplication for those patients with poor esophageal motility but no shortening.

C. Gastropexy Procedures

The Hill repair was first introduced in 1967 by Lucius Hill as an alternative to the Nissen and Belsey fundoplications. It, like the other procedures, has undergone several modifications and refinements. As opposed to all other antireflux operations, the Hill procedure is not a fundoplication. Instead, it attempts to recreate a normal angle of entry of the esophagus into the stomach by anchoring the gastroesophageal junction in the abdomen at the level of the crural decussation just anterior to the aorta, and thereby reestablish normal geometry to the gastroesophageal junction. By suturing the gastroesophageal junction posteriorly to the preaortic fascia, the normal angle of His is reconstructed and the gastroesophageal reflux barrier is restored. An important adjunct to the operation is the use of intraoperative manometry to calibrate the repair. Using this technique, Low and Hill reported subjective good or excellent results in 88% of patients a mean of 17 years after the open Hill procedure (28). In 1994 Hill and colleagues described their early results with the laparoscopic Hill procedure in 40 patients (29). After a mean follow-up of 10 months, subjective good or excellent results were obtained in 92% of patients, and 24-hour pH monitoring showed no abnormal reflux in 91% of patients. In this series, nine patients with pulmonary symptoms including aspiration, asthma, pulmonary fibrosis, or chronic laryngitis underwent a laparoscopic Hill procedure. Improvement or resolution of symptoms occurred in six (67%). Early dysphagia was common, and 15% of patients required one or more postoperative dilatations.

D. Esophageal Lengthening Procedure

In some patients, chronic inflammation has so shortened the body of the esophagus that despite complete intrathoracic mobilization there is insufficient length to allow construction of a tension-free fundoplication. The esophagus in these patients can be lengthened by means of a gastroplasty, described by J. Leigh Collis in 1961. This procedure creates 3–5 cm of neo-esophagus utilizing the lesser curve of the stomach around which a fundoplication is placed. The antireflux repair can then be placed below the diaphragm without tension. This segment of neo-esophagus, created from the lesser curve and gastrocardial junction, lacks peristalsis. We therefore favor a Belsey partial fundoplication in combination with the Collis gastroplasty, although others combine a Nissen fundoplication with Collis gastroplasty and report good results (30).

Traditionally, creation of a Collis gastroplasty required a transthoracic approach; however, techniques have recently evolved for the construction of a transabdominal Collis gastroplasty utilizing a combination of stapling devices. Only limited experience with this approach is available, yet early results of this procedure in combination with a Nissen or Toupet fundoplication done via an open abdominal or laparoscopic technique have been encouraging. Given the inability to adequately mobilize the esophagus with an abdominal approach, it is probably best if the transabdominal Collis procedure is utilized only in those patients thought to have sufficient esophageal length preoperatively, but intraoperatively were found to have a shortened esophagus such that an antireflux procedure alone would be under excessive tension.

V. Surgical Complications

Important operative complications include gastroparesis from vagal nerve injury, dysphagia, recurrent reflux, chest pain from gastric ischemia caused by herniation of the repair into the chest, and the gas bloat syndrome.

A. Gastroparesis

Vagal nerve injury is usually well tolerated provided it is unilateral. Bilateral disruption is known to produce gastric stasis, and, if recognized at the time of the operation, a gastric drainage procedure should be added to the fundoplication. Typically, vagal nerve injury is not a significant problem at the first operation, but in redo fundoplications it can be very difficult to identify and preserve the vagi.

B. Dysphagia

Postoperative dysphagia is a significant source of concern for both the patient and the surgeon when it occurs. There are a number of factors to consider when analyzing this problem. Abnormal esophageal motility and dysphagia are both frequently associated with reflux disease. Our group reported a preoperative prevalence of dysphagia to some degree in 65% of 100 consecutive patients with reflux who underwent a Nissen fundoplication (21). Forty-four of the 100 patients had abnormal esophageal body motility. Postoperatively, with elimination of reflux and repair of any associated hiatal hernia, the prevalence and severity of dysphagia was markedly improved in these patients (Fig. 9). Mild dysphagia may be present for up to 3 months after an antireflux operation and is likely related to postoperative tissue edema. However, persistent postoperative dysphagia in a patient without dysphagia preoperatively implies a mechanical problem.

Dysphagia induced by a fundoplication typically results either from not matching the fundoplication performed to the patient's physiology, or from a technical failure in constructing the fundoplication. Patients with marked loss of esophageal function who have contraction amplitudes of less than 20 mmHg

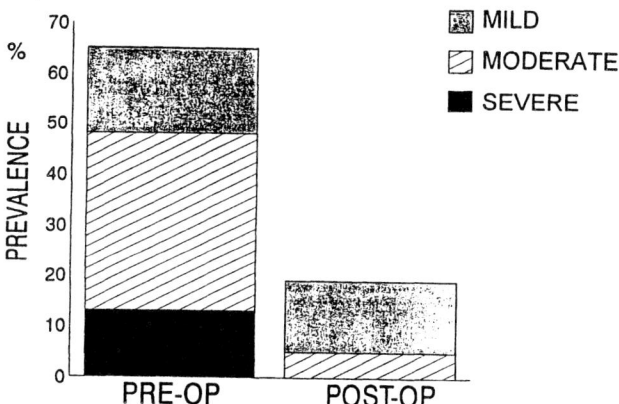

Figure 9 Prevalence and severity of dysphagia for all patients before and after Nissen fundoplication. Approximately half of the patients had moderate to severe dysphagia before operation. Both prevalence and severity markedly improved after Nissen fundoplication.

throughout the lower three-fifths of the esophageal body on preoperative manometry are at risk for dysphagia after a Nissen fundoplication. In this setting we prefer a partial fundoplication, since a complete fundoplication may prove to have too much outflow resistance for the severely impaired esophagus. Dysphagia can also be induced by an improperly constructed or herniated fundoplication. A Nissen fundoplication misplaced around the stomach (the so-called "slipped Nissen"), or a fundoplication that is too long or too tight, or one that has herniated into the chest as a consequence of disruption of the hiatal closure can produce dysphagia. These are all technical mishaps that should be rare but are important to look for in evaluating the postfundoplication patient with persistent dysphagia. Table 1 reviews the reasons for a failed antireflux procedure in 65 patients who underwent a repeat operation. To minimize the occurrence of dysphagia related to a Nissen that is too long or tight, we recommend a very short (1 cm) fundoplication that is very loose or "floppy," as it is performed over a 60 Fr bougie. Using these techniques, persistent or intermittent dysphagia of a degree that does not require bougienage has been reduced to 3% after Nissen fundoplication (31). Dysphagia requiring bougienage following the procedure is extremely rare.

C. Recurrent Reflux

Recurrent reflux implies disruption of the fundoplication. Typically, excessive tension secondary to an unrecognized short esophagus is the major culprit for

Table 1 Reasons for Failure of Prior Antireflux Procedure in 65 Patients Who Underwent Remedial Surgery

Reasons for failure	No. of procedures (%)
Placement of wrap around stomach	22 (31)
Disrupted fundoplication	17 (24)
Herniation of repair into chest	12 (17)
Too long or too tight a wrap	5 (7)
Operative damage to lower esophagus	4 (6)
Primary motility disorder of the esophagus	5 (7)
Ineffective but intact repair	5 (7)
Total	70

both herniation of the repair into the chest and disruption of the fundoplication. In some patients with herniation of an intact fundoplication into the chest, no hiatal closure was performed as part of the antireflux repair. Several series have reported a high incidence of this complication without hiatal closure, and thus crural closure should be a standard part of an antireflux procedure in all patients. Previously, in patients with a short esophagus the antireflux repair was deliberately left within the chest. Patients in whom the repair herniated into the chest or was deliberately placed in the chest have a 20% incidence of gastric ischemia and perforation as a consequence of the inability to belch. This leads to intrathoracic distension of the stomach, as well as tissue ischemia caused by the compression and stretching of the gastric vessels as they pass through the hiatus. As a consequence, any repair left in the chest is in a precarious state and should be revised.

D. Gas Bloat Syndrome

Gas bloat syndrome refers to a condition whereby patients, typically after a complete fundoplication, feel bloated and are unable to belch and relieve gastric distension. We have found that mild gastric bloating is present in 11–23% of patients after antireflux surgery (31). However, this symptom has likely been overemphasized as a surgical complication, since others have found that the prevalence of bloating was similar in medically treated GERD patients. This complaint is probably related to the habit of excessive air swallowing learned by many patients with GERD in an attempt to clear the esophagus of refluxed acid. Most patients are unable to belch after a Nissen procedure and are likely to notice some mild bloating as well as increased flatus, but this tends to decrease with time as the habit of air swallowing is unlearned.

E. Comparison of Complications in Open Versus Laparoscopic Antireflux Surgery

Laparoscopic antireflux surgery is well known to have an associated learning curve during which there is a higher incidence of complications including the need for conversion to an open procedure. This learning curve lasts for about 25 cases, after which laparoscopic antireflux surgery has an extremely low incidence of morbidity and mortality. Importantly, every effort is made to perform the fundoplication similarly to how it is performed in the open procedure. Thus, it is hoped that rate and nature of complications will be similar or less frequent than after an open procedure. Probably the most common complication, if it can be called that, of laparoscopic antireflux surgery is the need to convert to an open procedure. Often the need to open is based on poor visualization due to a large left lobe of the liver, adhesions, or obesity. Rarely is it related to bleeding or perforation of the esophagus, stomach, or bowel. Conversion rates in the published major series range from 0.5 to 14% but decrease to less than 1% in most centers as experience increases. Intraoperative splenic injury necessitating splenectomy in reported series of open procedures averages 2%, while it is 0% in several reported laparoscopic series. Likewise, mortality in open series is 0.5–1% and is 0% in reported laparoscopic series. Wound complications are reported in 4% of open procedures and <1% of laparoscopic procedures. One complication peculiar to laparoscopic surgery is gastric perforation related to traction with Babcock clamps; however, in most cases the perforation was repaired laparoscopically. The incidence of other complications, including atelectasis, pneumonia, urinary tract infection, and postoperative bleeding are quite similar between open and laparoscopic series of patients. Recurrence of reflux was noted in 3% of patients in one series of 100 open Nissen procedures followed for 10 years (31). Among 198 patients who underwent laparoscopic Nissen fundoplication, 92% of patients were free of reflux symptoms, 7% had mild symptoms, and 1% had moderate reflux symptoms a median of 12 months after the operation. In this series, the reoperation rate for failed Nissen fundoplication was 1.5% (22).

VI. Results of Surgery

Antireflux repairs are in general effective and durable. When surgically treated patients are compared to medically treated patients, they have better symptom relief and more consistent healing of esophagitis (32,33). The best studied repair is the Nissen, and several long-term follow-up studies suggest good to excellent results at 10 years in 90% of patients (Fig. 10). Partial fundoplications are not as durable. Ten-year follow-up on the Belsey Mark IV procedure suggests that symptomatically, 85% of patients have a good to excellent long-term result. Other partial repairs are less well studied, but likely will demonstrate outcomes similar

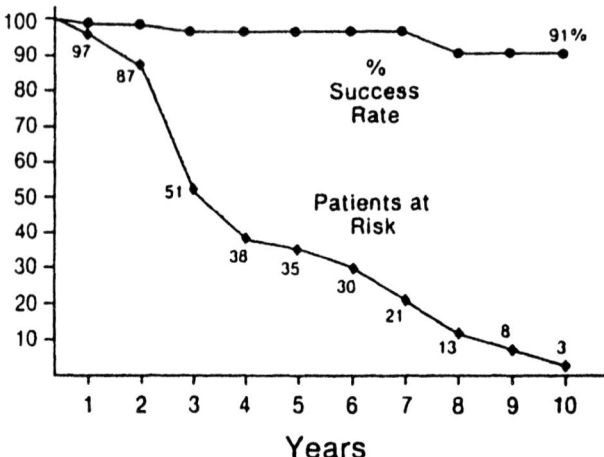

Figure 10 Actuarial success rate of the Nissen fundoplication in the control of reflux symptoms. The numbers on the lower curve represent the patients at risk for each subsequent yearly interval from which the actuarial curve was calculated.

to the Belsey. Table 2 outlines our reported results in 82 consecutive antireflux procedures that were tailored to each patient's preoperative esophageal function and length according to the algorithm shown in Figure 11 (23). Results with a Belsey partial fundoplication alone in our series are worse than when combined with a Collis gastroplasty. This perhaps indicates that patients with poor esophageal motility without shortening have intrinsic body dysfunction as opposed to dysfunction secondary to ongoing gastroesophageal reflux. An important consideration in the outcome of an antireflux procedure is that the success rate decreases incrementally with each attempt, and thus it is critical to do it right the first time (34).

In patients with gastroesophageal reflux documented by a positive 24-hour pH monitoring test, a Nissen fundoplication will abolish reflux symptoms in 91% of patients over a 10-year period (31). Relief of respiratory symptoms after an antireflux procedure, while overall better than with medical therapy, is less reliable than relief of reflux symptoms. This is because improvement is dependent upon the status of the esophageal body and the presence of normal esophageal motility. Previously, we reviewed the outcome after antireflux surgery in 50 patients with classic symptoms of reflux disease who had, in addition, a significant respiratory complaint consisting of one or more of the following: cough, shortness of breath, choking, chronic throat clearing, pleuritic chest pain, wheezing, voice change, hiccups, or frank aspiration. Antireflux surgery resulted in the complete

Table 2 Improvement in the Primary Symptom Responsible for Operation After the Various Tailored Antireflux Procedures

	N	No. of patients cured	No. of patients failed	% cured
Abdominal Nissen	49	44	5	90
Thoracic Nissen	20	19	1	95
Belsey	6	4	2	67
Collis-Belsey	10	8	2	80
Total	85	75	10	89

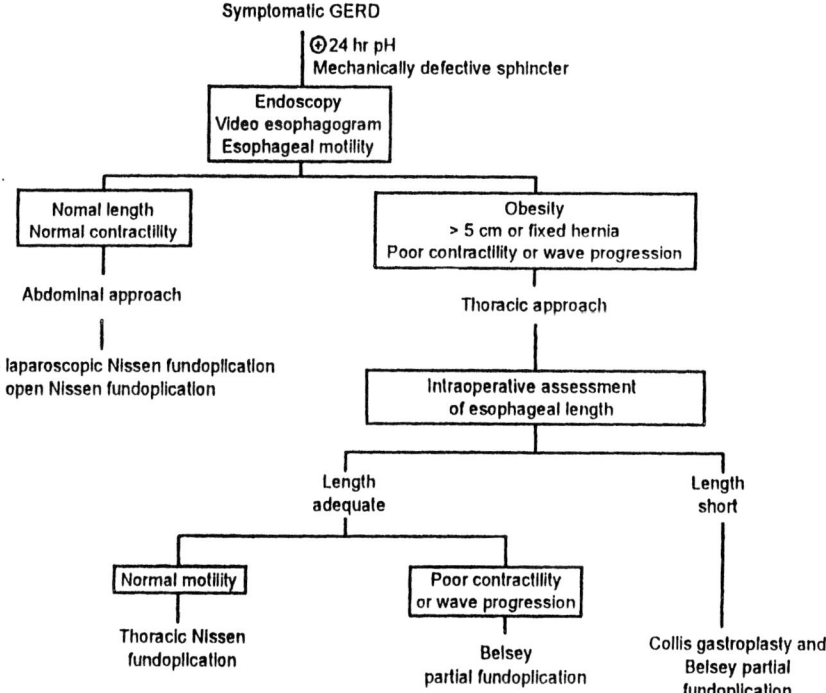

Figure 11 Algorithm for selection of antireflux procedures on the basis of clinical and functional evaluation.

alleviation or marked improvement of cough in 83%, choking in 86%, shortness of breath in 83%, throat clearing in 69%, voice change in 90%, wheezing in 64%, pleuritic chest pain in 100%, hiccups in 100%, and frank aspiration in 83%. Of the 12 patients with one or more symptoms that were not improved after surgery, nine of them (80%) had an esophageal body motor abnormality before surgery. Thirty-eight patients had normal preoperative esophageal motility, and respiratory symptoms were completely relieved after antireflux surgery in 29 of these patients (Fig. 12). Consequently, the improvement of respiratory symptoms in patients with overt gastroesophageal reflux disease treated surgically depends on two factors: whether a competent antireflux mechanism is reestablished and whether an esophageal body motor abnormality present before surgery persists after surgery (35).

An even more complex group of patients are those with pure respiratory symptoms and occult reflux. Among 17 such patients we found that while 82% were improved by an antireflux operation, only 53% of patients had their symptoms completely relieved by surgery (18). Careful analysis of these patients demonstrates that the best results were obtained in the subgroup of patients with normal esophageal motility and respiratory symptoms that occurred during or within 3 minutes after a reflux episode or were unrelated to a reflux episode in a patient with increased esophageal acid exposure (Table 3). Antireflux surgery fails to improve patients who have respiratory symptoms that precede a reflux episode. In addition, surgery is unlikely to alleviate respiratory symptoms in patients with abnormal esophageal body motility regardless of the relationship of

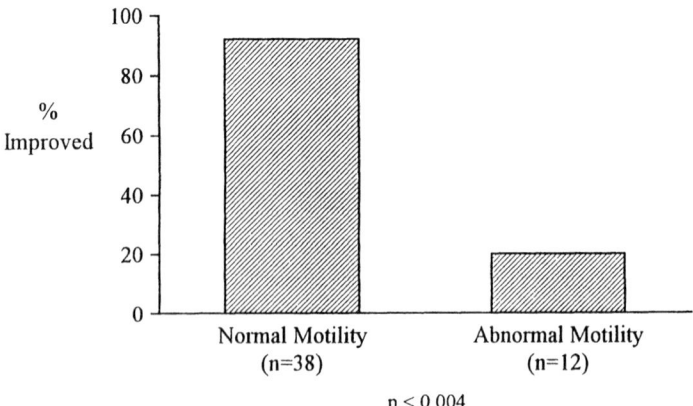

Figure 12 The outcome of antireflux surgery on respiratory symptoms in patients with overt gastroesophageal reflux disease, stratified according to the presence of a motility abnormality.

Table 3 Results of Antireflux Surgery[a]

	Success rate		
Relationship of symptoms to reflux episodes	Normal motility	Abnormal motility	Total
Related during or after an episode	2/2	2/4	4/6
Related before an episode	0/2	0/1	0/3
Unrelated to an episode	5/5	0/3	5/8
Total	7/9 (78%)	2/8 (25%)	9/17 (53%)[b]

[a] In 17 patients with respiratory symptoms found to have increased esophageal acid exposure on 24-hour pH monitoring using a single probe located 5 cm proximal to the upper border of the lower esophageal sphincter. Abnormal motility was considered present when there were >20% simultaneous or repetitive contractions during a stationary motility study.

[b] Fourteen (82%) of the patients had their symptoms improved by the operation, but for purposes of analysis only the nine patients who were completely free of symptoms after operation were considered successful.

the symptoms to reflux episodes. As a consequence of the abnormal esophageal body motility, these patients continue to aspirate esophageal contents postoperatively, and their respiratory symptoms persist.

VII. Summary

Respiratory symptoms can occur in conjunction with overt as well as occult gastroesophageal reflux. Patients with overt reflux seek medical attention for typical reflux symptoms like heartburn and regurgitation, and their respiratory complaints are secondary. Surgical fundoplication relieved the reflux symptoms in 86% of these patients, and in the majority of patients (76%) the respiratory symptoms were relieved as well. However, in patients whose respiratory symptoms are the primary reason for presentation to medical attention, occult reflux may be present and requires a high index of suspicion to diagnose. Frequently, neither typical reflux symptoms nor endoscopic esophagitis are present in these patients, and making the diagnosis requires 24-hour pH-monitoring techniques. The use of dual probes increases the likelihood of detecting abnormal reflux causing the respiratory symptoms since approximately 12% of patients with respiratory symptoms and abnormal esophageal acid exposure at an upper probe have normal acid exposure at the lower probe on 24-hour pH monitoring. Following antireflux surgery, 82% of these patients are improved, but respiratory symptoms were abolished only in those patients who had normal esophageal motility. Thus, the probability of relief of respiratory symptoms with an antireflux procedure is directly dependent upon the patient's esophageal motor function. There is also a direct correlation between the number of respiratory symptoms a patient experiences and the presence of abnormal esophageal body motility. Therefore, efforts should be made to carefully assess the esophageal motility of patients with primary respiratory symptoms secondary to occult gastroesophageal reflux. Left untreated, repetitive aspiration can lead to progressive pulmonary dysfunction and ultimately bronchiectasis, pulmonary fibrosis, and death.

References

1. Richter JE. Atypical manifestations of gastroesophageal reflux disease: pulmonary and ear, nose, and throat. Gastrointest Dis Today 1996; 5:1–7.
2. Peters JH, DeMeester TR. Gastroesophageal reflux. Surg Clin North Am 1993; 73: 1119–1144.
3. Sontag SJ, O'Connell S, Khandelwal S, Miller T, Nemchausky B, Schnell TG, Serlovsky R. Most asthmatics have gastroesophageal reflux with or without bronchodilator therapy. Gastroenterology 1990; 99:613–620.
4. Kauer WK, Peters JH, DeMeester TR, Ireland AP, Bremner CG, Hagen JA. Mixed reflux of gastric and duodenal juices is more harmful to the esophagus than gastric juice alone. Ann Surg 1995; 222:525–533.
5. DeMeester SR. Management of Barrett's esophagus free of dysplasia. Semin Thorac Cardiovasc Surg 1997; 9:279–284.
6. Fein M, Ireland AP, Ritter MP, Peters JH, Hagen JA, Bremner CG, DeMeester TR. Duodenogastric reflux potentiates the injurious effects of gastroesophageal reflux. J Gastrointest Surg 1997; 1:27–33.
7. Fein M, Ritter MP, DeMeester TR, Vos M, Hagen JA, Peters JH. Isolated upright gastroesophageal reflux is not a contraindication for antireflux surgery. Surgery 1997; 122:829–835.
8. Ortiz A, Martinez de Haro LF, Parrilla P, Morales G, Molina J, Bermejo J, Liron R, Aguilar J. Conservative treatment versus antireflux surgery in Barrett's oesophagus: long-term results of a prospective study. Br J Surg 1996; 83: 274–278.
9. Sagar PM, Ackroyd R, Hosie KB, Patterson JE, Stoddard CJ, Kingsnorth AN. Regression and progression of Barrett's oesophagus after antireflux surgery. Br J Surg 1995; 82:806–810.
10. Hetzel DJ, Dent J, Reed WD, Narielvala FM, Mackinnon WD, McCarthy JH, Mitchell B, Beveridge BR, Laurence BH, Gibson GG, Grant AK, Shearman DJC, Whitehead R, Buclke PJ. Healing and relapse of severe peptic esophagitis after treatment with omeprazole. Gastroenterology 1988; 95:903–912.
11. Bremner RM, Bremner CG, DeMeester TR. Gastroesophageal reflux: the use of pH monitoring. Curr Probl Surg 1995; 22:434–558.
12. Donnelly RJ, Berrisford RG, Jack CIA; Tran JA, Evans CC. Simultaneous tracheal and esophageal pH monitoring: investigating reflux-associated asthma. Ann Thoracic Surg 1993; 56:1029–1034.

13. Jack CIA, Walshaw MJ, Tran J, Hind CRK, Evans CC. Twenty-four-hour tracheal pH monitoring-a simple and non-hazardous investigation. Respir Med 1994; 88: 441–444.
14. Katz PO. Ambulatory esophageal and hypopharyngeal pH monitoring in patients with hoarseness. Am J Gastroenterol 1990; 85:38–40.
15. Dobhan R, Castell DO. Normal and abnormal proximal esophageal acid exposure: results of ambulatory dual-probe pH monitoring. Am J Gastroenterol 1993; 88:25–29.
16. Schnatz PF, Castell JA, Castell DO. Pulmonary symptoms associated with gastroesophageal reflux: use of ambulatory pH monitoring to diagnose and to direct therapy. Am J Gastroenterol 1996; 91:1715–1718.
17. Wynne JW, Ramphal R, Hood CI. Tracheal mucosal damage after aspiration. Am Rev Respir Dis 1981; 124:728–732.
18. DeMeester TR, Bonavina L, Iascone C, Courtney JV, Skinner DB. Chronic respiratory symptoms and occult gastroesophageal reflux. Ann Surg 1990; 211:337–345.
19. Pellegrini CA, DeMeester TR, Johnson LF, Skinner DB. Gastroesophageal reflux and pulmonary aspiration: incidence, functional abnormality, and results of surgical therapy. Surgery 1979; 86:110–119.
20. Sontag SJ, O'Connell S, Khandeleval S. Antireflux surgery in asthmatics with reflux (GER) improves pulmonary symptoms and function. Dysphagia 1991; 6:62–63.
21. Bremner RM, DeMeester TR, Crookes PF, Costantini M, Hoeft SF, Peters JH, Hagen JA. The effect of symptoms and nonspecific motility abnormalities on outcomes of surgical therapy for gastroesophageal reflux disease. J Thorac Cardiovasc Surg 1994; 107:1244–1250.
22. Hinder RA, Filipi CJ, Wetscher G, Neary P, DeMeester TR, Perdikis G. Laparoscopic Nissen fundoplication is an effective treatment for gastroesophageal reflux disease. Ann Surg 1994; 220:472–483.
23. Kauer WKH, Peters JH, DeMeester TR, Heimbucher J, Ireland AP, Bremner CG. A tailored approach to antireflux surgery. J Thorac Cardiovasc Surg 1995; 10:141–147.
24. Orringer MB, Skinner DB, Belsey R. Long-term results of the Mark IV operation for hiatal hernia and analyses of recurrences and their treatment. J Thorac Cardiovasc Surg 1972; 63:25–53.
25. Horbach JMLM, Masclee AAM, Lamers CBHW, Gooszen HG. Prospective evaluation of 24 hour ambulatory pH metry in Belsey Mark IV antireflux surgery. Gut 1994; 35:1529–1535.
26. Bensoussan AL, Yazbeck S, Carceller-Blanchard A. Results and complications of Toupet partial posterior wrap: 10 years experience. J Pediatr Surg 1994; 29:1215–1217.
27. Mosnier H, Leport J, Aubert A, Kianmanesh R, Idrissi MSS, Guivarc'h M. A 270 degree laparoscopic posterior fundoplasty in the treatment of gastroesophageal reflux. J Am Coll Surg 1995; 81:220–224.
28. Low DE, Hill LD. Fifteen to 20-year results following the Hill anti-reflux operation. J Thorac Cardiovasc Surg 1989; 98:444–450.

29. Kraemer SJM, Aye R, Kozarek RA, Hill LD. Laparoscopic Hill repair. Gastrointest Endosc 1994; 40:155–159.
30. Orringer MB, Sloan H. Combined Collis-Nissen reconstruction of the esophagogastric junction. Ann Thorac Surg 1978; 25:16–21.
31. DeMeester TR, Bonavina L, Albertucci M. Nissen fundoplication for gastroesophageal reflux disease. Ann Surg 1986; 204:9–20.
32. Spechler SJ, Department of Veteran Affairs Gastroesophageal Reflux Study Group. Comparison of medical and surgical therapy for complicated gastroesophageal reflux disease in veterans. N Engl J Med 1992; 326:786–792.
33. Isolauri J, Luostarinen M, Viljakka M, Isolauri E, Keyrilainen O, Karvonen A. Long-term comparison of antireflux surgery versus conservative therapy for reflux esophagitis. Ann Surg 1997; 25:295–299.
34. Law SKY, Hagen JA, Kauer WKH, DeMeester TR. Reoperation for failed antireflux procedures. In: Bremner CG, DeMeester TR, Peracchia A, eds. Modern Approach to Benign Esophageal Disease. St. Louis: Quality Medical Publishing, Inc., 1995: 183–190.
35. DeMeester TR, Johnson WE. Outcome of respiratory symptoms after surgical treatment of swallowing disorders. Semin Respir Crit Care Med 1995; 16:514–519.

10

GERD and Airways Disease in Children and Adolescents

STEPHEN J. McGEADY

Thomas Jefferson University
Philadelphia, Pennsylvania

I. Introduction

Investigators have recognized that some gastroesophageal reflux (GER) is a normal phenomenon in all individuals. When GER causes any symptomatic condition or histopathologic change, however, it is designated as gastroesophageal reflux disease (GERD) (1). This definition applies to children and adolescents as well as to adults. It is to those instances where GERD causes extraesophageal disease involving the respiratory tract that this chapter pertains. Technological advances have begun to elucidate the role of GERD in a variety of upper and lower respiratory diseases of childhood, and it seems likely that when more extensive data are available GERD will be shown to play a role in some of the most vexing and recalcitrant diseases of the pediatric airways. Clinicians may be able to prevent or control some cases of such diverse diseases as chronic asthma and recurrent otitis media by treatment of GERD. This chapter will review what is known of the role of GERD in these diseases as they pertain to the older child and the adolescent, as well as the contemporary methods of diagnosis and treatment of GERD in this age group. There are no available epidemiologic data on the prevalence of GERD in childhood and adolescence, but it is known that the prevalence of GER is greatly decreased from what is observed in the infant (2). There are factors in young children that might make them more vulnerable to GERD, but other features of their lives would seem to make them less severely affected. Among the protective features, it is found that children and adolescents are less apt to have the type of abdominal obesity that appears to aggravate GER in the adult. They are also less likely to smoke tobacco and to drink alcohol and strong caffeine-containing beverages, all of which are known to facilitate GER in the adult. Among factors that might aggravate GERD in the child are the anatomically shorter esophagus, which facilitates access of the refluxed material to the upper airway and surrounding structures. The longer sleep time of the child can also contribute to GERD in that upper esophageal sphincter pressure is decreased during sleep, permitting access of refluxed material to the pharynx (3), and it is known that refluxed material is cleared less efficiently during sleep (4). The volume of food intake per kilogram of body weight beginning in infancy is three times that of the adult, and this undoubtedly places stress on the mechanisms that protect against GER (5). While this ratio of food intake to body weight decreases throughout childhood, it may remain a factor in children. Added to these factors is the common custom of children to take a bedtime snack, which may include milk or ice cream. The child eating such a meal goes to bed with a full stomach, the high fat content of which may delay gastric emptying considerably. The result may be that the child develops symptoms similar to an adult with GER (6), with belching, water brash, and heartburn (7) or the GER may be silent.

II. Upper Airway Manifestation of GERD

When a connection between GER and extraesophageal disease was first noted, it was from recognition of the effects of GERD on the lower airways of children, but GERD is known to cause upper airway disease as well. In the past decade, the ability of GERD to produce upper airway disease in younger patients has received more attention. Table 1 lists the upper airway conditions that have been reported to be caused or aggravated by GERD. Advances in the technology of pH probe monitoring have led to studies in children in which the pH of the esophagus and pharynx are monitored for acid reflux simultaneously. Although single electrode studies had found decreases in pharyngeal pH in children with upper airway diseases (8), it was the simultaneous monitoring of the esophagus and pharynx that showed convincingly that GER into the esophagus led to the pharyngeal acidity associated with upper airway diseases (9). An important observation from this study was that pharyngeal pH of less than 6 was indicative of significant acidity, whereas esophageal pH of less than 4 has been considered indicative of gastric acid reflux into the esophagus. The connection between gastroesophago-pharyngeal reflux and upper airway disease is a fertile area for inves-

Table 1 Upper Respiratory Tract Disease

A. Laryngeal disease
   1. Structural—vocal cord ulcers and granulomas
   2. Functional/inflammatory
      a. Laryngomalacia
      b. Laryngitis and hoarseness
      c. Croup/spasmotic croup
      d. Stridor
B. Rhinitis and rhinopharyngitis
C. Sinusitis
D. Pharyngitis/dysphagia/throat clearing
E. Globus pharyngeus
F. Otalgia/recurrent otitis
G. Subglottic and supraglottic stenosis
H. Chronic cough

tigation, and it seems likely that in future studies this degree of reflux will be found to play a role in a number of diseases affecting the upper airway as well as upper digestive tract (10,11) (see Chap. 12).

A. Laryngeal Disease and GERD

It has been shown that refluxed acid peptic material may access the larynx in some children. Investigators have reported that GERD may lead to both structural damage to the larynx as well as milder inflammatory changes that produce a variety of functional impairments.

Structural Vocal Cord Ulcers and Granulomas

Both vocal cord ulcers and granulomas have been attributed to GERD in adult patients (12,13), and it seems likely that similar injury occurs in children. These lesions are particularly prone to occur in intubated patients where mucosal disruption from the endotracheal tube may be followed by recurrent exposure to refluxed gastric contents (14). Pediatric otolaryngologists consider it imperative to diagnose and treat GERD before undertaking surgical repair of laryngeal stenosis lest ongoing GERD cause further injury to the newly repaired larynx or delay decannulation (14–16) (see Chap. 4).

Inflammatory and Functional Laryngeal Diseases

Laryngomalacia is a condition observed almost always in infancy initially, but it may persist until later in childhood (17). The cause of laryngomalacia is floppy and redundant tissues in the area above larynx. These tissues, particularly the aryepiglottic folds, prolapse into the glottis during inspiration, causing stridorous breathing. There are several reports that associate laryngomalacia with GER. In one report 80% of a group of 20 children with laryngomalacia were shown to have GER by barium swallow studies (18). A second study of children with laryngomalacia severe enough to require surgical excision of the aryepiglottic folds showed that 50% of these children had GER, as demonstrated by barium swallow and esophagoscopy (19). Both of these authors proposed that the GERD played a role in the genesis of laryngomalacia in their subjects, suggesting that there was direct contact between refluxed acid-peptic material and the supraglottic tissues.

Laryngitis and hoarseness have often been reported in the adult literature associated with GERD (20,21). The physical finding of red inflamed vocal cords in a patient with demonstrated GER suggests acid-peptic reflux to be the cause of these changes. There is also evidence that GERD can cause hoarseness and laryngitis in children. In one case report, a child with GERD demonstrated by pH probe and esophageal biopsy had resolution of hoarseness when the reflux was treated medically (22). Other reports in pediatric subjects have described this association as well (23) and one group has recommended that reflux be considered in any case of hoarseness in a child in which the workup, including laryngoscopy, is otherwise negative (24).

Recurrent croup and acute spasmotic croup are also suspected of being caused by GERD. Most croup observed in infants and very young children is viral in etiology. This disease follows the pattern of presenting with an upper respiratory infection, which evolves into croup-like symptoms over several days. Another group of children who fit the profile of acute spasmotic croup develop croup-like symptoms but show no evidence of viral infection. In some of this latter group GERD has been thought to play a causative role (25). Children with acute spasmotic croup develop the croup-like symptoms spontaneously, tend to have frequent recurrences of these symptoms, and are sometimes suspected of being allergic. In several reports, evaluation of children with recurrent croup has revealed that a high percentage of these patients have GER. A study that evaluated reflux by several different modalities documented GER in 47% of 32 children with recurrent croup (26). Another study found no evidence of GER or pharyngeal reflux in the normal control subjects, but found both in each of the eight children who had two or more hospitalizations for croup (9).

Laryngospasm and stridor are considered together since laryngospasm may lead to stridor. Complete laryngospasm produces total occlusion of the airway, but lesser degrees produce a variably narrowed glottis, and stridor may result (27). Stridor is unlike hoarseness as the latter occurs only during speech (22), while stridor, in contrast, consists of the "crowing" respirations that are particularly noticeable on inspiration. It has been shown that stridor can be provoked by GERD in some children (28). Mechanisms by which this could occur are either laryngospasm due to vagal reflexes from acid injury to an inflamed esophagus or direct acid injury to upper airway structures. It has been shown that acid applied to the esophagus in some subjects can elicit stridorous breathing (29,30), and studies in experimental animals suggest that reflexes are an important cause of laryngospasm (31). Other reports indicating that gastric acid can reach the pharynx suggest that direct acid-peptic injury to the larynx and surrounding structures might also cause stridor from glottic narrowing (9). An underlying anatomic abnormality may be a cofactor in the development of stridor. Treatment of GERD can, in some instances, lead to elimination of stridor, thereby establishing this connection quite clearly (28,30). Stridor and laryngospasm associated with GER are observed most often in infancy, but may persist until later in childhood. Neurologically impaired children are especially prone to these problems, and GERD should always be considered when such children develop stridor.

B. Chronic Rhinitis and Rhinopharyngitis

Chronic rhinitis and rhinopharyngitis constitute a relatively unexplored complication of GER. In considering the high prevalence of these symptoms in the general pediatric population, it would be very useful to know the frequency with which they are caused by GERD. That GERD can be the cause of chronic rhinopharyngitis is shown by studies reported recently. Using a nasopharyngeal pH probe, investigators have shown that in 10 children with chronic rhinopharyngitis there was a significantly increased prevalence of low pharyngeal pH compared with 18 control subjects. These authors suggested that reflux of gastric contents into the nasal cavity was responsible for the inflammation observed (18). Less is known about the association of GERD and chronic sinusitis. It seems likely, however, that if gastric contents gain access to the nasal cavity, significant inflammation of the osteomeatal complex might ensue, leading to impaired mucus clearance from the sinuses and resulting disease. Further studies on this association will be of considerable interest.

C. Otitis Media and Otalgia

Otalgia is a common pediatric problem and is most often associated with recurrent otitis media. In some cases, however, there is otalgia without otitis media, and this has been associated with GER in infants, children, and adults (32). The mechanism of this symptom is thought to be that of referred pain resulting from inflammation of the pharynx due to the refluxed acid-peptic gastric contents (33,34). The physical findings in these patients include a normal ear examination and variable degrees of erythema in the pharynx. Treatment of the GERD has been reported to lead to resolution of the otalgia (35). Recurrent otitis media has also been reported to result from GERD (8). Otitis is thought to be caused by refluxed material gaining access to the eustachian tube, which in some young children is unusually patulous and straighter than it is in the older child or adult (36). Awareness of the possibility that GERD can contribute to recurrent otitis media in some cases should lead to consideration of this preventable cause in evaluating children with recurrent otitis.

D. Pharyngitis and Chronic Throat Clearing

The complaint of persistent sore throat or chronic pharyngitis is sometimes heard in children. If cultures prove negative and physical findings suggest inflammation of the pharynx, as evidenced by erythema of the pharynx, uvula, and tonsils, consideration should be given to GERD as a cause (33,34). These patients often have worse throat pain in the morning upon awakening, since GER may be more damaging during sleep (4). Chronic throat clearing in children may suggest the presence of airway disease including allergic diseases and sinusitis. If these conditions can be ruled out, however, by history, physical finding, and the appropriate laboratory studies, GERD should be considered as a possible cause. A case report of a 15-year-old boy with ''heavy drainage'' in the throat during exercise found GER to be the cause. Treatment of the GER resulted in complete resolution of the patient's symptoms (33).

E. Globus Pharyngeus

This is the sensation of having a lump in the throat. This same symptom, formerly referred to as ''globus hystericus,'' has been attributed to a psychoneurosis. However, it has been shown that GERD causing reflux pharyngitis may produce the symptom as well (37). Cases of globus pharyngeus due to GERD have been reported in adults, but they can occur in younger individuals as well. Awareness of GERD as a possible cause of this symptom will prevent the clinician from attributing it to psychological causes when a treatable physical problem is the true etiology (38).

F. Subglottic and Supraglottic Stenosis

Subglottic stenosis has been reported in children with GERD. The role of GERD in causing subglottic stenosis is complex, particularly since many children developing this problem have a history of prolonged endotracheal intubation, which is known to cause the condition. In some children with this complication, however, GER can be shown to be present and is thought to play a role in causing stenosis (39). It is thought that the initial subglottic injury is from the endotracheal tube and that variable degrees of aspiration of refluxed gastric contents may serve as a cofactor in producing the subglottic insult ultimately leading to stenosis (1,40). It is known that endotracheal intubation disturbs the function of the upper esophageal sphincter so that the likelihood of GERD may be increased in the intubated child, and it has been found that pharyngeal reflux of gastric contents is common in supine intubated patients (1). It is also known from work in experimental animals that airway obstruction, which is often the indication for intubation, results in a powerful pressure gradient between the chest and the abdomen, which may lead to GER (14).

Supraglottic stenosis/collapse is a condition identified in infants and children in which the supraglottic larynx is abnormally narrowed. In a recent report of 17 infants and children with this diagnosis, 53% were found to have a history of GER (41). As is the case for subglottic disease, the fact that an airway obstruction exists in supraglottic stenosis makes it difficult to know whether the reflux is a result of the airway obstruction or if the reflux may be causing or contributing to the supraglottic obstruction.

H. Chronic Cough

The mechanism of chronic cough associated with GERD has been reviewed in Chapter 5. Chronic cough due to GERD has been documented in a large cohort of infants and children presenting with this symptom. Overall the investigators documented that GERD alone was the cause of cough in 15% of these subjects and appeared as an etiology most often in children aged 6–15 years (42). A similar study evaluating 88 older adolescents and adults found that among subjects with chronic cough who were nonsmokers and had a normal chest x-ray, GERD along with asthma and postnasal drip were the most common causes of the cough (43). Several authors have noted that coughing due to GERD in children is likely to present with nocturnal symptoms (44,45). Other authors have listed GERD as among the most common causes of chronic cough in the child and noted that the list of causes is remarkably similar in both children and adults (46). One study of subjects with chronic cough symptoms examined the interaction between coughing and episodes of GER using prolonged esophageal pH probe monitoring. Those investigators found that in some instances the GER and coughing were unrelated, in others the cough preceded the reflux episode, and in some the reflux could trigger coughing. It was suggested from this study that a vicious cycle of cough, reflux, and more coughing is seen in some subjects (47). Although not known to be caused by upper airway irritation, cough variant asthma is thought to be provoked in some patients by GERD. Cough variant asthma is seen primarily in children and consists of persistent coughing paroxysms in the absence of wheezing, with the cough having nocturnal predominance. The cough is relieved by bronchodilators (48,49). Cough variant asthma was the most common cause of chronic cough in the large study of infants and children described above (33) and is prominently listed by other authors in the differential diagnosis of chronic cough (46).

III. GERD and Lower Respiratory Tract

Table 2 lists the diseases of the lower respiratory tract that have been associated with GERD. Most of these are relatively uncommon diseases or are seen primarily in special populations, such as neurologically impaired or developmentally delayed children. In contrast, asthma is quite common in the general population. The likely role of GERD in each is considered.

A. Aspiration Pneumonia

This condition occurs most often in children with some predisposing factor, such as neurologic injury or developmental delay (50–53). It is also described in otherwise neurologically normal children in association with depressed consciousness; aspiration during general anesthesia or CPR has been described (27,53,54). In both neurologically impaired and depressed patients, there is presumed to be dysfunction of the neural mechanisms that protect the upper airway when it is exposed to refluxed material. Developmentally delayed children may be prone to recurrent aspiration pneumonia (51,55), and these patients may develop some of the more serious complications. In addition to the neurologically impaired or depressed child, those who have had repair of esophageal atresia are at considerable risk for recurrent aspiration of refluxed material (56,57). These latter patients have abnormal motility of their esophagus, and the majority of them also have GER (27,57). Children with bronchopulmonary dysplasia (BPD) have likewise been identified as a high-risk group for GERD with aspiration. Since BPD often produces downward displacement of the diaphragm from air trapping, frequent coughing, and abdominal breathing due to airway obstruction, the condition is thought to favor occurrence of GER by overwhelming antireflux mechanisms (58). The tendency to aspiration of refluxed material in children with BPD may reflect neurological incoordination. The clinical signs of aspiration usually involve coughing and choking with food intake or during emesis.

Table 2 Lower Respiratory Tract Disease

A. Aspiration pneumonia
B. Lung abscess
C. Recurrent granulomatous pneumonia
D. Bronchiectasis
E. Chronic bronchitis
F. Bronchiolitis obliterans
G. Pulmonary fibrosis
H. Bronchial asthma

B. Lung Abscesses

These serious infections are believed to occur secondary to repeated aspiration of foreign material into the lungs (59). While material other than refluxed gastric contents may cause abscesses, the latter is known to do so often (60). Although mechanisms that have been reported to cause pulmonary abscesses include hematogenous spread of organisms and extensive bronchopneumonia, the possibility of repeated aspiration due to GERD should always be considered, especially in patients with developmental delay, depressed consciousness, or esophageal dysfunction, which, as noted above, favor aspiration pneumonias. Since lung abscesses are quite rare with foreign body aspiration, repeated episodes of aspiration may be needed to provoke this complication (59).

C. Recurrent Granulomatous Pneumonia

This rare condition is manifested as a persistent infiltrate on x-ray and demonstrates diffuse granulomas on histologic examination of the lung. Recurrent aspiration of small quantities of regurgitated vegetable food materials has been found to be the cause. Evaluation of the lesions has implicated the cellulose fraction of the vegetable as opposed to the starch in the aspirated foods as the cause of the granulomas (61). As suggested with lung abscesses, individuals having any condition predisposing to recurrent aspiration should be considered to be at risk for developing granulomatous pneumonia.

D. Bronchiectasis

This destructive pulmonary condition has been attributed to GERD resulting from the often severe and recurring pneumonias that occur with GERD and aspiration (62). Infection is the most common cause of bronchiectasis (14), and the persistent and recurrent nature of aspiration pneumonias in some children with GERD makes them vulnerable to such infections. The risk of developing bronchiectasis, which has a poor prognosis, is one of the principal reasons that GERD must be diagnosed and aggressively treated.

E. Chronic/Recurrent Bronchitis

The persistence of signs and symptoms of tracheobronchitis beyond 3 weeks or their recurrence more than 4 times per year (the definition of chronic bronchitis) may occur as a result of GERD (27,53). When this syndrome occurs it reflects the continued exposure of the airways to the noxious effects of often small quantities of aspirated gastric contents (63). As with the other pulmonary complications of GERD, bronchitis represents one of the problems associated with reflux that should be treated aggressively, lest it lead to progressive structural lung damage.

F. Bronchiolitis Obliterans

This condition represents a chronic persistent form of bronchiolitis that has been reported following a variety of insults to the lower airway (64). Prominent among these causes in children is GERD (65). Because of the chronic nature of bronchiolitis obliterans and its uncertain and at times poor prognosis, it is a pernicious complication of GERD with aspiration. Bronchiolitis obliterans is a problem that underscores the need to anticipate GER in the at-risk child and treat it aggressively when possible.

G. Pulmonary Fibrosis

This serious pulmonary disease has often been reported in adults in connection with gastroesophageal reflux (66). More recently the potential for the condition to occur in children with GERD has been recognized (27,53). The presumed mechanism for development of fibrosis is the repeated exposure of the lungs to small quantities of refluxed acid-peptic material. The resulting lesions are indistinguishable from those seen in idiopathic pulmonary fibrosis in the adult (66).

H. Bronchial Asthma and GERD

Of all the airway diseases in children and adolescents that may be due to GERD, asthma is by far the most prevalent, and thus arguably the most important. Recent epidemiologic estimates indicate that approximately 5% of children in the United States have bronchial asthma, and the prevalence appears to be increasing in recent years (67). The economic impact of this disease on American health care expenditures is very large, and there is evidence that a subpopulation of asthmatic patients with particularly severe disease account for a disproportionate share of these expenditures (68). If these negative trends are to be reversed, it is essential that all of the significant factors contributing to severe asthma be identified, and therefore it is particularly important that the contribution of GERD to severe bronchial asthma be defined. Unfortunately, despite a connection between GERD and asthma having been suggested over a century ago (69). The relationship remains unclear. The mechanisms by which GERD could adversely affect bronchial asthma are considered in detail in Chapter 7. The putative mechanisms usually cited in adults, microaspiration of refluxed acid-peptic materials, evocation of vagally mediated esophagobronchial reflexes, and increase in bronchial hyperreactivity secondary to esophageal acid exposure, are thought to be operative in children as well. It has also been suggested that a fourth mechanism might be an increase in IgE production. Denuding of the esophagus by acid reflux with enhanced allergen access to immunocompetent cells might lead to this outcome (66). Since most asthmatic children are atopic, this hypothesis may be worthy of consideration.

Does Childhood Asthma Cause GER?

In childhood asthma, as in the adult disease, virtual universal agreement exists that there is an increased incidence of virtual gastroesophageal reflux (70–72). The pathophysiologic features of asthma that contribute to GER include coughing, which produces bursts of increased intra-abdominal pressure, abdominal breathing patterns contributing a sustained pressure increase, the powerful negative intrathoracic pressures during breathing with bronchospasm, and the downward displacement of the diaphragm during asthmatic episodes. These changes are similar in both adult and pediatric asthma.

Do Bronchodilator Medications Explain GER in Asthmatic Children?

A number of reports have made note of the fact that bronchodilator medications diminish the pressure of the lower esophageal sphincter (LES). Both β_2-agonists (73–75) and methylxanthines (76,77) have been reported to have this effect. In contrast, clinical studies that have evaluated the impact of these pharmacologic agents have usually not seen an increase in the number of episodes of GER in patients receiving them. In one very large study of adult asthmatics and non-asthmatic control subjects, it was found that compared to normal control subjects, asthmatics had considerably more GER. Among asthmatic subjects taking theophylline, β-agonists or both, however, there was no difference noted in LES pressure, the percent of time with decreased esophageal pH, or the number of GER episodes as compared to asthmatics taking none. The authors concluded that GER is a common feature of bronchial asthma rather than a medication side effect (78). Supporting the absence of a drug effect was a study of 16 children evaluated for GER during sleep. This report actually noted fewer episodes of GER in the 9 asthmatic subjects who had therapeutic serum theophylline levels than in the 7 control subjects who received no medications (79). Similar findings were reported in a study of 18 asthmatic children of whom 13 were receiving bronchodilators and 5 were not. The two groups had a similar prevalence of GER (80). Recent discoveries of how antireflux barriers normally work may reconcile the observations that bronchodilators decrease LES pressure but do not increase the occurrence of clinical GER. It has been found that reduction of LES pressure even to zero does not permit GER if the contraction of the crural diaphragm is preserved (81). Theophylline is known to enhance diaphragmatic contractibility (82,83) and may thereby actually inhibit GER even in the face of decreased LES pressure. Theophylline does, however, increase gastric acid secretion and thus may not be totally benign in the GERD prone asthmatic (84). Overall, there seems little reason to avoid most bronchodilators for fear of exacerbating GERD. However, theophylline dosage must be carefully titrated to balance its clinical benefits and side effects, and serum theophylline levels can be helpful.

Does GERD Cause Childhood Asthma?

This is the crucial question to which there is as yet no final answer. Numerous studies have been carried out in adult asthmatics examining this question by attempting to recreate the conditions of GERD. The results have been conflicting. Table 3 shows data from five studies carried out in children and adolescents examining the question of whether recreating the conditions during GER, either by instillation of acid or by spontaneous GER, can result in asthma. The studies are small, most are uncontrolled, and diverse outcome measures of asthma are examined, with some reports relying on physical signs of bronchospasm. The two reports in this series that examine bronchial hyperreactivity (BHR) pursuant to esophageal acid exposure both found airway reactivity to be increased (80,87), a phenomenon that has also been suggested from studies in adults (88). There is a suggestion in several of these reports that reflux is most likely to cause nocturnal asthma (80,85,86), an observation that was made many years ago (89) and which may reflect both the more virulent nature of GER occurring during sleep (4) and the greater likelihood of asthmatics to develop bronchospastic episodes while asleep (90). Some reports of esophageal acid provocation including some of those listed in Table 3 and some performed in adult subjects, have failed to demonstrate any kind of airway response following provocation. Those studies, however, have not looked for increased BHR, so no comment can be made on that outcome measure (91,92). It would seem then that these ostensibly negative studies do not truly negate an effect of GERD on asthma. It is notable in Table 3 that acid-provocation studies in children and adolescents were all performed nearly a decade ago and that research in the importance of GERD in childhood and adolescent asthma has moved in a different direction. There are two principal reasons for the shift in focus of inquiry. The first reason is recognition of the fact that the interaction between asthma and GERD is quite complex. It has been noted, for example, that GERD does not cause bronchospasm or BHR in all asthmatics; it appears to do so only in those with preexisting esophagitis (85,93). In addition to this observation, GERD may not cause bronchospasm whenever it occurs, but may only do so at certain times of the day or night (85,94). Alternatively, it has been proposed that laryngeal exposure to irritant material is the stimulus most likely to elicit bronchospasm (95). To add complexity, none of the proposed mechanisms by which GERD might cause or aggravate asthma need exclude the others, and different ones may be operative in different patients or at various times in the same patient. One investigator has concluded that "it is very difficult to document a diagnosis of reflux-induced asthma. The only way to establish a causal relation is to demonstrate that the control of acid reflux by medical or surgical means ameliorates asthma" (96). The second reason for seeking an alternative investigative approach relates to the limitation of currently available technology. It has been stated that there is no acceptable diagnostic method available

Table 3 Studies of Esophageal Provocation in Children

Ref.	Subject/Control	Method of provocation	Method of documenting GER	Pulmonary parameter measured	% Change observed in PFT	Evidence of BHR	% of subjects reacting to provocation	Authors' conclusion
Wilson (80)	18/0	Spontaneous GER in sleep Ingest HCl 0.001 N & 0.01 N	pH probe N.A.	Histamine PC_{20} PEFR	No change	↓ Histamine PC_{20}	11/18	↓ PC_{20} at 90 min post–acid ingestion. No significant change in PEFR. If subject had GER and response to acid ingestion nocturnal asthma likely to be ↑ by GER.
Hughes (79)	9/7	Spontaneous GER during sleep	pH probe	Tidal volume O_2 sat Physical status	No significant changes observed	Not evaluated	0%	Patients with chronic asthma do not have ↑ GER at night. Reflux plays little if any role in nocturnal asthma.
Davis (85)	9/0	Intraesophageal acid installation	Tuttle test Bernstein test pH probe	Inductance plethysmography Physical status	75% change in mean inspiratory flow. 40% ↓ inspiratory time seen only at 4 a.m.	Not evaluated	4/9 (all with +Bernstein)	Patients with +Bernstein may be highly susceptible to nocturnal wheezing from GERD
Martin (86)	25/0	Spontaneous GER during sleep	Barium swallow pH probe	Physical status assessment	N.A.	Not evaluated	3/16 wheezed with GER episodes	Cause and effect between GER and wheezing suggested in 3/8 patients with nocturnal asthma
deBlic (87)	15/0	Intraesophageal acid instillation Spontaneous GER	Not stated	S Raw Carbachol PC_{20}	No change S Raw	↓ Carbachol PC_{20}	Not stated	Spontaneous GER appeared to aggravate asthma by ↑ bronchial hyperreactivity

to confirm the presence of GERD-induced asthma (97). Treatment outcome studies of sufficient size to resolve the questions of whether GERD can cause asthma do not exist. To adequately address this issue, studies will have to be large enough to ensure sufficient statistical power to detect modest differences. Prior to examining any asthma treatment outcomes, there should be adequate control of GERD for a sufficient duration to allow healing of esophagitis. These proposed studies should not rely solely on improvement in pulmonary functions as a treatment outcome, since these improvements are known to occur slowly (98). Failure to demonstrate adequate suppression of GERD with usual doses of proton pump inhibitors has recently been demonstrated (99). Documentation of adequate acid suppression will clearly be needed in future studies. We all eagerly await this future research.

What Can We Conclude About Asthma and GERD?

While the final answer to this question is not available, the preponderance of evidence supports a role for GERD in the cause and/or perpetuation of asthma in the child or adolescent. The known occurrence of GERD in the majority of asthmatics, the occurrence of reflux esophagitis in many, the studies showing that esophageal acidification can elicit bronchospasm or BHR, and reports claiming improvement in asthma with medical or surgical treatment, all support a role for GERD in causing or perpetuating asthma. It is also notable that virtually all investigators who have examined the problem of GERD and asthma have concluded that there is a connection (1,96). While some investigators have held that a causative role of GERD in bronchial asthma is unproven, few would deny its existence.

IV. Diagnosis of GERD

The methods available for the diagnosis of GERD are considered in detail with their indications and shortcomings in Chapter 3. Considered here will be the applicability of these tests to the child and adolescent whose size and ability to cooperate with testing will differ from that of the adult patient. Evaluation of the child and adolescent for GERD is based on identifying the best tests to define the cause of a specific set of symptoms. Since there are a large number of testing methods available, the testing is best done with input from a pediatric gastroenterologist if one is available.

A. History

Obtaining a history suggestive of GERD in the child and the adolescent presents a challenge to the clinician. The symptoms of GERD in the infant are considered in the previous chapter; with rare exceptions the symptoms in the older child and adolescent are similar to those in the adult (6). That is to say, children will have substernal burning most often but may have dysphagia, regurgitation, water brash, and belching as well (7). Unfortunately, many of these symptoms are beyond the vocabulary of the younger child, and the clinician must inquire carefully and in simple terms when eliciting this history. Adolescents may present a special challenge since they often have a need to deny illness and an aversion to any medical or parental intervention into their lives. Several visits and a friendly, nonconfrontational interviewing technique with attention to the amount of over-the-counter antacids being taken may be needed to learn the extent of the GERD-related symptoms in the teenager. Despite the clinician's best efforts it is sometimes the physical sequelae involving either the upper or lower airway that first draw attention to the presence of GERD.

B. Physical Examination

In most instances of GERD associated with respiratory disease there are few physical signs supporting a connection on ordinary examination. In cases of GERD involving reflux to the pharynx, there may be redness in the throat, but even this sign is not reliable. Since some physicians have become proficient in performing rhinopharyngoscopy as part of a specialty evaluation, they may find inflammation of the larynx or surrounding tissues from GERD. Rarely the physician may see the peculiar head-cocking behavior associated with severe GERD that has been called Sandifer's syndrome (100).

C. Diagnostic Testing

When making a choice of diagnostic tests in the child or adolescent, the clinician balances the need for specific information against the invasiveness of the test and the child's ability to cooperate. Ideally, sedation and anesthesia are avoided, but practically, these may be necessary.

D. Scintigraphy

This is the most physiologic method of all testing for GER in children. A dose of radioactive technetium 99 proportional to the child's weight is administered in a feeding. As milk is used for the vehicle in younger children, it is sometimes called a "milk scan." After variable periods of time (such as 1, 4, and 24 hours) the upper abdomen and chest are scanned for radioactivity. The presence of radioactivity in the esophagus would indicate GER, while presence in the lungs would reflect aspiration. Aspirated material can be detected by this method many hours after the event has occurred. Although some authors have proposed scinitscan as a sensitive detector of GER in children (101), others find this study is insensitive in detecting GER when compared to esophageal pH probe monitoring (102). One authority has suggested that the diagnostic capability of scintigraphy is underdeveloped at most institutions and that much better information could be gathered with further development (53).

E. Barium Swallow

This study is also well tolerated in children, and sedation is seldom necessary. It is usually done as part of an upper gastrointestinal series, and fluoroscopic examination of the swallowing process is carried out to rule out aspiration during deglutition. This study is an important part of any evaluation when GERD is suspected to be associated with airway disease, since it both demonstrates the swallowing process and rules out anatomic defects in the upper gastrointestinal tract (103,104). As a means of demonstrating reflux, however, the barium swallow is relatively insensitive(24,53,102). Occasionally, particularly if done with air contrast, barium studies will demonstrate mucosal changes of esophagitis, but the ability to do so is limited to the more florid cases of inflammation.

F. Esophageal Manometry

This study of esophageal pressures is usually performed prior to surgery for fundoplication to exclude esophageal dysmotility which might affect the surgical result (53). Since there is no strong correlation between reflux and LES pressure, the information gained from this study is of limited value in the overall assessment of GER (105).

G. pH Probe

Often described as the "gold standard" for the demonstration of GER (106), this study is very effective in evaluating patients with suspected GERD. While children and adolescents dislike passage of the monitor electrode via the nose into the esophagus, a staff member who is skilled in working with children can accomplish this without sedating the child, and once in place the probe is well tolerated even for a 24-hour study. The primary value of esophageal pH monitoring is the quantitative data that is generated on reflux. One can detect reflux into the upper esophagus using two channel pH recorders and may be able to correlate respiratory or other symptoms with reflux episodes (107). The limitations of pH probe monitoring are that the technique will not reflect reflux of neutral or alkaline gastric contents such as those that occur after meals. This study also fails to detect esophageal disease, recording only reflux episodes, which are not necessarily correlated with disease. A logistical problem is that although esophageal pH monitoring is available in medical centers, it may not be in remote areas. Overall, pH monitoring provides important information in diagnosis of GERD, and, as noted above, modification of the technique to monitor pharyngeal pH has begun to yield useful insights into several previously unrecognized complications of GERD (8).

H. Esophageal Biopsy

Biopsy provides the definitive diagnosis of esophagitis. This is a critical piece of information since quantitatively abnormal reflux can occur without injury to the esophagus in some instances (4). In children, methods have been established to perform suction biopsies of the esophagus without endoscopy from a suction capsule passed to the appropriate level of the esophagus. The level of biopsy is determined from standard regression equations (53,108), or manometrically. Large series have demonstrated the safety and effectiveness of this procedure (109). Biopsy may and should be obtained during endoscopy, and the procedure permits visual selection of the biopsy site as well as overall assessment of the status of the esophageal mucosa. While suction biopsy can be performed with the child fully awake, endoscopy requires the child to be under sedation.

I. Bernstein Test and Tuttle Test

The Bernstein test involves the alternating infusion of acid and saline into the esophagus through a nasogastric tube, with pain or discomfort upon acid infusion considered a positive result. Most often the test is used to determine whether esophagitis is present, but for this it is less sensitive than esophageal biopsy (53). The Bernstein test is occasionally able to reproduce the respiratory symptoms suspected of resulting from GER, and in that situation it is diagnostic. The Tuttle test for acid reflux places a standard amount of acid in the stomach and monitors esophageal pH for an hour following the instillation to determine whether reflux has occurred. This test has largely been replaced by esophageal pH monitoring (110).

J. Ultrasonography

A new and promising method for diagnosis of GER is the use of ultrasound. The technique is not yet widely accepted for diagnosing GER, but it has the advantages of being noninvasive, not exposing to radiation, and not requiring sedation of the child being studied. A recent report described completion of the study in 209 of 220 infants and children in which it was attempted, indicating that most children can cooperate well enough to permit a valid study (111). The ultrasound can detect reflux episodes in children as well as anatomic conditions such as hiatus hernia that may predispose to GER (112). It has been reported that ultrasonography compares favorably to other methods used to diagnose GER in children, including barium swallow (113) and pH monitoring (114). The use of color-coded

Doppler ultrasonography in children has recently been described as a method to detect very small amounts of gastroesophageal reflux (115). The authors claimed that the color-coded Doppler increased sensitivity of the method to 94% using comparison with 24-hour pH monitoring. Despite these impressive findings, the authors suggested use of the technique as a supplement to pH probe monitoring in evaluating children with suspected GER. Other investigators have described the use of endoscopic ultrasonography in which the ultrasound probe is passed into the esophagus. This technique has been said to be a method for staging the degree of severity of reflux esophagitis as well as its response to therapy (116). Overall, ultrasonography appears to have many advantages compared to some older technologies used to diagnose GER in children, although additional studies are needed to confirm the claims made and to compare it to more traditional tests. It seems likely that the technology of ultrasonography will improve in the future and that refinements will be made that will enhance the power of this test to diagnose GER and the attendant abnormalities.

V. Treatment of GERD

A detailed consideration of the available medical and surgical treatment of GERD is presented in Chapters 8 and 9. The discussion in this chapter will be limited to therapies for GERD in children and to the consideration of their special needs. In planning GERD therapy in children, it is important to view the child as a young person whose life can be expected to span seven or eight decades. This fact emphasizes the need to consider the likely duration of treatment for GERD and any attendant airway disease. Second, the developmental aspects of the child or adolescent need to be considered in devising a treatment plan. Since children are in their formative years, it is important that they be enabled, to the extent possible, to carry out the educational, athletic, and playtime activities that their peers do. Children unable to do so may develop a self-image of being sickly or inadequate. Finally, the cost of therapy of GERD in purely economic terms needs to be considered (117). Many families are devastated by the costs of a chronic illness in a child, and GERD is no exception. Unfortunately, at this time there is still insufficient information to respond to all of the considerations delineated above and to recommend optimal therapy for each child. The available information must be synthesized, and future studies carefully designed, in order to define the treatment of choice for GERD in children and adolescents with airway disease associated with this condition. Some of what is known of GERD therapy is described below.

A. Conservative Management of GERD

While it is common for GERD in the infant to resolve spontaneously, there is evidence that as many as 50% of older children diagnosed with GERD will have persistent disease requiring chronic therapy (118,119). Simple, cost-effective measures for treatment of GERD include avoiding food intake for at least 3 hours before bedtime (107). As noted above, the bedtime snack is a common and pleasurable custom of many children in the United States. Adolescents, who may eat continually, seldom stop grazing as bedtime approaches. However, in the child or teenager with a diagnosis of GERD, this activity should be discouraged so that the stomach is relatively empty when the patient becomes recumbent. Tight clothing and obesity increases intra-abdominal pressure and thereby GER episodes, and these risks should be avoided. The sleeping position that best avoids reflux is not known with certainty, but some authors have suggested that sleeping prone is beneficial (6). Propping the head of the bed by about 6 inches has been recommended by some (2,6), however, a recent report did not find benefit in this practice (120). The avoidance of foods such as chocolate, peppermint, coffee, citrus, fats, and carbonated beverages (which cause bloating) has likewise been recommended as a means of controlling gastric acidity and LES tone (53,121). Cigarette smoke has been shown to adversely affect GER in smokers. Avoidance of secondhand smoke in the young child and avoidance of smoking or smoke exposure for the adolescent are well advised. Since respiratory diseases such as asthma, BPD, and cystic fibrosis are known to aggravate GER by the mechanisms described above, it may be difficult to successfully treat GER while the effects of the coexisting respiratory disease are at work. It is important then to employ all of the therapies available to bring these respiratory conditions under optimal control while treating the GERD. If a vicious cycle exists of a respiratory disease affecting GERD, which in turn aggravates the respiratory disease further, the cycle may need to be broken at several points. Despite all of these precautions being carried out, many children with GERD will continue to have symptoms, and for these patients pharmacologic therapy is indicated.

B. Pharmacologic Treatment of GERD

A large number of drugs are used for treatment of GERD, and the pharmacology and relative efficacy of these agents are discussed in Chapter 8. The drugs used in children are used in adults, with the dosages made proportionate to the size of the child. In addition, there are some caveats on the long-term effects of some of these agents in children. Therapeutic agents used to treat GERD in children are divided into the three categories of acid reducing agents, prokinetic agents, and mucosal protecting agents.

Acid-Reducing Agents

Acid-neutralizing agents are the historical mainstay of therapy to reduce gastric acidity. They are usually given as a liquid to the younger child but may be given as tablets to the older child or adolescent. Dosage guidelines are vague, but usually 0.5–1.0 ml/kg/dose is prescribed three to eight times daily. Drawbacks include the unpalatability of the drugs, the side effects of diarrhea or constipation (53), and the need for frequent administration, which may be difficult in a school-age child. Overdosing with these agents is possible and should be avoided. Alginic acid combined with an antacid is said to offer extra benefit, forming a viscous solution in the stomach that acts as a mechanical barrier to acid. Indications are that its effect is comparable to the antacids alone (121).

H_2 blockers are used in children of all ages, although none are currently FDA approved for pediatric use. The number of these agents available in the United States is continually increasing, and there is no firm experimental evidence to recommend one compound over another on the basis of drug efficacy (122). There is a difference in recommended frequency of administration, however, and this feature may lead to greater compliance as well as less interference in the daily activities of school-aged or older children. Ranitidine (Zantac) and famotidine (Pepcid) are usually recommended to be given three times per day versus cimetidine (Tagamet), which is given four times per day. The author's experience and that of others is that treatment failures, as judged by esophageal pH probe monitoring, are common with H_2 blockers. Follow-up studies while the patient is receiving the H_2 blocker to demonstrate suppression of gastric acid secretion are necessary even when maximum recommended doses are given (102). One report of ranitidine given as a single bedtime dose to a group of asthmatic children and adolescents described a 30% reduction in nocturnal asthma symptoms (123). The authors were unimpressed with this result, although it was statistically significant, and they stated that acid suppression had not been demonstrated in their study. They urged additional, better controlled studies of asthmatic subjects using these drugs. Apart from this report, however, there are no data by which to judge the efficacy of H_2 blockers in pediatric asthma associated with GERD.

Proton pump inhibitors have been used in the United States for several years—initially, omeprazole (Prilosec) and, more recently, lansoprazole (Prevacid). These agents are recognized as being more effective acid suppressors than are H_2 blockers. Dosages of omeprazole ranging from 0.7 to 3.3 mg/kg/day were required to suppress gastric acidity in one study (124). This nearly fivefold range in dosage required to achieve acid suppression is reflected by observations in two studies of this drug in adults, where very high doses were needed in some subjects to achieve acid suppression (99,125). It appears that in treatment with omeprazole, as is true for the H_2 blockers, treatment failures are common. Verification of acid suppression in the individual patient is essential regardless of the dose administered. Pediatric studies have demonstrated elevated gastrin levels in children treated with omeprazole. The effect over the long term is unknown, but there is concern that the persistently elevated gastrin might lead to argyrophyll cell neoplasia (124). There are no data on treatment of pediatric airway disease with proton pump inhibitors, but preliminary reports of treatment of adult asthmatics with omeprazole are very encouraging (99,126). Experience with lansoprazole in children is limited and awaits further exploration.

Prokinetic Agents

Prokinetic agents have been successfully used for treatment of GERD in some children. These agents are thought to increase LES pressure, improve esophageal clearance, and facilitate gastric emptying. Bethanecol was the first prokinetic agent used. It has not been shown to be consistently successful in treatment of reflux (127). There are also concerns that the use of bethanecol, which is a cholinergic agonist, might be aggravating in children with reactive airway disease. The drug is used infrequently in treating GER in children at present. Metoclopramide (Reglan) has been used for over a decade in the United States in the treatment of GER, but has not been identified as a drug of choice due to reports that question its efficacy (128,129). The side effect profile of metoclopramide includes CNS symptoms including irritability, extrapyramidal effects, and tardive dyskinesia. The author's experience is that metoclopamide in usual doses, even when combined with an H_2 blocker, does not reliably abolish GER in asthmatic children (102). Cisapride (Propulsid) has been used in children with GER for several years in the United States. The drug appears to be effective and to have fewer undesired side effects than other prokinetic agents. Some authorities consider cisapride to be the prokinetic drug of first choice for GER in children and adolescents. Domperidone is an experimental prokinetic drug but is available in Europe. One study of 55 children with cough comparing cisapride and domperidone found domperidone to be superior in preventing GER by scintiscan, although differences were slight (130).

Several studies have evaluated the effect of prokinetic agents in airway disease of children. The above-cited study comparing cisapride and domperidone involved children with chronic cough and showed that with either agent the cough cleared in approximately two thirds of patients (130). An uncontrolled report describing use of cisapride therapy for 3 months in 36 children with uncontrolled asthma revealed that there were highly significant improvements in both the clinical asthma scores and in the pharmacologic score of asthma medications (131). Some authors have described combination of prokinetic drugs with acid-reducing agents, either H_2 blockers or proton pump inhibitors being an effective antireflux regimen (109). These combinations, given in dosages sufficient to achieve suppression, may prove to be quite effective in treatment of GERD with airway disease. At present, however, every known acid-suppressive regimen requires a follow-up assessment by pH probe to ensure that suppression has actually been achieved (102).

Mucosal-Protecting Agents

Mucosal-protecting agents consist only of sucralfate (carafate), although some have suggested that alginic acid (see above) behaves as a mucosal protector as well. Sucralfate has been reported to be an effective agent in treatment of reflux esophagitis in children (132). The agent is relatively nontoxic and is minimally absorbed from the gastrointestinal tract.

C. Surgery for GERD

The decision to undertake surgery in GERD with airway disease is made only after other remedies have failed or proved impractical. Considerations include the surgical risk involved, the impact of the procedure on the child, the cost, and the likelihood that the surgery will be beneficial for a prolonged period. Often considerations focus on the effectiveness of current therapy and the impact of the child's GERD and its treatment on him or her and on the family. In considering the latter, relevant questions address days of school absenteeism, ability to play with friends or to play sports, and overall quality of life. If the decision to proceed with surgery is made, there are a number of procedures described. Recently the use of laparoscopic surgery has been introduced as a means to perform surgery with reduced risk, cost, and morbidity. Complete description of these surgical procedures is provided in Chapter 9. The surgical procedures that have been advocated for children balance the need to decrease reflux with that to preserve other functions of the upper gastrointestinal tract including swallowing, belching, or vomiting. The complications that have been observed postoperatively in children have been the result of the fundoplication either being too obstructing, not preventing GER, or breaking down over time with recurrence of GER. Experience in both adult and pediatric patients has emphasized the need to evaluate the total upper GI tract, including the status of the motility of esophagus and the ability of stomach to empty, before deciding which surgical repair to undertake (123,124).

Common Surgical Repairs

Nissen fundoplication is the single most commonly used procedure in children today. The postoperative complications in children include gas bloat, dysphagia, and need for dilation (133). There is a small but significant failure rate of the fundoplication wrap following surgery, and it has been reported that failure in children is most often due to the stress placed on the wrap by persistent airway disease (134,135). It is necessary therefore to treat the airway disease vigorously postoperatively to minimize this problem. The long-term integrity of the wrap of gastric fundus around the esophagus seems to determine the success of the outcome in adults with Nissen repairs who have been followed longitudinally

(136). This determinant applies to children as well. It is recognized that children with cystic fibrosis, asthma, BPD, and chronic pulmonary infections have an increased propensity for wrap disruption (137). Usually, a temporary gastrotomy tube is placed at time of surgery to decompress the stomach during early healing. Depending on preoperative findings, a pyloroplasty or gastric antroplasty may be indicated to facilitate stomach emptying (137).

The Thal procedure is preferred in children in whom there is esophageal dysmotility, since it only wraps the fundus three fourths of the way around the esophagus and is said to permit the esophagus to empty more easily into the stomach. This procedure is often used in neurologically impaired children (137). Some experienced surgeons feel, however, that recurrence of GER is more common with the Thal procedure than with the Nissen fundoplication, and therefore it is less often used (137). The recurrence of GER following Nissen fundoplication has been reported as being between 0 and 12%, with a 12% recurrence rate being reported in one large series of 242 children followed for an average of 30 months (138). Data on comparable series following Thal procedure are not available.

Other procedures include the Borema anterior gastropexy, the Hill posterior gastropexy, the Belsey Mark IV, and a number of other procedures. In general they are less often used then the Nissen and Thal procedures and may have a higher failure rate (136,137). In one other procedure a silastic elastomer prothesis in the form of a c-shaped ring, called the Angelchik prosthesis, is placed around the esophagogastric junction as an antireflux device. This device has been reported to work effectively in children, performing comparably to Nissen fundoplication (139). However, some authors have expressed concern that complications such as including migration of the prosthesis occur too often and urge more experience with the device before general adoption (133).

Laparoscopic Nissen fundoplication has been used by pediatric surgeons for the past 6 years, and results in adults have been reported to be comparable to those with the open surgical procedures (140). The applicability to children remains to be more fully evaluated, but one experienced pediatric surgeon has recommended that, at this time, the procedure seems best suited for children with GER who are over 5 years of age and who are not neurologically impaired (137).

The Role of Surgery

It has generally been held that most children and adolescents with GERD do not need surgery (6). Indications for surgical intervention have included the development of Barrett's esophagus in which the squamous epithelium of the esophagus is replaced by columnar epithelium and strictures of the esophagus resulting from GERD. Intractable symptoms, including respiratory disease, caused by reflux are also accepted as an indication for surgery. Recent studies in adult patients have proposed that with use of laparoscopic fundoplication, surgery is preferable to long-term medical treatment of GERD (141,142). Insofar as GERD may be part of a vicious cycle in airway disease like asthma, it may be time to reconsider the role of surgery. When it is recognized that the asthmatic child may have the disease for many years or throughout his or her life span, the cost of GERD in personal as well as economic terms can be considerable. Sufficient data to define the indications and effectiveness of surgery for GERD in chronic diseases of the pediatric airways do not exist at present. The problem of severe childhood asthma is great enough, that carefully controlled, multicenter studies of patients matched for disease severity and randomized to receive medical or surgical treatment would be quite helpful. A report of adult asthmatics randomized to receive medical or surgical treatment has favored surgical therapy as providing the best long-term control of asthma (143). Similar studies in children are lacking and much needed.

D. Complications of GERD

The role of GERD in pediatric airway disease is often difficult to define. As noted above, there is evidence that some airway diseases such as asthma or BPD may contribute to GER and that the refluxed gastric contents could then in turn contribute to further airway disease. Some are skeptical of the contribution of GERD to ongoing airway disease, and the connection, while strongly suspected, is unproven (144). Apart from its role in airway disease, GERD is a pernicious condition itself and deserves vigorous treatment and ongoing follow-up wherever it exists. Among the complications of GERD in the pediatric age group are development of peptic esophageal strictures, bleeding, intractable heartburn, anemia, and Barrett's esophagus (53). Although it occurs rarely, Barrett's esophagus may undergo malignant transformation in the child as well as in the adult (144). Thus, GERD must be diagnosed in the child with chronic airway disease and aggressively treated where it is found.

References

1. Kahrihas PJ. Gastroesophageal reflux disease. JAMA 1996; 276:983–988.
2. Herbst JJ, Hilman BC. Gastroesophageal reflux and respiratory sequelae. In: Hilman BC, ed. Pediatric Respiratory Disease: Diagnosis and Treatment. Philadelphia: WB Saunders Company 1993:521–532.
3. Kahrilas PJ, Dodds WJ, Dent J, et al. Effect of sleep, spontaneous gastroesophageal reflux, and a meal on upper esophageal sphincter pressure in normal human volunteers. Gastroenterology 1987; 92:466–471.
4. Orenstein SR, Orenstein DM. Gastroesophageal reflux and respiratory disease in children. J Ped 1988; 112:847–858.

5. Herbst JJ. Development of gastroesophageal reflux. In: Lebenthal E, ed. Textbook of Gastroenterology and Nutrition in Infancy. 2d ed. New York: Raven Press, 1989: 803–813.
6. Orenstein SR. Gastroesophageal reflux disease. Semin Gastrointest Dis 1994; 5:2–14.
7. Richter JE. Typical and atypical presentations of gastroesophageal reflux disease. Gastroenterol Clin North Am 1996; 25:75–102.
8. Contencin P, Narcy P. Nasopharyngeal pH monitoring in infants and children with chronic rhinopharyngitis. Int J Pediatr Otorhinolaryngol 1991; 22:249–256.
9. Contencin P, Narcy P. Gastropharyngeal reflux in infants and children. A pharyngeal pH monitoring study. Arch Otolaryngol Head Neck Surg 1992; 118:1028–1030.
10. Gadmundsson K, Kristleifsson G, Theodors A, Holbrook WP. Tooth erosion, gastroesophageal reflux and salivary buffer capacity. Oral Surg Oral Med Oral Pathol Oral Radiol Endod 1995; 79:185–189.
11. Neurna JH, Toskala J, Nutinen P, Klemetti E. Oral and dental manifestations in gastroesophageal reflux disease. Oral Surg Oral Med Oral Pathol Oral Radiol Endod. 1994.
12. Kambie V, Radsel Z. Acid posterior laryngitis aetiology, diagnosis and treatment. J Laryngol Otol 1984; 98:1237–1240.
13. Cherry J, Margulies SI. Contact ulcer of the larynx. Laryngoscope 1967; 77:1937–1940.
14. Koufman JA. The otolaryngologic manifestations of gastroesophageal reflux disease. Laryngoscope 1991; 10 (suppl 53):1–78.
15. Jiminez-Isabel MA, Matute-Cardenas JA, Delagado-Munoz MD, et al. Surgical treatment versus tracheostomy of laryngeal stenosis in children. Chir Pediatr 1997; 10:38–41.
16. Prescott CA. Factors that influence successful decannulation after surgery for laryngo-tracheal stenosis in children. Int J Pediatr Otorhinolaryngol 1994; 30:183–188.
17. Bierman CW, Pearlman DS. Asthma. In: Chernick V, ed. Kendig's Disorders of the Respiratory Tract in Children. Philadelphia: WB Saunders, 1990:557–601.
18. Belmont JR, Grundfast K. Congenital laryngeal stridor (laryngomalacia). Etiologic factors and associated disorders. Ann Otol Rhinol Laryngol 1984; 93:430–437.
19. Polonovski JM, Contencin P, Viala P, Narcy P. Aryepiglottic fold excision for the treatment of severe laryngomalacia. Ann Otol Rhinol Laryngol 1990; 99:625–627.
20. Hanson DG, Kamel PL, Kahrilas PJ. Outcomes of antireflux therapy for the treatment of chronic laryngitis. Ann Otol Rhinol Laryngol 1995; 104:550–555.
21. Shaker R, Milbrath M, Pen J, Toohill R, Hogan NJ, LiQ, Hoffman CL. Esophagopharyngeal distribution of refluxed gastric acid in patients with reflux laryngitis. Gastroenterology 1995; 109:1575–1582.
22. Putnam PE, Orenstein SR. Hoarseness in a child with gastroesophageal reflux. Acta Pediatr Scand 1992; 81:635–636.
23. Buts JP, Barundi C, Moulin D, Claus D, Cornu G, Otte JB. Prevalence and treatment of silent gastroesophageal reflux in children with recurrent respiratory disorders. Eur J Pediatr 1986; 145:396–400.

24. Putnam PE, Ricker DH, Orenstein SR. Gastroesophageal reflux. In: Beckerman RC, Brouilette RF, Hunt CE, eds. Respiratory Control Disorders in Infants and Children. Baltimore: Williams and Wilkins, 1992:322–341.
25. Grad R, Taussig LM. Acute infections producing upper airway obstruction. In: Chernick V, ed. Kendig's Disorders of the Respiratory Tract in Children. Philadelphia: WB Saunders, 1990:336–359.
26. Waki EY, Madgy DM, Belenky WM, Gower VC. The incidence of gastroesophageal reflux in recurrent croup. Int J Pediatr Otorhinolaryngol 1995; 32:223–232.
27. Nielson DW, Heldt GP, Tooley WH. Stridor and gastroesphageal reflux in infants. Pediatrics 1990; 85:1034–1039.
28. Orenstein SR, Orenstein DM, Whitington PF. Gastroesophageal reflux causing stridor. Chest 1983; 84:301–302.
29. Orenstein SR, Kocoshis SA, Orenstein DM, Proujansky R. Stridor and gastroesophageal reflux: diagnostic use of intraluminal esophageal acid perfusion (Bernstein test). Pediatr Pulmonol 1987; 3:420–424.
30. Henry RL, Mellis CM. Resolution of inspiratory stridor after fundoplication: case report. Austr Pediatr J 1982; 18:126–127.
31. Harned HS, Myracle J, Ferriero J. Respiratory suppression and swallowing from introduction of fluids into the laryngeal region of the lamb. Pediatr Res 1978; 12:1003–1009.
32. Gibson WS, Cochran W. Otalgia in infants and children—a manifestation of gastroesophageal reflux. Int J Pediatr Otorhinolaryngol 1994; 28:213–218.
33. Bain WM, Harrington JW, Thomas PE. Head and neck manifestations of gastroesophageal reflux. Laryngoscope 1983; 93:175–179.
34. Dechner WK, Benjamin SB. Extraesophageal manifestations of gastroesophageal reflux disease. Am J Gastroenterol 1989; 84:1–5.
35. Bernstein J. Otalgia: it's not always what it seems to be. J Respir Dis 1987; 8:71–82.
36. Bluestone CD. Recent advances in the pathogenesis diagnosis and management of otitis media. Pediatr Clin North Am 1981; 28:727–755.
37. Ott DJ, Ledbetter MS, Koufman JA, Chen MY. Globus pharyngeus: radiographic evaluation and 24 hour pH monitoring of the pharynx and esophagus in 22 patients. Radiology 1994; 191:95–97.
38. Ravich WJ, Wilson RS, Jones B, Donner MW. Psychoogenic dysphagia and globus: re-evaluation of 23 patients. Dysphagia 1989; 4:35–38.
39. Little FB, Kolut RI, Koufman JA, Marshall RB. Effect of gastric acid on the pathogenesis of subglottic stenosis. Ann Otol Rhinol Laryngol 1985; 94:516.
40. Orenstein DM. Subglottic stenosis. In: Behrman RE, Kliegman RM, Arvin AM, eds. Nelson Textbook of Pediatrics. 15th ed. Philadelphia: WB Saunders, 1996: 1208–1209.
41. Walner DL, Holinger LD. Supraglottic stenosis in infants and children. A preliminary report. Arch Otolaryngol Head Neck Surg 1997; 123:337–341.
42. Holinger LD, Sanders AD. Chronic cough in infants and children. An update. Laryngoscope 1991; 101:596–605.
43. Mello CJ, Irwin RS, Curley FJ. Predictive values of the character, timing and com-

plications of chronic cough in diagnosing its cause. Arch Intern Med 1996; 156: 997–1003.
44. Alland S, Casimir G. Chronic cough in a 22 month old girl. Rev Med Brux 1994; 15:202–203.
45. DeVita C, Berni Canani J, Cirillo B, Della Rotandi GM, Berni Canani R. Silent gastroesophageal reflux and upper respiratory pathologies in childhood. Acta Otorhinolaryngol Ital 1996; 16:407–411.
46. Corrao WM. Chronic persistent cough: diagnosis and treatment update. Pediatr Ann 1996; 25:162–168.
47. Ing AJ, Ngu MC, Breslin ABX. Chronic persistent cough and gastroesophageal reflux. Thorax 1991; 46:479–483.
48. Cloutier MM, Loughlin GM. Chronic cough in children a manifestation of airway hyperactivity. Pediatrics 1981; 67:6–12.
49. Hanaway PJ, Hoffer DK. Cough variant asthma in children. JAMA 1982; 247:206–210.
50. Byrne WJ, Campbell M, Ashcraft E, Seibert J, Euler AR. A diagnostic approach to vomiting in severely retarded patients. Am J Dis Child 1983; 259–262.
51. Sondheimer JM, Morris BA. Gastroesophageal reflux among severely retarded children. J Pediatr 1979; 94:710–714.
52. Cadman D, Richards J, Feldman W. Gastroesophageal reflux in severely retarded children. Dev Med Child Neurol 1978; 20:95–98.
53. Orenstein SR. Gastroesophageal reflux. In: Wyllie R, Hyams JS, eds. Pediatric Gastrointestinal Disease: Pathophysiology Diagnosis Management. Philadelphia: WB Saunders, 1993:337–369.
54. Euler AR, Byrne WJ, Ament ME, Fonkalsrud EW, Strobel CF, Siegel SC, Katz RM, Rachelefsky GS. Recurrent pulmonary disease in children. A complication of gastroesophageal reflux. Pediatrics 1979; 63:47–51.
55. Wesley JR, Coran AG, Sarahan TM, Klein M White SJ. The need for evaluation of gastroesophageal reflux in brain damaged children referred for feeding gastrostomy. J Pediatr Surg 1981; 16:866–870.
56. Fonkalsrud EW. Gastroesophageal fundoplication for reflux following repair of esophageal atresia: experience with nine patients. Arch Surg 1979; 114:48–51.
57. Werlin SL, Dodds WJ, Hogan WJ, Glicklich M, Arndorfer R. Esophageal function in esophageal atresia. Dig Dis Sci 1981; 26:796–800.
58. Hazinski TA. Bronchopulmonary dysplasia. In: Chernick V, Kendig EL Jr, eds. Disorders of the Respiratory Tract in Children. Philadelphia: WB Saunders, 1990: 300–320.
59. Asher MI, Beaudy PH. Lung abscess. In: Chernick V, Kendig EL Jr, eds. Disorders of the Respiratory Tract in Children. Philadelphia: WB Saunders, 1990:429–436.
60. Perlman LV, Lerner E, D'Esopo W. Clinical classification and analysis of 97 cases of lung abscess. Am Rev Respir Dis 1969; 99:390–398.
61. Knoblich R. Pulmonary granulomatosis caused by vegetable particles. Am Rev Respir Dis 1969; 99:380–389.
62. Brown MA, Lemen RJ. Bronchiectasis. In: Chernick V, Kendig EL Jr, eds. Disorders of the Respiratory Tract in Children. Philadelphia: WB Saunders, 1990:416–429.

63. Laughlin GM. Bronchitis. In: Chernick V, Kendig EL Jr, eds. Disorders of the Respiratory Tract in Children. Philadelphia: WB Saunders, 1990:349–359.
64. Wohl MEB. Bronchiolitis. In: Chernick V, Kendig EL Jr, eds. Disorders of the Respiratory Tract in Children. Philadelphia: WB Saunders, 1990:360–370.
65. Hardy KA, Schidlow DV, Zaeri W. Obliterative bronchiolitis in children. Chest 1988; 93:460–466.
66. Perrin-Fazolle M. Gastroesophageal reflux and chronic respiratory disease in adults. Clin Rev Allergy 1990; 8:457–469.
67. Adams PF, Marano MA. Current estimates from the National Health Interview Survey, 1994. Vital Health Stat 1995; 10:94–106.
68. Weiss KB, Gergen PJ, Hodgson TA. An economic evaluation of asthma in the United States. N Engl J Med 1992; 326:862–866.
69. Osler W. The Principles and Practice of Medicine. New York: D. Appleton and Co., 1892:501.
70. Hozoux C, Forget P, Lambrects L. Chronic bronchopulmonary disease and gastroesophageal reflux in children. Pediatr Pulmonol 1985; 1:149–153.
71. Gustaffson PM, Kjellman NI, Tibbling L. Oesophageal function and symptoms in moderate and severe asthma. Acta Pediatr Scand 1986; 75:729–736.
72. Shapiro GG, Christie DL. Gastroesophageal reflux in steroid dependent asthmatic youths. Pediatrics 1979; 63:207–212.
73. Shindlbeck NE, Heinrich C, Huber RM, Muller-Lissirer SA. Effects of albuterol on esophageal motility and gastroesophageal reflux in healthy volunteers. JAMA 1988; 260:3156–3158.
74. Zfasa AM, Prince R, Allen FW, Farrar JF. Inhibitory beta-adrenergic receptors in the human distal oesophageal. Am J Dig Dis 1970; 15:303–310.
75. DiMarino AJF, Cohen S. Effect of an oral beta 2 adrenergic agonist on lower esophageal sphincter pressure in normals and in patients with achalasia. Dig Dis Sci 1982; 27:1063–1066.
76. Stein MR, Towner TG, Weber RW, Mansfield TE, Jacobson KW, McDonnell JT, Nelson HS. The effect of theophylline on the lower esophageal sphincter pressure. Ann Allergy 1980; 45:238–239.
77. Berquist WE, Rachelefsky GS, Kadden M, Siegel SC, Katz RM, Mickey MR, Ament ME. Effect of theophylline on gastroesophageal reflux in normal adults. J Allergy Clin Immunol 1981; 67:407–411.
78. Sontag SJ, O'Connell S, Khandelwal S, Miller T, Nemchansky B, Schrell TG, Sherloosky R. Most asthmatics have gastroesophageal reflux with or without bronchodilator therapy. Gastroenterology 1990; 99:613–620.
79. Hughes DMN, Spier S, Rivein J, Levinson H. Gastroesophageal reflux during sleep in asthmatic patients. J Pediatr 1983; 102:666–672.
80. Wilson NM, Charette L, Thomson AH, Silverman W. Gastro-oesophageal reflux and childhood asthma: the acid test. Thorax 1985; 40:592–597.
81. Mittal RK, Balaban DH. The esophagogastric junction. N Engl J Med 1997; 336:924–932.
82. Aubier M, Frazer A, Sampson M, Macklem P, Rossos E. Aminophylline improves diaphragmatic contractibility. N Engl J Med 1981; 305–249–252.

83. Munciano D, Aubier M, Lecocguic Y, Pariente R. Effects of theophylline on diaphragmatic strength and fatigue in patients with chronic obstructive pulmonary disease. N Engl J Med 1984; 311:349–353.
84. Weinberger M. The pharmacology and therapeutic use of theophylline. J Allergy Clin Immunol 1984; 73:525–540.
85. Davis RS, Larsen GL, Grunstein MM. Respiratory response to intraesophageal acid infusion in asthmatic children during sleep. J Allergy Clin Immunol 1983; 72:393–398.
86. Martin ME, Grunstein MM, Larsen GL. The relationship of gastroesophageal reflux to nocturnal wheezes in children with asthma. Ann Allergy 1982; 49:318–322.
87. deBlic Y, Revillon Y, Seheinmann P. The relationship between gastroesophageal reflux and chronic respiratory disease. Clin Rev Allergy 1990; 8:427–441.
88. Herve P, Denjean A, Jian R, Simmoneau G, Duroux P. Intraesophageal perfusion of acid increases the bronchomotor response to methacholine and to isocapneic hyperventilation in asthmatic subjects. Am Rev Respir Dis 1986; 134:986–989.
89. Dees SC. The role of gastroesophageal reflux in nocturnal asthma in children. NC Med J 1974; 35:230–233.
90. Barnes P, Fitzgerald G, Brown M, Dollery C. Nocturnal asthma and changes in circulating epinephrine, histamine and cortisol. N Engl J Med 1980; 303:263–267.
91. Wessling G, Brummer RJ, Wouters EFM, ten Valde GPM. Gastric acid? No change in respiratory impedance during intraesophageal acidification in adult asthmatics. Chest 1993; 104:1733–1736.
92. Tan WC, Martin RJ, Pondez R, Ballard RD. Effects of spontaneous and simulated gastroesophageal reflux on sleeping asthmatics. Am Rev Respir Dis 1990; 141:1394–1399.
93. Mansfield LE, Stein MR. Gastroesophageal reflux and asthma: a possible reflex mechanism. Ann Allergy 1978; 41:224–226.
94. Ekstrom F, Tibbling L. Esophageal acid perfusion, airway function, and symptoms in asthmatic patients with marked bronchial hyperreactivity. Chest 1989; 96:995–998.
95. Nadel JA, Salem H, Tamplin B, Tokiwa Y. Mechanisms of broncho constriction during inhalation of sulfur dioxide. J Appl Physiol 1965; 20:164–167.
96. Pope CE II. Acid-reflux disorders. N Engl J Med 1994; 331:656–660.
97. Sontag SJ. Gut feelings about asthma. Chest 1991; 99:1321–1323.
98. Perin P, McGeady SJ. Objective indicators of severity of asthma. J Allergy Clin Immunol 1994; 94:517–522.
99. Harding SM, Richter JE, Guzzo MR, Schan CA, Alexander RW, Bradley LA. Asthma and gastroesophageal reflux: acid suppressive therapy improves asthma outcome. Am J Med 1996; 100:395–405.
100. Kinsbourne M. Hiatus hernia with contortions of the neck. Lancet 1964; 1:1058–1060.
101. Gonzalez-Fernandez F, Arguelles-Martin F, Rodriquez de Quesada B. Gastroesophageal scintigraphy: a useful screening test for GE reflux. J Pediatr Gastroenterol Nutr 1987; 6:217–219.
102. Balson B, Kravitz E, McGeady SJ. Gastroesophageal reflux in childhood asthma (abstr). J Allergy Clin Immunol 1995; 95:201.

103. Meyers WF, Roberts CC, Johnson DG. Value of tests for evaluation of gastroesophageal reflux in children. J Pediatr Surg 1985; 20:515–520.
104. Ott DJ. Barium esophagram. In: Castell DO, Wm W, Ott DJ, eds. Gastro-Esophageal Reflux Disease: Pathogenesis, Diagnosis, Therapy. Mt. Kisco, NY: Future Publishing, 1985; 109–128.
105. Welch RW, Luckmann K, Ricks P. Lower esophageal sphincter pressure in histologic esophagitis. Dig Dis Sci 1980; 25:420–426.
106. Working Group of the European Society of Gastroenterology and Nutrition. A standardized protocol for the methodology of esophageal pH monitoring and interpretation of the data for the diagnosis of gastroesophageal reflux. J Pediatr Gastroenterol Nutr 1992; 14:467–471.
107. Nelson HS. Gastroesophageal reflux and pulmonary disease. J Allergy Clin Immunol 1984; 73:547–556.
108. Strobel CF, Byrne WJ, Avert ME. Correlation of esophageal lengths in children with height: application to the Tuttle test without prior manometry. J Pediatr 1979; 103:215–218.
109. Orenstein SR. Controversies in pediatric gastroesophageal reflux. J Pediatr Gastrenterol Nutr 1992; 14:338–348.
110. Euler AR, Bryne WJ. Twenty four hour esophageal intraluminal pH probe testing: a comparative analysis. Gastroenterology 1981; 80:957–961.
111. Westra SJ, Derkx, HHF, Taminiau JA. Symptomatic gastroesophageal reflux: diagnosis with ultrasound. J Ped Gastroenterol Nutr 1994; 19:58–64.
112. Westra SJ, Wolf BHM, Stealman CR. Ultrasound diagnosis of gastroesophageal reflux and hiatus hernia in young children. J Clin Ultrasound 1990; 18:477–485.
113. Naik DR, Bolio A, Moore DJ. Comparison of barium swallow and ultrasound in diagnosis of gastro-esophageal reflux in children. Br Med J 1985; 290:1943–1945.
114. Gomes H, Menanteau B. Gastroesophageal reflux: comparative study between sonography and pH monitoring. Pediatr Radiol 1991; 21:168–174.
115. Hirsch W, Preiss U, Kedan R. Color coded Doppler ultrasound in diagnosis of gastroesophageal reflux. Klin Pediatric 1997; 209:6–10.
116. Caletti GC, Ferrari A, Mattoli S, Zannoli R. Di Simone MB, Bocus P, Gozetti G, Barbara L. Endoscopy versus ultrasonography in staging reflux esophagitis. Endoscopy 1994; 26:794–797.
117. Stein MR. Simplifying the diagnosis and treatment of gastroesophageal reflux and airway disease. J Asthma 1995; 32:167–172.
118. Treem WR, Davis PM, Hyams JS. Gastroesophageal reflux in the older child: presentation, response to treatment and long term followup (abstr). Gastroenterology 1990; 98:139.
119. Pesendorfer P, Hollwarth ME, Uray E. Long term followup of infants with pathological gastroesophageal reflux. Klin Pediatr 1993; 205:363–366.
120. Pollmann H, Zillessen E, Pohl J, Rosemeyer D, Abucan A, Armbrecht U, Bornhofen B, Herz R. Effect of elevated head position in bed in therapy of gastroesophageal reflux. Gastroenterology 1996; 34 (suppl 2):93–99.
121. Richter JE, Castell DO. Gastroesophageal reflux: pathogenesis, diagnosis and therapy. Ann Intern Med 1982; 97:93–103.

122. Lambert J, Mobassaleh M, Grand R: Efficacy of cimetidine for gastric acid suppression in pediatric patients. J Pediatr 1992; 120:474–478.
123. Gustaffson PM, Kjellman WIM, Tibbling L. A trial of ranitidine in asthmatic children and adolescents with or without pathological gastroesophageal reflux. Eur Respir J 1992; 5:201–206.
124. Gunasekaren TS, Hassall EG. Efficacy and safety of omeprazole for severe gastroesophageal reflux in children. J Pediatr 1993; 123:48–54.
125. Katzka DA, Paoletti V, Leite L, Castell DO. Prolonged ambulatory pH monitoring in patients with gastroesophageal reflux disease symptoms: testing while on therapy identifies the need for more aggressive anti-reflux therapy. Am J Gastroenterol 1996; 91:2110–2113.
126. Depla AC, Bartelsman JF, Roos CM, Tytgat GN, Jansen HM. Beneficial effect of omeprazole in a patient with severe bronchial asthma and gastroesophageal reflux. Eur Respir J 1988; 1:966–968.
127. Orenstein SR, Loftor DW, Orenstein DM. Bethanechol for pediatric gastroesophageal reflux: a prospective, blind controlled study. J Pediatr Gastroenterol Nutr 1986; 5:549–555.
128. Tolia V, Calhoun J, Kuhns L. Randomized, prospective double blind trial of metoclopromide and placebo for gastroesophageal reflux in infants. J Pediatr 1989; 115:141–145.
129. Machida HM, Forbes DA, Gall DG, Scott RB. Metoclopramide in gastroesophageal reflux of infancy. J Pediatr 1988; 112:483–487.
130. Dordal MT, Baltazan MH, Roca I, Marques L. Nocturnal spasmotic cough. Evolution after antireflux treatment. Allerg Immunol 1994; 26:53–58.
131. Tucci, J, Resti M, Fontana R, Novembre E, Lami CA, Vierucci A. Gastroesophageal reflux and bronchial asthma: prevalence and effect of cisapride therapy. J Pediatr Gastroenterol Nutr 1993; 17:265–270.
132. Arguelles-Martin F, Gonzalez-Fernandez F, Gentles MG. Sucralfate versus cimetidine in the treatment of reflux esophagitis in children. Am J Med 1989; 86(suppl): 73–76.
133. Johnson DG, Current thinking on the role of surgery in gastroesophageal reflux. Pediatr Clin North Am 1985; 32:1165–1179.
134. Kauer WK, Peters JH, De Meester LR, Heimbuche J, Ireland AP, Bremmer CG. A tailored approach to antireflux surgery. J Thorac Cardiovasc Surg 1995; 110: 141–146.
135. Taylor LA, Weiner T, Lacey SR, Azizkhan RG. Chronic lung disease is the leading risk factor correlating with the failure (wrap disruption) of antireflux procedures in children. J Pediatr Surg 1994; 29:161–164.
136. Luostarinen M. Nissen fundoplication for reflux esophagitis. Long term clinical and endoscopic results in 109 of 127 consecutive patients. Ann Surg 1993; 217: 329–337.
137. Fonkalsrud EW, Ament ME. Gastroesophageal reflux in childhood. Curr Probl Surg 1996; 33:1–80.
138. Wheatley MJ, Coran AG, Wesley JR, Oldham KT, Turnage RH. Redo fundoplication in infants and children with recurrent gastroesophageal reflux. J Pediatr Surg 1991; 26:758–761.

139. Gourley GR, Pellett JR, Li BUK. A prospective randomized double blind study of gastroesophageal reflux surgery in pediatric-sized developmentally disabled patients. Nissen fundoplication versus Angelchik prosthesis. J Pediatr Gastroenterol Nutr 1986; 5:52–61.
140. Cuschieri A, Hunter J, Wolfe B. Multicenter prospective evaluation of laparoscopic antireflux surgery. Surg Endosc 1993; 7:505–510.
141. Cadiere GB, Himpens J, Rajan A, Muls V, Lemper JC, Bruyns J, Urbain D, Ham H. Laparoscopic Nissen fundoplication: laparoscopic dissection technique and results. Hepatogastroenterology 1997; 44:4–10.
142. Mosnier H, Leport J, Aubert A, Kianmanesh R, Sbai-Idrassi MS, Guivarch M. A 270 degree laparoscopic posterior fundoplasty in the treatment of gastroesophageal reflux. J Am Coll Surg 1995; 181:220–224.
143. Larrain A, Carrasco E, Galleguillos F, Sepulveda R, Pope CEII. Medical and surgical treatment of nonallergic asthma associated with gastroesophageal reflux. Chest 1991; 99:1330–1335.
144. Goldman JM, Bennett JR. Gastroesophageal reflux and asthma; a common association but of what clinical importance? Gut 1990; 31:1–4.
145. Hoeffel JC, Nihoul-Fekete C, Schmitt M. Esophageal adenocarcinoma after gastroesophageal reflux in children. J Pediatr 1989; 115:259–261.

11

Respiratory Complications of Reflux Disease in Infants

SUSAN R. ORENSTEIN

University of Pittsburgh School of Medicine
and Children's Hospital of Pittsburgh
Pittsburgh, Pennsylvania

Infantile apnea and stridor, exacerbations of bronchopulmonary dysplasia and cystic fibrosis, and the pulmonary disease associated with repaired esophageal atresia and diaphragmatic hernia are respiratory diseases affected by gastroesophageal reflux (GER) and presenting in infancy. Nasal regurgitation is a further airway manifestation of reflux essentially limited to infancy. These infantile forms of reflux-associated airway disease are the subject of this chapter.

I. Physiology: Infants Versus Older Children and Adults

Why are some manifestations of reflux-associated respiratory disease limited to infancy? The answers are to be found in the unique aspects of the infant's physiology, as well as in the occurrence of congenital disease. These unique aspects of physiology are to be found in the gastrointestinal tract, in the respiratory tract, at the intersection of the two tracts in the pharynx, and in the infant's body as a whole. They comprise both structural and functional immaturities.

A. Gastrointestinal

Similarities between infants and adults with regard to the pathophysiology of reflux are greater than previously suspected, despite marked differences in clinical manifestations of GER disease (GERD). These similarities include the gastroduodenal secretions that make up the refluxate, the lower esophageal sphincter (LES) tone, and the transient lower esophageal sphincter relaxations (TLESRs), which allow reflux to occur.

Soon after birth, term newborn infants are able to secrete enough HCl to drop their gastric pH to 2 and below; peptic activity is similarly mature (1–3). Bile acids and trypsin are also present in the infant's duodenal contents from birth (4). Lower esophageal sphincter tone is well developed even in premature infants (5).

As in adults, TLESRs are the major mechanism for reflux events in infants (6–9). They occur frequently enough that the daily duration of distal esophageal acid exposure is remarkably similar in normal infants and adults (10–12). However, because gastric contents are buffered by infant milk formula for about 2 hours after feedings, pH probe values for acid reflux may significantly underestimate the frequency and duration of total reflux in infants.

Despite all of the similarities enumerated above, there are marked differences in gastrointestinal physiology between infants and older people with regard to reflux. These differences include both structural and functional aspects, although much remains to be learned. Structurally, the ratio of esophageal to gastric volume is much less in the infant, so that the esophageal capacity is more easily overwhelmed by reflux (13). This favors regurgitation as a manifestation of reflux disease in infants, and it may make refluxate more accessible to the respiratory tract than in adults.

Functionally, gastric and esophageal compliance likely play a role in determining LES and upper esophageal sphincter (UES) relaxation. The much lower gastric compliance in infants than in adults (14) may promote LES relaxation at comparably lower intragastric volumes in infants than in adults.

The UES relaxes in infants in response to gastroesophageal reflux (15) and to air insufflation into the esophagus (16); information regarding developmental aspects of esophageal compliance and thresholds for this response are needed. It is possible that the prominence of regurgitation in infants is facilitated by lower-threshold relaxation of both the LES and UES.

Esophageal motor activity is less frequently peristaltic in premature infants than in adults; in the premature infants only about one fourth of esophageal body pressure waves are peristaltic, a finding also true in the near-term babies (5). Such immaturity of esophageal function would impair the return of refluxed material into the stomach and promote its supraesophageal migration.

Finally, the oropharyngeal function of infants is immature. The suck-swallow of the infant is different from the complex chewing and bolus manipulation of the mature human. Material regurgitated into the pharynx may thus be less effectively manipulated into a safe location, promoting airway manifestations of GERD in infants.

The differences in gastrointestinal physiology that provoke reflux-associated respiratory disease in infants are exacerbated by the infant's diet. This diet is largely liquid, which seems to induce more regurgitation than the thicker consistency of the masticated adult diet. Infants ingest a larger meal compared to their gastric volume than adults do, which also provokes more reflux (17). Furthermore, infants are more apt to manifest allergies to their dietary constituents, and cow milk or soy sensitivity may lead to vomiting and esophagitis, initiating the vicious cycle of esophagitis and reflux.

There are several ameliorating factors in the infant diet. It contains little in the way of acid material; infant milk formulas have a pH of nearly 7, compared to many adult beverages with pH < 3 (18). It is largely isotonic [compared to many adult beverages with osmolalities between 600 and 2600 mOsm/L (18)], and it does not include the refluxogenic effects of caffeine and first-hand tobacco smoke exposure, as many adult diets do.

B. Respiratory

The respiratory physiology of infants is also different from adults. The softer, more flexible upper respiratory structures in many babies represent a developmental laryngotracheomalacea, which resolves during infancy. Thus, babies are more susceptible to stridor induced by strong negative pressures during inspiration, a phenomenon that is exacerbated by reflux in some of them.

The smaller cross-sectional area of the airway, most exaggerated in the upper airway, is another factor making upper airway symptoms, like stridor, predominate over lower ones in infants, in contrast to the lower respiratory symptom predomination in older children.

The fact that young infants are obligate nose breathers makes nasal obstruction by nasal regurgitation or otherwise (e.g., by viral infections or by bedding) a far more hazardous phenomenon in babies than in older individuals.

Primitive reflexes are a further aspect of infant physiology that leads to distinct manifestations of reflux-associated respiratory disease. Prolonged apnea is a singular manifestation of reflux in young infants and virtually never occurs in adults.

C. Pharynx (Gastrointestinal-Respiratory Intersection)

The structure of the pharynx differs in the infant, in whom the soft palate extends nearly to the larynx, with complex possible effects on swallowing, reflux, and speech (19). This difference may underlie, for example, the frequency of nasal regurgitation in infants (20).

The function of the infantile oropharynx does not include the array of airway-protective abilities present in older children and adults. Throat-clearing and other automatic and volitional protections develop during childhood.

D. Other Effects

Other differences between infants and adults that impact on reflux are limited gross motor abilities and postural tone. The immature tone of the somatic musculature of the torso and extremities leads to a preponderance of time in the supine position and to slumping postures and increased abdominal pressure when seated. Both supine and slumped-seated positions provoke reflux and impair its gravitational clearance (21,22). Premature infants are particularly hypotonic and may be especially affected by the reflux-provoking effects of such postures. In addition to being unable to stand independently, or even to sit without support during much of infancy, babies are unable to change their position at will in response to symptoms suggesting GERD or respiratory compromise. The youngest infants are unable even to turn over, and premature babies cannot even lift their heads clear of regurgitated material. The ramifications for respiratory sequelae from reflux are obvious.

II. Gastroesophageal Reflux Disease in Infants

A. Disease Course

The course of reflux disease in infants differs considerably from that in older children and adults. Infantile reflux becomes symptomatic during the first months of life but often not until 2–4 months, the peak age of onset. However, it resolves by 12–24 months of age in at least 80% of afflicted babies (23,24). This is in contrast to reflux in older children and adults, which appears anew after infancy. It then tends to persist, waxing and waning symptomatically for years (25,26).

B. Epidemiology

The epidemiology of reflux disease is beginning to be clarified in infants. In the first year of life, nearly 7% of all infants come to medical attention for GER symptoms (27); most receive some treatment, and 1–2% undergo diagnostic evaluation. Less than 1% of infants undergoes antireflux surgery, and the number may be decreasing with improved understanding of nonsurgical therapies. The incidence of symptomatic GERD in very low birthweight infants is higher—3–10% of such infants have symptoms of reflux-associated apnea, bradycardia, or exacerbated bronchopulmonary dysplasia (28,29).

C. Symptoms

The symptoms of GERD are also different in infants. Many of the unique symptoms of infantile GERD, such as apnea and stridor, are airway manifestations.

These symptoms may be more acutely dangerous, as well as being more prevalent and more diverse, in infants than in adults.

D. Causes for Infant–Adult Differences in Clinical GERD

The differences in clinical presentation in infants have three likely causes: infants' developmental immaturity, infants' nonverbal nature, and the chronological brevity of infantile reflux. Developmental immaturity makes regurgitation, apnea, and stridor common manifestations of reflux in infants, whereas they rarely occur in adults (discussed above). The nonverbal nature of infants means that complaints of "heartburn" or other descriptions of esophageal pain do not occur, although intractable crying may be an analogous symptom (30–32). The limited chronicity of reflux in infants minimizes presentations that require chronicity of acid exposure to the esophagus itself, such as erosive esophagitis and stricture. One might even consider infants to manifest the primary pathophysiology of reflux disease more purely, before the vicious cycles and irreversible changes of esophagitis and dysmotility, esophageal shortening and hiatal hernia, scarring and stricture, supervene.

III. Vicious Cycles Between Reflux and Respiratory Disease

Reflux provokes respiratory disease by obstructing the respiratory tract. The most primitive conceptualization of how this happens attributed all of the obstruction to gastric material aspirated after being regurgitated into the pharynx. Our sophistication has grown since this concept was first introduced, and we now understand that the respiratory tract may be obstructed at a series of loci by multiple mechanisms, which may occur in concert (33).

A. Reflux Causing Respiratory Disease

Actual aspiration of a quantity of gastric material probably occurs only rarely. Even "microaspiration" may be a relatively infrequent event. The lumen of the respiratory tract may be obstructed by its own secretions, however, as well as by aspirated material. In addition, edema of the airway may participate in airway occlusion, and the airway-supporting musculature may contract, represented by laryngospasm or bronchospasm. Gastroesophageal reflux may participate by producing airway motor spasm, edema, or secretions on a reflex basis, as well as by allowing refluxate to reach and occlude the airway. Such reflexes, with afferents in the esophagus and efferents in the airway, have been indicated by pediatric and animal studies, as well as by adult studies (see Chap. 2) (34–40).

B. Respiratory Disease Causing Reflux

The other half of the cycle, in which respiratory disease can provoke reflux, involves the provocative effects of positive abdominal and negative intrathoracic pressures. These pressure changes are exaggerated during forced inspiration and expiration, as well as during stridor and coughing. These pressure relationships promote the movement of gastric contents into the esophagus. They are countered by the bolstering effect of the crural diaphragm, which contracts in support of the LES during such straining, if there is no hiatal hernia. Respiratory disease may also provoke reflux more indirectly by prompting the use of therapies that provoke reflux. These therapies include medications, postural drainage, and mechanical ventilation (21,41–49).

IV. Respiratory Diseases in Infants

The mechanics of infantile respiratory diseases that allow their participation in the vicious cycles indicated above are similar to those in adults. However, several respiratory disorders that are unique to infancy or have their most challenging manifestations during infancy will be briefly discussed individually.

A. Apnea

Apnea has been clearly demonstrated to be temporally correlated with some episodes of reflux and to be experimentally induced by acid infusion into the esophagus (34,35). A large series of infants presenting with apparent life-threatening events (ALTE) found reflux to be responsible for more cases than any other single cause (50). Such reflux-associated apnea usually involves laryngeal closure and can be viewed as an exaggerated protective response to hazardous material threatening the airway (51,52). The relative roles of microaspiration, laryngeal stimulation, and esophageal stimulation in producing apnea have been debated (34,35, 51,53,54).

Clinically, reflux-induced apnea is recognized as generally postprandial, occurring in the seated or supine position, apparently obstructive and associated with respiratory efforts, and sometimes associated with oral or nasal regurgitation (55–58). These episodes are generally survived, but occasional deaths have occurred (59).

The determination of whether reflux has provoked apnea is a common pediatric diagnostic dilemma. We generally proceed as follows. If a single episode is described as a classic reflux-related event (the infant is postprandial, seated or supine, struggling and turning red and then dusky or pale, and, particularly, if oral or nasal regurgitation is actually seen), we diagnose it without formal investigation. We treat by normalizing feeding volume and frequency, avoiding seated and supine positioning, and consider further empiric therapy with thickening of formula, prokinetic medication, and sometimes even empiric acid suppression. If there is recurrence despite such therapy, or if episodes are initially presented as recurrent or as ambiguous with regard to reflux, we perform pH probe with pneumocardiogram (including some measurement of nasal air flow to allow documentation of obstructive apnea). If a clear association is thus demonstrated between reflux and apnea, we augment therapy and consider fundoplication for persisting severe cases, although this is rarely required. If the initial presentation is of central apnea or if the pH probe demonstrates apnea that is clearly unassociated with reflux, we pursue other causes of apnea, such as metabolic or infectious ones, more vigorously (50).

B. Stridor

Stridor may represent an incomplete version of obstructive apnea in infants. Because laryngomalacia may be responsible for stridor without participation of reflux (60) clinicians are faced with the decision of whether individual infants with stridor may benefit by antireflux pharmacotherapy or even fundoplication in intractable cases (61–63). Otolaryngologists and pulmonologists have begun to recognize laryngeal changes attributed to GERD during laryngoscopy, although it is not yet absolutely clear that inflammatory changes are due to acid irritation rather than to mechanical trauma in the context of underlying laryngomalacia. While pH probe monitoring (63) or esophageal acid infusion (64) may disclose a temporal association with intermittent stridor, thus prompting therapy of reflux, the relative merits of this approach (evaluation for peptic esophagitis or laryngitis or empiric therapy) are as yet unclear.

C. Bronchopulmonary Dysplasia

The participation of chronic lung disease and its therapies in vicious cycles with GERD mandates consideration of reflux as contributing to difficult-to-manage bronchopulmonary dysplasia (BPD) (65–68). Evaluation for esophagitis will select a group for whom antireflux therapy is definitely indicated; in ambiguous cases scintigraphic or bronchoscopic evaluation for aspiration, or empiric pharmacotherapy, may be worthwhile.

D. Cystic Fibrosis

Many studies have indicated an increased proportion of infants and children with cystic fibrosis (CF) to have pathological GER (69–81). The underlying reasons for the association, as well as the approach to diagnosis and management, will be similar to infants with BPD. In addition, the increased gastric acidity and the malnutrition due to pancreatic insufficiency in CF pose additional problems for the clinician managing infants with CF and GERD.

E. Esophageal Atresia (Tracheoesophageal Fistula)

Esophageal atresia usually occurs with a distal tracheoesophageal fistula, although a small minority of infants may be born with isolated esophageal atresia, isolated tracheoesophageal fistula (''H-type''), or a proximal fistula. After repair, infants with these anomalies are likely to have GERD for a number of reasons. These are related both to the dysfunctional anatomy postrepair and to congenital disturbances of the antireflux barrier in these infants (82–89). The GERD may induce anastomotic strictures or participate in vicious cycles of reflux and respiratory disease. The difficulty of interrupting the vicious cycle in these children often prompts fundoplication, but fundoplication may be particularly problematic in them because of their esophageal shortening and peristaltic dysfunction due to the atresia itself.

F. Diaphragmatic Hernia

Infants born with congenital diaphragmatic hernia usually experience a difficult neonatal course with only about half of live-born infants surviving. They generally have associated pulmonary hypertension, lung hypoplasia, and intestinal malrotation. In addition to surgical repair, extracorporeal membrane oxygenation is often used for weeks before infants are able to wean, due to their associated pulmonary hypertension. Nearly all survivors have clinical GERD, with as many as 20% requiring fundoplication (90). Awareness of the possible contribution of GERD to their chronic lung disease will allow early recognition and a degree of prophylactic intervention.

V. Diagnosis of Reflux in Infantile Respiratory Disease

In addition to the specific diagnostic approaches indicated above, there are some general principles. If chronic or recurrent pneumonia suggests aspiration, the techniques used to diagnose aspiration depend on the institution's capabilities. Nuclear medicine's scintigraphy, bronchoscopy evaluating gross appearance and lipid-laden macrophages, or assessment of endotracheal tube for methylene blue instilled in the stomach by nasogastric or gastrostomy tube are all potentially useful.

When respiratory symptoms are discrete and recurrent, such as episodes of stridor or cough, one can monitor for the symptom during a 24-hour (or longer) pH probe test. The same phenomenon can be evaluated experimentally and perhaps more efficiently using the modified Bernstein test. A 24-hour pH probe alone, without documentation of symptom association, can also be used to define reflux quantity or score as abnormal (and thus both likely to be pathological and likely to warrant therapy).

At our institution we frequently use esophageal suction biopsy to diagnose pathologic reflux in infants. The test is rapid, safe, and relatively inexpensive, and in many cases defines the reflux as pathological and thus warranting treatment. Response to antireflux therapy is then used to support the association between the reflux and the respiratory disease.

The issue of whether to use empiric therapy for respiratory disease that is suspected to be reflux-associated is a difficult one. This is largely because of the intensity and duration of therapy that have been found to be required to ameliorate most such respiratory disease.

VI. Therapy of Reflux in Infantile Respiratory Disease

A. Conservative Therapy

Although nonpharmacologic therapy ameliorates reflux symptoms in the majority of infants with reflux symptoms, the addition of pharmacotherapy is necessary for most respiratory disease associated with reflux. Nonetheless, this "conservative therapy" is a crucial underpinning of all treatment.

Many infants are overfed at infrequent feedings; simply correcting this error will have dramatic effects on regurgitation. Similarly, thickening of infant feedings with a tablespoon of rice cereal per ounce of formula increases the caloric density by 50% and reduces regurgitation as well. A trial of hypoallergenic elemental formula will also ameliorate symptoms in the babies whose regurgitation initially had an allergic basis, and it might also benefit the occasional infant with an allergic component to the respiratory disease. Avoidance of thin liquids (juices) also benefits reflux, particularly because these juices are usually acidic.

Positioning is an important component of antireflux therapy, particularly in young infants, who are unable to change their own position at will in response to symptoms. Supine and slumped-seated positions provoke reflux; we recommend completely avoiding them. This recommendation is in accord with the American Academy of Pediatrics positioning recommendations for prevention of sudden infant death syndrome, which exempts infants with GERD from the "back-to-sleep" campaign.

B. Pharmacotherapy

Infants with respiratory disease associated with reflux will generally require both a prokinetic agent and acid suppression, and they may require more intensive therapy for longer durations than infants with simple regurgitation. This corre-

Table 1 Therapy of Reflux

I. Conservative
   A. Position: prone; or completely upright (avoid supine, semi-seated)
   B. Thicken infant feedings: 1 tbsp. rice cereal/oz. formula (= 30 cal/oz., if original formula is 20 cal/oz)
   C. Fast before bed; avoid large meals, obesity, tight clothing
   D. Avoid foods and medications that lower LES tone or increase gastric acidity:
      Fatty foods, citrus, tomato, carbonated or acid beverages, coffee, alcohol, smoke exposure
      Anticholinergics, adrenergics, theophylline, caffeine, calcium channel blockers, prostaglandins
II. Pharmacologic[a]
   A. Prokinetic:
      Cisapride (0.2 mg/kg/dose qid: AC, HS) {cramping, arrhythmias}
      {{concurrent macrolide or antifungal antibiotics—potentially serious arrhythmias}}
      Metoclopramide (0.1 mg/kg/dose qid: AC, HS)
      {restlessness, drowsiness, dystonic reactions—antidote; diphenhydramine}
      {{gastrointestinal obstruction; pheochromocytoma; extrapyramidal risk}}
      Bethanechol {{avoid in respiratory disease}}
   B. Antacid:
      Cimetidine (5–10 mg/kg/dose qid: AC, HS) {headache, pancytopenia, gynecomastia, cholestasis}
      Ranitidine (2–3 mg/kg/dose tid) {similar to cimetidine, less gynecomastia, more hepatitis}
      Famotidine (0.5 mg/kg/dose bid or tid; adult 40 mg HS)
      Omeprazole (0.7–3.3 mg/kg/dose qd or divide bid; adult 20 mg HS or bid)
      Antacid (0.5–1 cc/kg/dose, 3–8×/day: 1–2 hr PC,HS) {diarrhea, constipation, rickets, Al or Mg toxicity}
   C. Barrier or miscellaneous mechanism:
      Sucralfate slurry (1 g in 5–15 ml solution, qid: PC, HS)—protects against bile salts, trypsin, acid
      {constipation, gastric concretions, potential binding of other medications}
      Alaginic acid-antacid (2 g 3–8× a day: PC)
III. Surgical
   A. Fundoplication (complete vs. loose wrap; ±gastrostomy, ±pyloroplasty; laparotomy vs. laparoscopy)
   B. Gastrojejunostomy

(), Common doses; {}, partial list of side effects; {{}}, partial list of contraindications.
[a]Usual course is 8 weeks.
Source: Adapted from Ref. 97.

sponds to adult data suggesting the need for particularly vigorous therapy to interrupt the reflux-respiratory vicious cycles (91).

Table 1 indicates typical doses and other aspects of pharmacotherapy.

C. Surgical Therapy

Nissen fundoplication is the most effective antireflux therapy and thus is lifesaving for some children with intractable reflux-associated respiratory disease (92–95). Its long-term efficacy is incomplete, however, and a number of side effects and complications prevent it from being a panacea. Some of its problems are particularly pronounced in infants with respiratory disease, such as, herniation of the wrap due to exaggerated abdominothoracic pressure relationships or dysphagia in children who have the underlying esophageal dysmotility associated with repaired esophageal atresia.

Newer forms of surgical intervention in GERD have also been applied to infants: gastrojejunostomy (96) and laparoscopic fundoplication. Their advantages and disadvantages are debated, and their use must be individualized, both to the patient and to the surgeon. Gastrojejunostomy disrupts less of the normal anatomy and physiology but probably requires ongoing antireflux pharmacotherapy to be maintained as well.

VII. Conclusion

Increasing recognition of the association between a variety of respiratory diseases and gastroesophageal reflux in infants will permit us to better identify and treat it. Thus we can prevent morbidity and mortality in these individuals who have many decades of potential health ahead of them.

References

1. Hyman PE, Clarke DD, Everett SL, et al. Gastric acid secretory function in preterm infants. J Pediatr 1985; 106:467–470.
2. Sondheimer J, Clark D, Gervaise E. Continuous gastric pH measurement in young and older healthy preterm infants receiving formula and clear liquid feedings. J Pediatr Gastroenterol Nutr 1985; 4:352–355.
3. DiPalma J, Kirk CL, Hamosh M, Colon AR, Benjamin SB, Hamosh P. Lipase and pepsin activity in the gastric mucosa of infants, children, and adults. Gastroenterology 1991; 101:116–121.
4. Lebenthal E, Lee P. Development of functional response in human exocrine pancreas. Pediatrics 1980; 66:556–560.
5. Omari T, Miki K, Fraser R, Davidson G, Haslam R, Goldsworthy W, Bakewell M,

Kawahara H, Dent J. Esophageal body and lower esophageal sphincter function in healthy premature infants. Gastroenterology 1995; 109:1757–1764.
6. Cucchiara S, Staiano A, DiLorenzo C, DeLuca G, dellaRocca A, Auricchio S. Pathophysiology of gastroesophageal reflux and distal esophageal motility in children with gastroesophageal reflux disease. J Pediatr Gastroenterol Nutr 1988; 7:830–836.
7. Cucchiara S, Bartolotti M, Minella R, et al. Fasting and postprandial mechanisms of gastroesophageal reflux in children with gastroesophageal reflux disease. Dig Dis Sci 1993; 38:86–92.
8. Dent J, Davidson GP, Barnes BE, Freeman JK, Kirubakaran C. The mechanism of gastro-oesophageal reflux in children. Aust Paediatr J 1981; 17:125.
9. Werlin SL, Dodds WJ, Hogan WJ, Arndorfer RC. Mechanisms of gastroesophageal reflux in children. J Pediatr 1980; 97:244–249.
10. Johnson L, DeMeester T. Twenty-four-hour pH monitoring of the distal esophagus: a quantitative measure of gastroesophageal reflux. Am J Gastroenterol 1974; 62: 325–332.
11. Vandenplas Y, Sacre-Smits L. Continuous 24-hour esophageal pH monitoring in 285 asymptomatic infants 0–15 months old. J Pediatr Gastroenterol Nutr 1987; 6:220–224.
12. Orenstein SR. Gastroesophageal reflux. In: Stockman J, Winter R, eds. Current Problems in Pediatrics. Chicago: Mosby Year Book Medical Publishers, 1991; 193–241.
13. Roessle R, Roulet F. Mass und Zahl in der Pathologie und Klinik in Einzeldarstellungen. Vol. 5. Berlin: Springer, 1932; 144.
14. DiLorenzo C, Mertz H, Rehm D, Meyer E, Hyman P. Postnatal maturation of gastric response to distension in newborn infants. Gastroenterology 1994; 107:1222.
15. Willing J, Davidson G, Dent J, Cook I. Effect of gastro-oesophageal reflux on upper oesophageal sphincter motility in children. Gut 1993; 34:904–910.
16. Orenstein S, DiLorenzo C, Orenstein D, Shalaby T, Deneault L, Lutz J. Isolated lower esophageal sphincter relaxation (TLESR) as ''wave-suppressed'' secondary peristalsis. Dysphagia 1997; 12:207–211.
17. Sutphen JL, Dillard VL. Effect of feeding volume on early postcibal gastroesophageal reflux in infants. J Pediatr Gastroenterol Nutr 1988; 7:185–188.
18. Feldman M, Barnett C. Relationships between the acidity and osmolality of popular beverages and reported heartburn. Gastroenterology 1995; 108:125–131.
19. Laitman J, Reidenberg J. Specializations of the human upper respiratory and upper digestive systems as seen through comparative and developmental anatomy. Dysphagia 1993; 8:318–325.
20. Oestreich A, Dunbar J. Pharyngonasal reflux: spectrum and significance in early childhood. AJR 1984; 141:923–925.
21. Torres A, Serra-Batlles J, Ros E, Riera C, de la Bellacasa JP, Cobos A, Lomena F, Rodriguez-Roisin R. Pulmonary aspiration of gastric contents in patients receiving mechanical ventilation: the effect of body position. Ann Int Med 1992; 116:540–543.
22. Orenstein SR, Whitington PF, Orenstein DM. The infant seat as treatment for gastroesophageal reflux. N Engl J Med 1983; 309:760–763.
23. Shepherd RW, Wren J, Evans S, Lander M, Ong TH. Gastroesophageal reflux in

children. Clinical profile, course and outcome with active therapy in 126 cases. Clin Pediatr (Phila) 1987; 26:55–60.
24. Carre IJ. A historical review of the clinical consequences of hiatal hernia (partial thoracic stomach) and gastroesophageal reflux. In: Gellis S, ed. Gastroesophageal Reflux: Report of the 76th Ross Conference on Pediatric Research. Columbus, OH: Ross Laboratories, 1979:1–12.
25. Treem W, Davis P, Hyams J. Gastroesophageal reflux in the older child: presentation, response to treatment and long-term follow-up. Clin Pediatr 1991; 30:435–440.
26. Schindlbeck N, Klauser A, Berghammer G, Londong W, Muller-Lissner S. Three year follow up of patients with gastroesophageal reflux disease. Gut 1992; 33:1016–1019.
27. Aronow E, Silverberg M. Normal and abnormal GI motility. In: Silverberg M, ed. Pediatric Gastroenterology. New York: Medical Examination Publishing Co, Inc., 1983:214.
28. Hrabovsky EE, Mullett MD. Gastroesophageal reflux and the premature infant. J Pediatr Surg 1986; 21:583–587.
29. Campfield J, Shah B, Angelides A, Hirsch B. Incidence of gastroesophageal reflux (GER) in VLBW. Pediatr Res 1992; 31:106A.
30. Flores AF, Katz AJ. The crying baby syndrome: the role of gastroesophageal reflux. Pediatr Res 1984; 18:195A.
31. Ryan P, Lander M, Ong TH, Shepherd P. When does reflux oesophagitis occur with gastro-oesophageal reflux in infants? A clinical and endoscopic study, and correlation with outcome. Aust Paediatr J 1983; 19:90–93.
32. Berkowitz D, Naveh Y, Berant M. "Infantile colic" as the sole manifestation of gastroesophageal reflux. J Pediatr Gastroenterol Nutr 1997; 24:231–233.
33. Putnam PE, Ricker DH, Orenstein SP. Gastroesophageal reflux. In: Beckerman R, Brouilette R, Hunt C, eds. Respiratory Control Disorders in Infants and Children. Baltimore: Williams & Wilkins, 1992; 322–341.
34. Herbst JJ, Book LS, Bray PF. Gastroesophageal reflux in the "near miss" sudden infant death syndrome. J Pediatr 1978; 92:73–75.
35. Herbst JJ, Minton SD, Book LS. Gastroesophageal reflux causing respiratory distress and apnea in newborn infants. J Pediatr 1979; 95:763–768.
36. Downing SE, Lee JC. Laryngeal chemosensitivity: a possible mechanism for sudden infant death. Pediatrics 1975; 55:640–649.
37. Davis RS, Larsen GL, Grunstein MM. Respiratory response to intraesophageal acid infusion in asthmatic children during sleep. J Allergy Clin Immunol 1983; 72:393–398.
38. Mansfield L, Stein M. Gastroesophageal reflux and asthma: a possible reflex mechanism. Ann Allergy 1978; 41:224–226.
39. Mansfield L, Hameister H, Spaulding H, Smith N, Glab N. The role of the vagus nerve in airway narrowing caused by intraesophageal hydrochloric acid provocation and esophageal distention. Ann Allergy 1981; 47:431–434.
40. Spaulding H, Mansfield L, Stein M, Sellner J, Gremillion D. Further investigation of the association between gastroesophageal reflux and bronchoconstriction. J Allergy Clin Immunol 1982; 69:516–521.
41. Berquist WE, Rachelefsky GS, Kadden M, Siegel SC, Katz RM, Mickey MR, Ament

ME. Effect of theophylline on gastroesophageal reflux in normal adults. J Allergy Clin Immunol 1981; 67:407–411.
42. Berquist WE, Rachelefsky GS, Rowshan N, Siegel S, Katz R, Welch M. Quantitative gastroesophageal reflux and pulmonary function in asthmatic children and normal adults receiving placebo, theophylline, and metaproterenol sulfate therapy. J Allergy Clin Immunol 1984; 73:253–258.
43. Zfass A, Prince R, Allen F, Farrar J. Inhibitory beta-adrenergic receptors in the human distal esophagus. Am J Dig Dis 1970; 15:303–310.
44. DiMarino AJ, Cohen S. Effect of an oral $beta_2$-adrenergic agonist on lower esophageal sphincter pressure in normals and in patients with achalasia. Dig Dis Sci 1982; 27:1063–1066.
45. Ruzkowski C, Sanowski R, Austin J, Rohwedder J, Waring J. The effects of inhaled albuterol and oral theophylline on gastroesophageal reflux in patients with gastroesophageal reflux disease and obstructive lung disease. Arch Intern Med 1992; 152:783–785.
46. Lyrenas E, Sand C, Abrahamsson H. Inhibitory effects of terbutaline on human esophageal peristalsis and development of tolerance. Scand J Gastroenterol 1993; 28:907–910.
47. Button B, Heine R, Catto-Smith A, Phelan P, Olinsky A. Postural drainage and gastrooesophageal reflux in infants with cystic fibrosis. Arch Dis Child 1997; 76:148–150.
48. Stein M, Towner T, Weber R, Mansfield L, Jacobson K, McDonnell J, Nelson H. The effect of theophylline on the lower esophageal sphincter pressure. Ann Allergy 1980; 45:238–241.
49. Marino W, Pitchumoni C. Reversal of negative pressure ventilation-induced lower esophageal sphincter dysfunction with metoclopramide. Am J Gastroenterol 1992; 87:190–194.
50. Kahn A, Rebuffat E, Franco P, N'Duwlmana M, Blum D. Apparent life-threatening events and apnea of infancy. In: Beckerman R, Brouilette R, Hunt C, eds. Respiratory Control Disorders in Infants and Children. Baltimore: Williams & Wilkins, 1992: 178–189.
51. Thach BT, Menon A. Pulmonary protective mechanisms in human infants. Am Rev Respir Dis 1985; 131:
52. Ruggins NR, Milner AD. Site of upper airway obstruction in infants following an acute life-threatening event. Pediatrics 1993; 91:595–601.
53. Altschuler SM, Boyle JT, Nixon TE. Apnea: Does laryngeal microaspiration play a role? Pediatr Res 1984; 18:189A.
54. Bauman N, Sandler A, Schmidt C, Maher J, Smith R. Reflex laryngospasm induced by stimulation of distal esophageal afferents. Laryngoscope 1994; 104:209–214.
55. Spitzer AR, Boyle JT, Tuchman DN, Fox WW. Awake apnea associated with gastroesophageal reflux: a specific clinical syndrome. J Pediatr 1984; 104:200–205.
56. Menon AP, Schefft GL, Thach BT. Frequency and significance of swallowing during prolonged apnea in infants. Am Rev Respir Dis 1984; 130:969–973.
57. Menon AP, Schefft GL, Thach BT. Apnea associated with regurgitation in infants. J Pediatr 1985; 106:625–629.
58. Plaxico D, Loughlin G. Nasopharyngeal reflux and neonatal apnea. Am J Dis Child 1981; 135:793–794.

59. Jolley S, Halpern L, Tunnell W, Johnson D, Sterling C. The risk of sudden infant death from gastroesophageal reflux. J Pediatr Surg 1991; 26:691–696.
60. Belmont JR, Grundfast K. Congenital laryngeal stridor (laryngomalacia): etiologic factors and associated disorders. Ann Otol Rhinol Laryngol 1984; 93:430–437.
61. Henry RL, Mellis CM. Resolution of inspiratory stridor after fundoplication: case report. Aust Paediatr J 1982; 18:126–127.
62. Nielson DW, Heldt GP, Tooley WH. Stridor and gastroesophageal reflux in infants. Pediatrics 1990; 85:1034–1039.
63. Orenstein SR, Orenstein DM, Whitington PF. Gastroesophageal reflux causing stridor. Chest 1983; 84:301–302.
64. Orenstein SR, Kocoshis SA, Orenstein DM, Proujansky R. Stridor and gastroesophageal reflux: diagnostic use of intraluminal esophageal acid perfusion (Bernstein test). Pediatr Pulmonol 1987; 3:420–424.
65. Chen P-H, Chang M-H, Hsu S-O. Gastroesophageal reflux in children with chronic recurrent bronchopulmonary infection. J Pediatr Gastroenterol Nutr 1991; 13:16–22.
66. Sindel B, Maisels M, Ballantine T. Gastroesophageal reflux to the proximal esophagus in infants with bronchopulmonary dysplasia. Am J Dis Child 1989; 143:1103–1106.
67. Lew C, Keens T, O'Neal M, et al. Gastroesophageal reflux prevents recovery from bronchopulmonary dysplasia. Clin Res 1981; 29:149A.
68. Guiffre RM, Rubin S, Mitchell I. Antireflux surgery in infants with bronchopulmonary dysplasia. Am J Dis Child 1987; 141:648–651.
69. Bendig DW, Seilheimer DK, Wagner ML, Ferry GD, Barrison GM. Complications of gastroesophageal reflux in patients with cystic fibrosis. J Pediatr 1982; 100:536–540.
70. Dab I, Malfroot A. Gastroesophageal reflux: a primary defect in cystic fibrosis? Scand J Gastroenterol Suppl 1988; 143:125–131.
71. Feigelson J, Girault F, Pecau Y. Gastro-oesophageal reflux and esophagitis in cystic fibrosis. Acta Paediatr Scand 1987;76:989–990.
72. Scott RB, OLoughlin EV, Gall DG. Gastroesophageal reflux in patients with cystic fibrosis. J Pediatr 1985; 106:223–227.
73. Thomas D, Rothberg RM, Lester LA. Cystic fibrosis and gastroesophageal reflux in infancy. Am J Dis Child 1985; 139:66–67.
74. Vinocur CD, Marmon L, Schidlow DV, Weintraub WH. Gastroesophageal reflux in the infant with cystic fibrosis. Am J Surg 1985; 149:182–186.
75. Stringer D, Sprigg A, Juodis E, Corey M, Daneman A, Levison H, Durie P. The association of cystic fibrosis, gastroesophageal reflux, and reduced pulmonary function. Can Assoc Radiol 1988; 39:100–102.
76. Foster AC, Voyles JB, Murphy SA. Twenty-four-hour pH monitoring in children with cystic fibrosis: association of chest physical therapy to gastroesophageal reflux. Pediatr Res 1983; 17:118A.
77. Grand RJ. Esophageal complications in cystic fibrosis. Gastroenterology 1983; 85:477–482.
78. Cucchiara S, Santamaria F, Andreotti MR, Minella R, Ercolini P, Oggero V, de Ritis G. Mechanisms of gastro-oesophageal reflux in cystic fibrosis. Arch Dis Child 1991; 66:617–622.

79. Hassall E, Israel D, Davidson A, Wong L. Barrett's esophagus in children with cystic fibrosis: not a coincidental association. Am J Gastroenterol 1993; 88:1934–1938.
80. Smith H, Handy D, et al. Cisapride and cystic fibrosis. Lancet 1989; 338.
81. Prinsen J, Thomas M. Cisapride in cystic fibrosis. Lancet 1985; 512–513.
82. Fonkalsrud EW. Gastroesophageal fundoplication for reflux following repair of esophageal atresia. Experience with nine patients. Arch Surg 1979; 114:48–51.
83. Jolley SG, Johnson DG, Roberts CC, Herbst JJ, Matlak ME, McCombs A, Christian P. Patterns of gastroesophageal reflux in children following repair of esophageal atresia and distal tracheoesophageal fistula. J Pediatr Surg 1980; 15:857–862.
84. Koch A, Rohr S, Plaschkes J, Bettex M. Incidence of gastroesophageal reflux following repair of esophageal atresia. Prog Pediatr Surg 1986; 19:103–113.
85. Lindahl H, Rintala R, Louhimo I. Failure of the Nissen fundoplication to control gastroesophageal reflux in esophageal atresia patients. J Pediatr Surg 1989; 24:985–987.
86. Parker AF, Christie DL, Cahill JL. Incidence and significance of gastroesophageal reflux following repair of esophageal atresia and tracheoesophageal fistula and the need for anti-reflux procedures. J Pediatr Surg 1979; 14:5–8.
87. Pieretti R, Shandling B, Stephens CA. Resistant esophageal stenosis associated with reflux after repair of esophageal atresia: a therapeutic approach. J Pediatr Surg 1974; 9:355–357.
88. Ashcraft KW, Goodwin C, Amoury RA, Holder TM. Early recognition and aggressive treatment of gastroesophageal reflux following repair of esophageal atresia. J Pediatr Surg 1977; 12:317–321.
89. Wheatley MJ, Coran AG, Wesley JR. Efficacy of the Nissen fundoplication in the management of gastroesophageal reflux following esophageal atresia repair. J Pediatr Surg 1993; 28:53–55.
90. Stolar CJ, Berdon WE, Dillon PW, Reyes C, Abramson SJ, Amodio JB. Esophageal dilatation and reflux in neonates supported by ECMO after diaphragmatic hernia repair. Am J Roentgenol 1988; 151:135–137.
91. Larrain A, Carrasco E, Galleguillos F, Sepulveda R, Pope C. Medical and surgical treatment of non-allergic asthma associated with gastroesophageal reflux. Chest 1991; 99:1330–1336.
92. Follette D, Fonkalsrud EW, Euler A, Ament M. Gastroesophageal fundoplication for reflux in infants and children. J Pediatr Surg 1976; 11:757–764.
93. Turnage RH, Oldham KT, Coran AG, Blane CE. Late results of fundoplication for gastroesophageal reflux in infants and children. Surgery 1989; 105:457–464.
94. Sindel B, Maisels M, Ballantine T, Karl S. The effect of a Nissen fundoplication on infants with chronic lung disease. Pediatr Res 1985; 19:365A.
95. Ross A. Fundoplication for gastroesophageal reflux in infants and children. In: Sabiston D, ed. Atlas of General Surgery. Philadelphia: WB Saunders, 1994:316–322.
96. Albanese C, Towbin R, Ulman I, Lewis J, Smith S. Percutaneous gastrojejunostomy versus Nissen fundoplication for enteral feeding of the neurologically impaired child with gastroesophageal reflux. J Pediatr 1993; 123:371–375.
97. Orenstein SR. Gastroesophageal reflux. In: Wyllie R, Hyams JS, eds. Pediatric Gastrointestinal Disease: Pathophysiology, Diagnosis, Management. 2d ed. Philadelphia: WB Saunders, 1997.

12

Oral Manifestations of GERD

DAVID A. LAZARCHIK and STEVEN J. FILLER

University of Alabama School of Dentistry
Birmingham, Alabama

I. Introduction

A multitude of extraesophageal manifestations have been associated with gastroesophageal reflux disease (GERD). These include asthma (1), chronic coughing (2), dyspnea (3), laryngitis (4), recurrent pneumonitis, pharyngitis, and laryngeal carcinoma (5). Although the effects of various acidic substances on the oral cavity have been known for many years, only more recently has gastric acid been recognized as a cause of oral disease. Gastrointestinal disorders such as malabsorption syndrome in children (6), voluntary reflux phenomenon (rumination) (7), and subclinical regurgitation associated with chronic alcoholic gastritis (8) and eating disorders associated with chronic vomiting [anorexia nervosa and bulimia (9)] have been linked to damage to dental hard tissues. Howden (10) documented dental erosion in a patient suffering from hiatus hernia, one of the first reports of the effects of GERD on the oral cavity. Dental erosion can be considered to be the predominant oral lesion associated with GERD. Because of the subtle changes in the early stages of erosion, the multifactorial etiology of the lesion, and the many factors that may modify the effects of gastric acid, diagnosis of GERD-associated erosion can be problematic. Early intervention is very important in avoiding chronic damage to the dentition. Such damage can be severe and debilitating and require extensive and formidable dental rehabilitation.

II. Oral Soft Tissue Manifestations

A. Mucosal Lesions

Damage to the esophageal mucosa as a result of gastric reflux can lead to erosive esophagitis and the development of strictures (11). Extension of such injury to the oral mucosa might be expected but has not been extensively documented. In one study (12) the orodental status of 109 patients with upper gastrointestinal symptoms was examined. Approximately 55% of patients with reflux esophagitis reported mouth symptoms such as burning mouth sensation, sensitivity in the tongue, and painful ulcers. Pathognomonic oral lesions were not observed in the patients studied. In another study (13) oral, dental, and salivary parameters in 117 patients with reflux disease were evaluated. The majority of patients reported frequently suffering from dry mouth, dentinal hypersensitivity, nonspecific itching/burning sensations in the mouth, and/or pharyngeal symptoms. Again, pathognomonic lesions were not reported, and no significant differences existed between dental erosion and erosion-free groups. Because of the lack of studies in this area and the many possible etiologies of the mucosal lesions and symptoms, one cannot make firm conclusions regarding such lesions in GERD patients.

B. Periodontal Manifestations

Other oral soft tissue manifestations such as gingivitis and periodontitis have also received little or no study. No correlation has been found between PI (plaque index, an indicator of oral hygiene status commonly used in clinical dental studies) or GI (gingival index, a measure of gingival inflammation) and GERD as diagnosed by 24-hour esophageal pH levels (14). In other groups suffering from chronic oral acid exposure (bulimics and anorexics), CPITN (Community Periodontal Index of Treatment Needs, an indicator of periodontal health and extent of therapy indicated) and PI were measured as part of a larger study of other oral and dental complications (15). The study group actually showed lower plaque scores than the control group but had significantly more gingival recession and periodontal bleeding sites. There was no difference between groups in the presence of destructive periodontal disease as characterized by deeper periodontal pockets.

C. Salivary Gland Manifestations

Salivary gland enlargement, especially enlargement of the parotids, is a complication seen in chronic regurgitation which might potentially be seen in GERD patients. Brady (16) noted parotid enlargement in up to 10% of bulimics, especially frequent in those bingeing and vomiting one or more times per day. Fifty percent showed elevated serum amylase levels, the significance of which has not been explained. Proposed mechanisms for salivary enlargement include "work hypertrophy" due to intense repeated glandular stimulation and irritation of the epithelial linings of the salivary ducts by repeated exposure to gastric acid. One might expect similar, though possibly less severe, enlargement in patients suffering from the most severe forms of chronic GERD. Such patients should be carefully examined for such a finding.

III. Hard Tissue Manifestations

A. Tooth Erosion

In contrast to the limited documentation of soft tissue manifestations, tooth erosion as a manifestation of chronic GERD has been more extensively studied. Dental erosion, the primary oral manifestation of chronic GERD, is defined as the loss of tooth substance by chemical process (usually acid exposure) not involving bacteria (17). The initial stages of erosion are extremely difficult to detect. The earliest change is a loss of surface sheen with the development of a frosted glass appearance of the enamel surface of the tooth. This initial finding can best be detected when the teeth are completely dry. Gradually, as the erosion process continues over years, the developmental features on the enamel surface are corroded away. Pits, fossae, and primary and secondary grooves normally found on the occlusal (biting) surfaces of molars and bicuspids become rounded out and lose their characteristic definition. The facial (outside) and lingual (inside) surfaces of exposed teeth begin to erode, leaving a smooth, cupped-out lesion with well-defined borders. Once the outer layer of enamel is eroded through, the softer and less acid resistant dentinal layer is exposed (Fig. 1). This layer deteriorates more rapidly, and exposure of the dentin often results in hypersensitivity to thermal change, sweets, and dietary acids. Such hypersensitivity is frequently refractory to treatment. As the erosive process continues, tooth substance is lost around existing restorations, and the appearance of amalgam fillings "standing proud" is characteristic of the process (Fig. 2). Severe cupping of occlusal and incisal surfaces can result in the appearance of an enamel shell surrounding a dished out dentinal surface (18) (Fig. 3). Diagnosis of erosion can be complicated by the presence of other lesions such as abrasion and attrition, which also result in a gradual loss of enamel and dentin.

B. Classification System

One of the difficulties in comparing different studies of dental erosion is the lack of standardization of classification systems for judging the severity of the lesions.

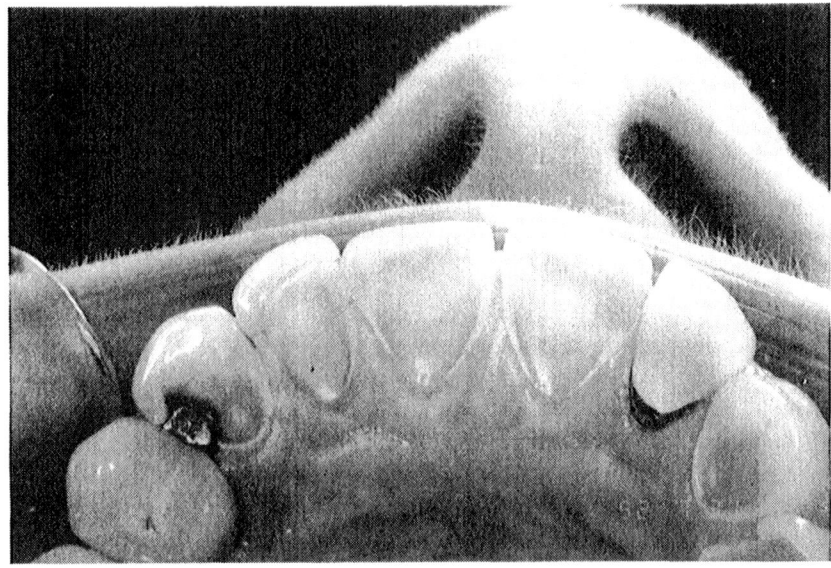

Figure 1 Lingual view of maxillary incisors. Dished-out lesions with enamel eroded through to dentin surface.

The most widely used system was developed by Eccles and Jenkins in 1974 (19). It is based on clinical appearance and involves evaluating the loss of surface characteristics and the depth of lesions for each tooth surface judged (Table 1). Numerical grades are assigned based on the following criteria: Grade 0 = no detectable erosion; Grade 1 = loss of normal surface features with resulting smooth, glazed surface, but lesion confined to enamel; Grade 2 = enamel eroded exposing dentin on less than one third of the surface; Grade 3 = exposure of dentin on more than one third of surface. Use of this system has allowed consistency in evaluation among studies.

C. Etiology/Prevalence in the General Population

Tooth erosion has been recognized in the dental literature for over 200 years and has been associated with a multitude of causes both extrinsic and intrinsic. One of the earliest identified extrinsic causes was exposure to acids used in chemical and manufacturing industries. Other extrinsic factors include dietary acids found in citrus fruits, soft drinks, vinegar, and sports drinks, certain medicines such as vitamin C and iron tonic preparations (20), gas chlorinated swimming pool water (21), and even certain types of oral hygiene swab-sticks intended for institutional

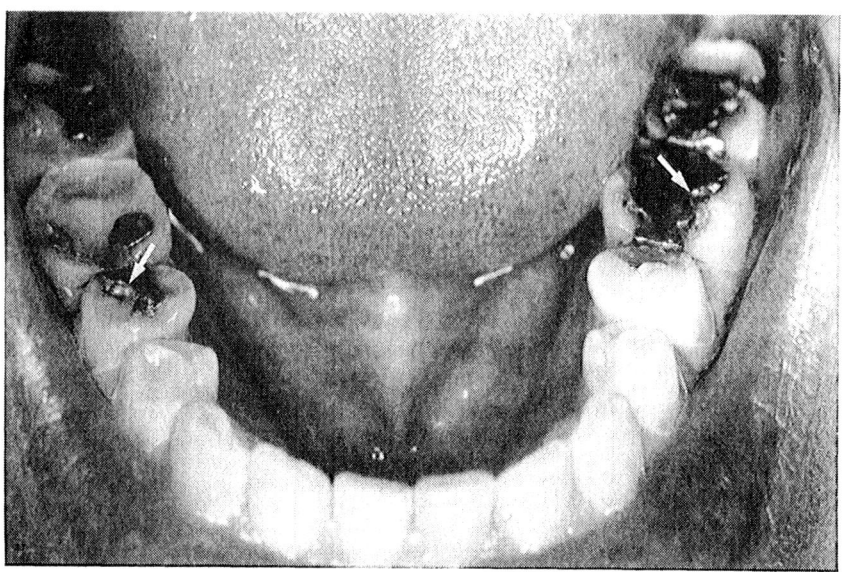

Figure 2 Erosion on occlusal surfaces of mandibular posterior teeth. Loss of tooth structure surrounding restorations gives appearance of amalgams "standing proud" (arrows).

use (22). As previously mentioned, intrinsic causes of dental erosion can include any gastrointestinal or psychological disorder associated with chronic vomiting or gastric reflux.

The reported prevalence of dental erosion in the general population varies widely. Pindborg (13) reported in 1970 that 2% of 1345 U.S. males examined had erosion. Brady and Wood (23) examined the labial tooth surfaces of 900 dentists and reported 5.3% with cervical erosions. Sognnaes et al. (24) examined 10,000 extracted teeth and reported an 18% incidence of erosion-like lesions. A more recent study of 391 Swiss adults (25) showed an overall prevalence of 16% with at least one tooth demonstrating evidence of facial erosion. The variation in reported results of these studies can be explained by the different populations studied, the lack of a clear distinction between erosion and other similar lesions, the differences in tooth surfaces studied, and the differences in erosion grading systems used.

D. Erosion in GERD Patients

A few studies have attempted to establish a relationship between dental erosion and GERD. In one, erosion was detected in 20% of patients diagnosed with either

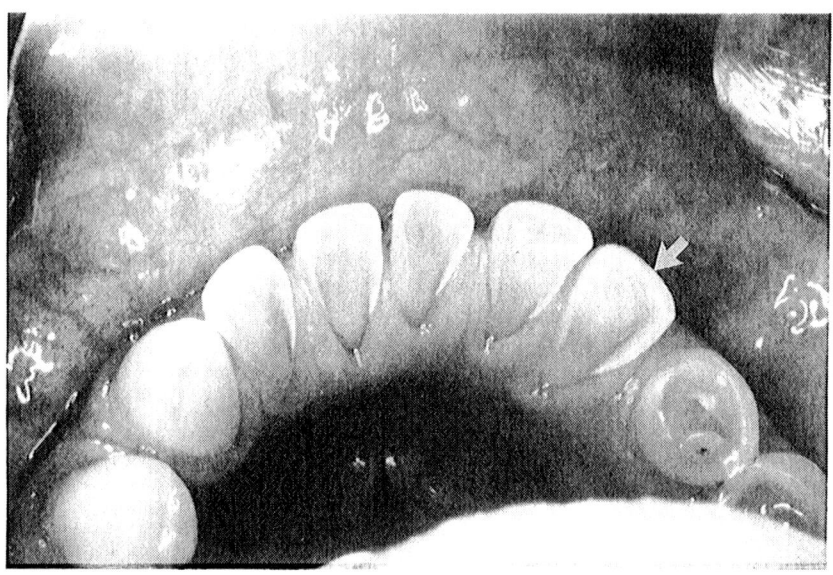

Figure 3 Lingual view of mandibular incisors. An enamel shell surrounds the cupped-out remaining dentin surface (arrow).

reflux esophagitis or duodenal ulcer. It was concluded that dental erosion might be linked with gastrointestinal disorders, which result in increased gastric acid output (12). Interestingly, no erosions were found in patients with duodenogastric reflux in the study group who had undergone cholecystectomy. The authors surmised that alkaline duodenogastric reflux in these patients may have reduced

Table 1 Eccles and Jenkins Erosion Grading System

Rating	Definition	Clinical appearance
Grade 0	No erosion	Normal; enamel shiny with normal surface characteristics
Grade 1	Enamel only	Loss of surface characteristics; glazed appearance
Grade 2	Dentin exposure less than 1/3 surface	Concavities at tooth cervix; smooth, dished-out lesions more wide than deep
Grade 3	Dentin exposure more than 1/3 surface	Cupping of incisal edges and cusp tips; amalgams "stand proud" above adjacent tooth structure

Source: Ref. 19.

the acidity of gastric contents. The medical diagnosis in this study was done by gastroscopy. Other studies using esophagogastroduodenoscopy with biopsy to diagnose reflux disease detected a similar rate of dental erosion (24%) (13). Patients with erosion were older and the mean duration of their reflux disease was longer as compared to those without erosion.

A more direct link between acid reflux and tooth erosion has been explored using 24-hour esophageal pH monitoring (26). Fifty-five percent of patients with reflux as diagnosed by pH testing had dental erosion. Eighty-three percent of patients with idiopathic dental erosion referred by dentists for pH testing had abnormal reflux. The authors of this study felt that the connection was so strong that dental erosion should be considered an atypical manifestation of GERD. Others have attempted to further strengthen the association by proving the presence of acid in the oral cavity at the same time gastric reflux episodes were occurring (27). Intraesophageal and intraoral pH were simultaneously monitored for 24 hours in patients with tooth erosion of unknown etiology. Unexpectedly, changes in oral pH were not detected concurrent with reflux even during long supine reflux episodes. However, only 21% of the patients who underwent pH monitoring were judged to have pathologic acid reflux. Eighty percent who had severe erosion also had low salivary buffer capacity. It was suggested that dietary acids in this study group of young males and their low salivary buffer capacity may have been the cause of erosion, not reflux episodes. The conflicting results in these studies can be attributed to variations in study group size and composition and the multitude of possible causes of erosion (especially extrinsic sources) and modifying factors such as saliva quantity and quality. It has also been suggested that erosion only becomes evident in patients with severe, long-duration (over 15 years) reflux disease. With milder GERD, acid reflux either is not propelled all the way to the oral cavity or is rapidly cleared or neutralized by normal physiologic mechanisms.

IV. Relationship of Dental Erosion to Salivary Parameters

Enamel dissolves at a critical pH of approximately 5.5, well above the estimated pH of less than 2.0 of gastric refluxate (28). Because of the loss of ameloblasts (enamel-forming cells) upon eruption of the tooth into the mouth, dental enamel has no capacity to repair itself when damaged by the propulsion of gastric refluxate into the oral cavity. However, the same salivary parameters that have been shown to play a protective role against acid challenge in the esophagus may modify the effects of gastric acid on oral tissues. It has been shown that saliva flow can double in esophagitis patients with the onset of heartburn and may play an important role in clearing refluxed gastric acid from the esophagus (29) and presumably from the oral cavity. Chemical and mechanical stimulation of esophageal mucosa results in a dramatic increase in salivary flow, pH, and viscosity, all factors related to a protective mechanism in the esophagus (30). Thus, saliva may play a protective role in the oral cavity by the maintenance of a neutral pH via physical flow and resulting lavage of acid. Saliva may also help maintain tooth integrity by remineralization of early subsurface lesions from its supersaturated solution of calcium phosphate salts (31). Whether dental erosion occurs in the GERD patient may depend on whether the balance of acid challenge versus protective salivary factors is upset. Some studies have shown that patients with severe idiopathic erosion have dramatically lower unstimulated salivary flow rates (32) and a higher mucin content. It has been estimated that patients with low unstimulated salivary flow rate are at a five times greater risk of suffering dental erosion than those with normal flow rates (20). Elevated mucin levels may prevent the precipitation of calcium phosphate salts, which repair enamel demineralization (33). Others have shown that a significantly greater number of erosion patients have a lower saliva buffer capacity than controls (34). It has been suggested that abnormal buffer capacity allows greater injury to oral tissues by gastric acid. This theory of the protective role of saliva against the effects of gastric acid on the oral cavity remains untested; erosion patients in some studies have had normal salivary parameters (35).

V. Differential Diagnosis of Dental Erosion

As mentioned previously, the most prominent oral condition noted in some GERD patients is that of tooth erosion. Unfortunately, the clinician is often faced with considerable difficulty in differentiating dental erosion from other similar appearing oral hard tissue lesions. Additionally, once the diagnosis of dental erosion is made, tying the condition to GERD may not be as simple as one would wish. Because a variety of internal and external factors may also cause dental erosion, a rather detailed dental examination as well as a nutritional and medical history must be gathered from the patient to establish the etiology. In the patient with severe, extensive dental erosive lesions, the diagnosis is usually much easier, but the etiology may still remain obscure. With good examination techniques, proper patient questioning, and appropriate testing, the astute clinician can usually obtain a reliable diagnosis.

A. Dental Caries

Like dental erosion, dental caries is also caused by acidic attack on tooth structure. The acid in this case is produced by colonies of bacteria (*Streptococcus mutans*, *Lactobacillus*, and some species of *Actinomyces*), which attach to the tooth. The appearance of caries differs considerably from patient to patient and location to location, but it is generally not difficult to differentiate caries from dental erosion. Caries (Fig. 4) will usually present as irregular, cavitated areas found predominantly between teeth and on their chewing surfaces. These areas are soft, sticky when probed, and frequently exhibit some type of colored debris. The colors range from the usual tans and browns to the less-seen greens, oranges, and black. Patients with easily observed caries will also tend to exhibit signs of poor dental hygiene such as inflamed, hemorrhagic, and receded gingiva, as well as plaque and calculus accumulation. Although caries may involve extensive areas of the tooth, the lesions are generally more limited than those of erosion, which will be seen broadly covering the tooth surface with a smoother, more uniform loss of tooth substance.

B. Attrition

Attrition (Fig. 5) can be defined as the natural, physiological, and sometimes pathological wearing down of teeth over time. As such, it can only be seen in areas where teeth touch. This is unlike dental erosion, which will be seen on any tooth area sufficiently exposed to acidic substrate. A frequent feature in older dentitions, attrition is often seen in combination with tooth erosion. Where areas of attrition and erosion overlap, it will be difficult, if not impossible to differenti-

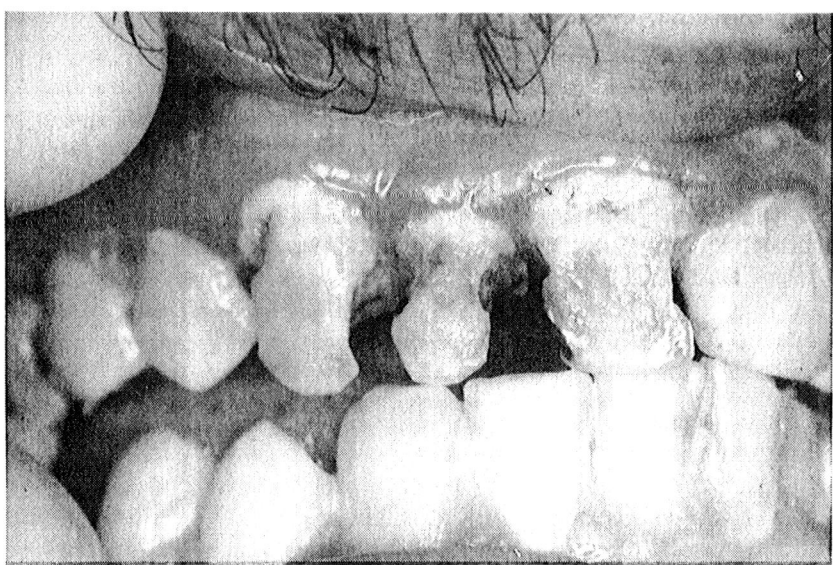

Figure 4 Dental caries. Note rough irregular margins of debris-filled lesions as opposed to clean, smooth erosion lesions of previous figures.

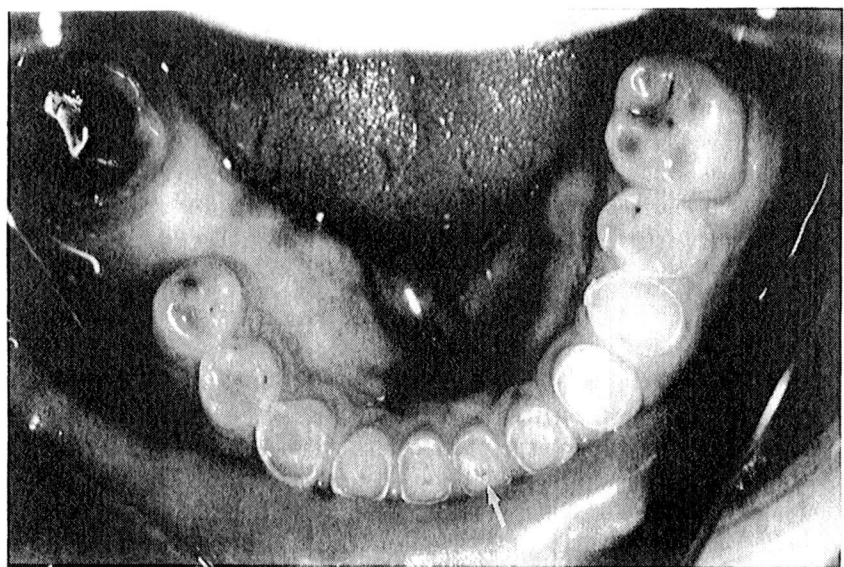

Figure 5 Attrition on occlusal and incisal surfaces of mandibular teeth. Enamel layer has been completely lost on incisors exposing dentin. Pulp chambers are visible on some teeth (arrow).

ate between the two. To establish erosion as a diagnosis, the clinician should look for areas that exhibit those lesions exclusive of areas of occlusion. Attrition can be expedited by pathological habits. This may occur as the result of habitual clenching, grinding, or repetitive tapping of teeth together. The oral results of habits of forced clenching and bruxing (Fig. 6) are frequently confused with those of dental erosion.

C. Abrasion

Abrasion is defined as the pathologic wearing away of tooth substance (36) and is most often secondary to harmful habits involving various materials such as metal, plastic, and wood. This includes the improper use and oral manipulation of toothpicks, toothbrushes, pencils, pens, bobby pins, and other items. Tooth abrasion is generally not confused with dental erosion because it tends to be very localized on specific teeth and usually takes the form of grooves, chips, and wedges (Fig. 7). Abrasion, attrition, and erosion often appear together as a triad of similar, difficult-to-separate conditions. However, they can often be distinguished

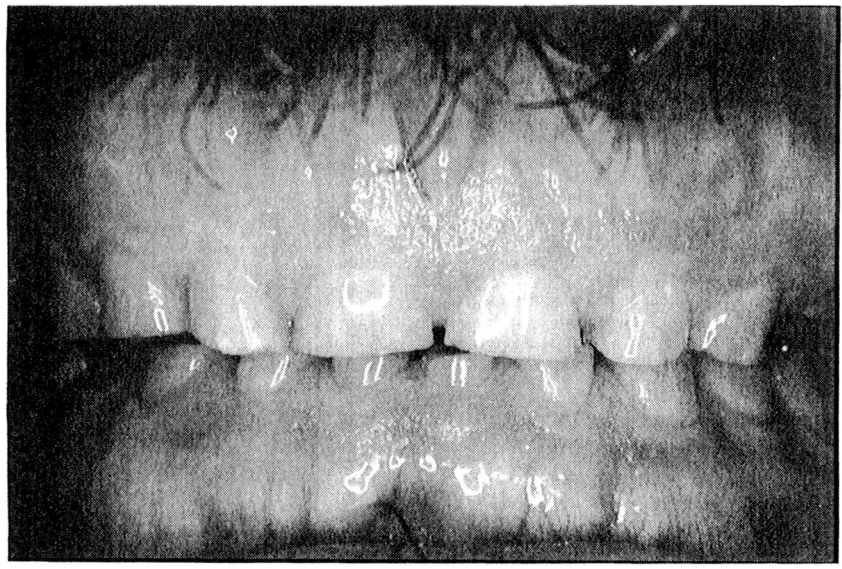

Figure 6 Effects of bruxism. Note wear of incisal edges in a straight line establishing flat plane of occlusion. Teeth have lost 50% or more of their normal incisal length.

from each other by detailing the dental history and carefully noting the location of the lesions.

D. Relationship of Etiology to Location

The position and surfaces of teeth affected by erosion can provide valuable clues as to the origin of the problem. Anatomical considerations, such as conformity of the cheek to the teeth as well as the size and positioning of the tongue, may protect some tooth surfaces from attack. This varies from patient to patient, but with intrinsically produced erosions (e.g., GERD, bulimia, and chronic vomiting) one would expect to find more significant erosions on the lingual and occlusal surfaces of teeth (37) (Table 2). Because of protection from the tongue, the lingual of the maxillary arch (particularly behind the incisors) is often affected to a greater extent than the mandibular arch. Dental erosion produced by extrinsic sources (e.g., overuse of citrus fruits and their products and environmental acid exposures) tends to be most visible on the facial surfaces of teeth or the occlusal surfaces. Although possible, lingual erosions are much less likely. In severe cases (intrinsic or extrinsic) the entire dentition will show signs of erosion (Fig. 8). Since specific tooth erosions are indistinguishable from each other, any link to

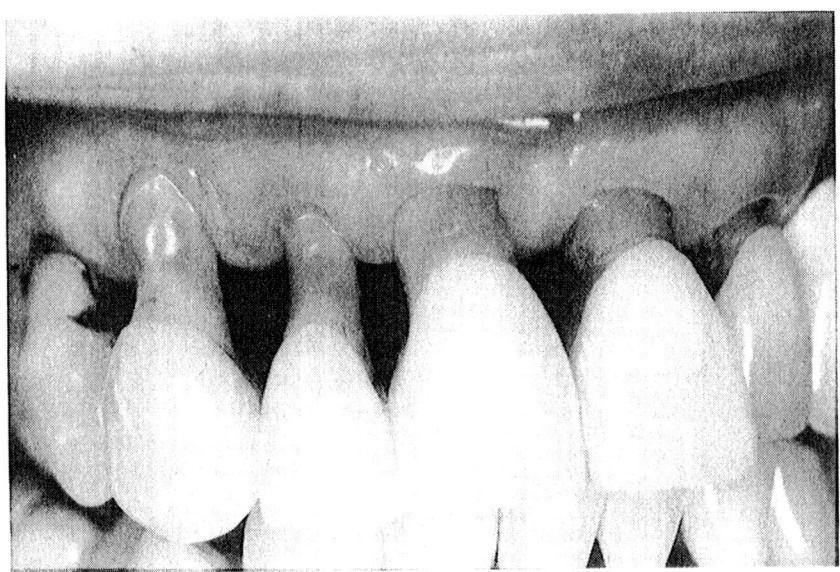

Figure 7 Abrasion. Overvigorous use of hygiene aids has worn grooves into root surfaces of teeth after exposure by gingival recession secondary to periodontal disease.

Table 2 Erosion Etiology Related to Oral Location

Erosion source	Teeth/surfaces most affected
Intrinsic:	
GERD	Lingual surfaces of anterior maxillary and mandibular
Bulimia	teeth; occlusal surfaces of all teeth
Chronic vomiting	
Extrinsic:	
Overuse of citrus products	Facial surfaces of maxillary teeth; occlusal surfaces of all teeth
Environmental/ occupational	

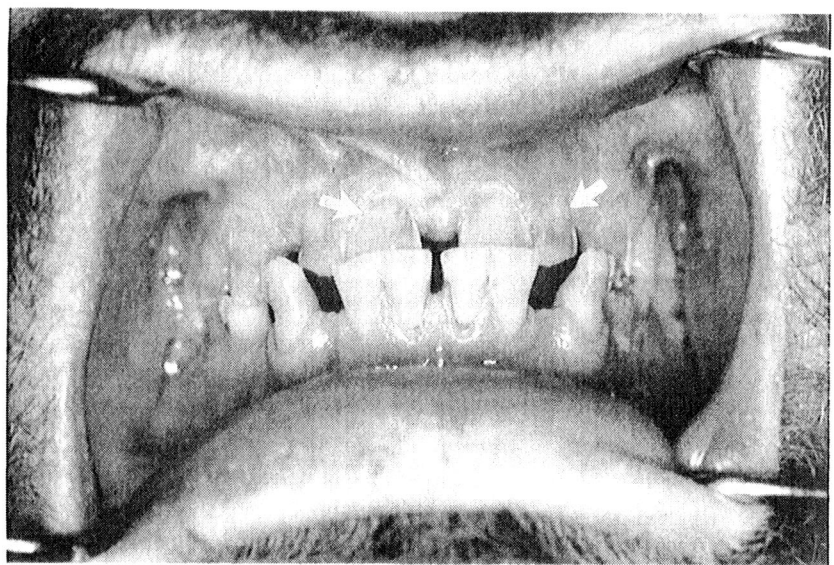

Figure 8 Severe erosion with resulting loss of entire plates of enamel (arrows) on the facial surfaces of maxillary anterior teeth.

a cause, such as GERD, is made by noting location, taking a thorough dental and medical history, and carrying out appropriate medical testing.

VI. Prevention of Oral Manifestations

Over the years, dentists and others have developed a number of methods in an attempt to prevent loss of tooth material due to reflux of gastric acids. It should be obvious to the reader that these methods are temporary measures or are utilized when adequate medical control of the condition is not accomplished. The preferred method for preventing oral manifestations of GERD is medical control of the disease. Without that control, dental methods meet with limited success, and progression of the erosion, although frequently slowed, will continue.

A. Acid Neutralization

In those individuals with GERD who are immediately aware of symptoms subsequent to a reflux episode, there may be value in attempting to neutralize the acidic refluxate orally. This can be accomplished by encouraging the patient to quickly rinse with a solution of sodium bicarbonate or magnesium hydroxide or by immediately taking antacid tablets. It has been suggested that allowing antacids to slowly dissolve in the mouth before swallowing them may better neutralize acid and protect the oral tissues (38). Care should be taken to select sugar-free products. Toothbrushing should be delayed for at least one hour after a reflux episode as it may damage acid-weakened enamel. Since masticatory stimulation has been shown to cause profound increases in salivary pH and bicarbonate levels (39), chewing sugar-free gum may help stimulate salivary flow and neutralize oral acid.

B. Physical Barriers

Various materials (e.g., acrylic, vinyl, silicone, and polyethylene) can be utilized to construct a physical barrier to prevent as much refluxate as possible from contacting teeth. These "mouth guards" fit snugly over the tooth surfaces and when properly monitored by dental personnel can be worn over long periods of time. They should especially be worn during reflux episodes and at night, when diurnal variations cause a decrease in salivary flow and buffering capacity (40). An additional benefit to the patient is the ability of the device to function as a carrier for tooth-protective fluoride gel (1.1% neutral sodium fluoride).

C. Saliva Stimulation

Decreased amounts of saliva jeopardize the patient's oral health in many ways. Saliva not only provides a lubricating effect, thereby reducing tooth-to-tooth friction and resulting in tooth substance loss, but it also serves to dilute and buffer acidic attack from any source, including the bacteria of dental caries. Xerostomia in the patient with significant GERD problems will increase oral complications and hasten the process of dental erosion. Artificial salivas are available (e.g., Xero-Lube, Salivart, Moi-stir), but patient compliance is critical and often difficult to maintain over time. Since many medications contribute to decreased saliva flow, it is recommended that patients be queried about dry mouth and, wherever possible, alternative medications utilized. Of drugs used to treat GERD, omeprazole has been shown to cause reduced salivary flow in some patients (41). Salivary stimulants such as pilocarpine may be appropriate to utilize with some patients.

VII. Treatment of Oral Manifestations

A. Soft Tissue Lesions

Palliative measures can be taken for patients who complain of burning mouth sensations or painful ulcers. Various combinations of coating agents and topical anesthetics have been used: a 50/50 mix of diphenhydramine and attapulgite (Kaopectate), 2% viscous lidocaine, and 0.5% dyclonine hydrochloride. Oral ulcers can be treated with Orabase with benzocaine or Zilactin gel.

B. Dental Erosion

Indication for Treatment

Dental restorative treatment is indicated in those GERD patients with sufficiently affected dentitions to produce tooth pain and/or sensitivity, functional, or cosmetic problems. Not all affected teeth require treatment, and when restoration is necessary, a conservative treatment approach is recommended. If the patient's reflux problem is under good medical control and the patient does not report pain, function, or cosmetic concerns, dental treatment should be limited. On the other hand, continued progression of the loss of tooth structure will require active intervention on the part of a dentist. The extent of this treatment will depend on the nature of the problem and the extent of the destruction. Patients with a history of GERD should be monitored for dental erosion throughout their life and dental treatment instituted when appropriate.

Dental Treatment Options

Patients exhibiting less severe tooth erosion often do well with simple tooth-colored dental restorations (glass ionomers, composites, or "bonding") that restore tooth contours and serve to protect the underlying structure from further acidic attack. Some of these materials contain fluoride, which provides additional protection for the tooth. Teeth that have lost large amounts of enamel and dentin often require more extensive and aggressive dental care. Following additional shaping of the teeth, a dentist will prepare partial or complete metal and/or porcelain coverings for the teeth (crowns). If the tooth pulp has been compromised, endodontic treatment (root canal therapy) will be required or the tooth may require extraction. For severe dental erosion cases, patients will require full mouth rehabilitation with multiple crown units and perhaps bridges. Unfortunately, the financial burden of such extensive dental care necessitates that many patients seek extraction of teeth and construction of a removable prosthetic appliance.

VIII. Conclusion

Although dental erosion has been studied for years, we are just beginning to understand its relationship to GERD. Little data exist about the effects of gastric refluxate on the oral soft tissues, and the data about hard tissue manifestations are often confusing. This is because of the many possible etiologies of erosion, the difficulty of diagnosing erosion in the presence of other lesions of hard tooth structure, and the interplay of modifying factors such as salivary parameters, the duration and severity of reflux, and exposure to extrinsic causes of erosion. The combined efforts of physicians (in controlling or minimizing reflux) and dentists (in preventing and treating oral lesions) are necessary if the patient is to avoid the devastating dental consequences of chronic GERD.

References

1. Simpson WG. Gastroesophageal reflux disease and asthma: diagnosis and management. Arch Intern Med 1995; 155(8):798–803.
2. Ludviksdottir D, Bjornsson E, Janson C, Boman G. Habitual coughing and its associations with asthma, anxiety and gastroesophageal reflux. Chest 1996; 109(5):1262–1268.
3. Field SK, Underwood M, Brant R, Cowie RL. Prevalence of gastroesophageal reflux symptoms in asthma. Chest 1996; 109(2):316–322.
4. Pope CE. Current concepts: acid-reflux disorders. N Engl J Med 1994; 331(10):656–660.
5. Kahrilas PJ. Gastroesophageal reflux disease. JAMA 1996; 276(12):983–988.
6. Ansaldi N, Morabito A, Balocco P, Galleano E. Dental changes in children with malabsorption. Minerva Pediatr 1989; 41:581–585.
7. Gilmour AG, Beckett HA. The voluntary reflux phenomenon. Br Dent J 1993; 175:368–372.
8. Smith BGN, Robb ND. Dental erosion in patients with chronic alcoholism. J Dent 1989; 17:219–221.
9. Roberts MW, Shou-Hua L. Oral findings in anorexia nervosa and bulimia nervosa: a study of 47 cases. J Am Dent Assoc 1987; 115:407–410.
10. Howden GF. Erosion as the presenting symptom in hiatus hernia. Br Dent J 1971; 131:455–456.
11. Brown CM, Rees WD. Review article: factors protecting the oesophagus against acid-mediated injury. Alim Pharm Ther 1995; 9:251–262.
12. Jarvinen V, Meurman JH, Hyvarinen H, Rytomaa I, Murtomaa H. Dental erosion and upper gastrointestinal disorders. Oral Surg Oral Med Oral Pathol 1988; 65:298–303.
13. Meurman JH, Toskala J, Nuutinen P, Klemetti E. Oral and dental manifestations in gastroesophageal reflux disease. Oral Surg Oral Med Oral Pathol 1994; 78:583–589.
14. Schroeder PL, Filler SJ, Ramirez B, Lazarchik DA, Vaezi MF, Richter JE. Dental erosion and acid reflux disease. Ann Intern Med 1995; 122:809–815.
15. Touyz SW, Liew VP, Tseng P, Frisken K, Williams H, Beumont PJV. Oral and dental complications in dieting disorders. Int J Eating Disord 1993; 14:341–348.
16. Brady JP. Parotid enlargement in bulimia. J Fam Pract 1985; 20(5):496–502.
17. Pindborg JJ. Chemical and physical injuries. In: Pindborg JJ, ed. Pathology of the Dental Hard Tissues. Philadelphia: WB Saunders, 1970:312–325.
18. Bevenius J, L'Estrange PL. Chairside evaluation of salivary parameters in patients with tooth surface loss: a pilot study. Aust Dent J 1990; 35:219–221.

19. Eccles JD, Jenkins WG. Dental erosion and diet. J Dent 1974; 2:153–159.
20. Jarvinen VK, Rytomaa II, Heinonen OP. Risk factors in dental erosion. J Dent Res 1991; 70:942–947.
21. Filler SJ, Lazarchik DA. Tooth erosion: an unusual case. Gen Dent 1994; 42:568–569.
22. Meurman JH, Sorvari R, Pelttari A, Rytomma I, Franssila S, Kroon L. Hospital mouth-cleaning aids may cause dental erosion. Spec Care Dent 1996; 16(6):247–250.
23. Brady JM, Wood RD. Scanning microscopy of cervical erosion. J Am Dent Assoc 1977; 94:726–729.
24. Sognnaes RF, Wolcott RB, Xhonga FA. Dental erosion I. Erosion-like patterns occurring in association with other dental conditions. J Am Dent Assoc 1972; 84:571–576.
25. Lussi A, Schaffner M, Hotz P, Suter P. Dental erosion in a population of Swiss adults. Commun Dent Oral Epidemiol 1991; 19:286–290.
26. Schroeder PL, Filler SJ, Ramirez B, Lazarchik DA, Vaezi MF, Richter JE. Dental erosion and acid reflux disease. Ann Intern Med 1995; 122:809–815.
27. Gudmundsson K, Kristleifsson G, Theodors A, Holbrook WP. Tooth erosion, gastroesophageal reflux, and salivary buffer capacity. Oral Surg Oral Med Oral Pathol Oral Radiol Endod 1995; 79: 185–189.
28. DeMeester TR, Johnson LF, Joseph GJ, Toscano MS, Hall AW, Skinner DB. Patterns of gastroesophageal reflux in health and disease. Ann Surg 1976; 184:459–470.
29. Helm JF, Dodds WJ, Hogan WJ. Salivary response to esophageal acid in normal subjects and patients with reflux esophagitis. Gastroenterology 1987; 93:1393–1397.
30. Namiot Z, Rourk RM, Piascik R, Hetzel DP, Sarosiek J, McCallum RW. Interrelationship between esophageal challenge with mechanical and chemical stimuli and salivary protective mechanisms. Am J Gastroenterol 1994; 89(4):581–587.
31. Mandel ID. The role of saliva in maintaining oral homeostasis. J Am Dent Assoc 1989; 119:298–304.
32. Wolgtens JHM, Vingerling P, de Blicck-Hogervorst JMA, Bervoets D. Enamel erosion and saliva. Clin Prev Dent 1985; 7:8–10.
33. Mannerberg F. Saliva factors in cases of erosion. Odont Revy 1963; 14:156–166.
34. Gudmundsson K, Kristleifsson G, Theodors A, Holbrook WP. Tooth erosion, gastroesophageal reflux, and salivary buffer capacity. Oral Surg Oral Med Oral Pathol Oral Radiol Endod 1995; 79:185–189.
35. Schroeder PL, Filler SJ, Ramirez B, Lazarchik DA, Vaezi MF, Richter JE. Dental erosion and acid reflux disease. Ann Intern Med 1995; 122:809–815.
36. Shafer WG, Hine MK, Levy BM. A Textbook of Oral Pathology. 3d ed. Philadelphia: WB Saunders, 1974.
37. Jarvinen V, Rytomaa I, Meurman JH. Location of dental erosion in a referred population. Caries Res 1992; 26:391–396.
38. Meurman JH, Kuittinen T, Kangas M, Tuisku T. Buffering effect of antacids in the mouth—a new treatment of dental erosion? Scan J Dent Res 1988; 96(5):412–417.

39. Sarosiek J, Scheurich CJ, Marcinkiewicz M, McCallum RW. Enhancement of salivary esophagoprotection: rationale for a physiological approach to gastroesophageal reflux disease. Gastroenterology 1996; 110:675–681.
40. Jenkins GN. The Physiology and Biochemistry of the Mouth. 4th ed. Oxford: Blackwell Scientific Publications, 1978.
41. Teare JP, Spedding C, Whitehead MW, Greenfield SM, Challacombe SJ, Thompson RPH. Omeprazole and dry mouth. Scand J Gastroenterol 1995; 30:216–218.

13

Odds and Ends and the State of the Art

MARK R. STEIN

University of South Florida College of Medicine
Tampa, Florida

This final chapter will initially focus on information not covered elsewhere. It includes a review of gastroesophageal reflux disease (GERD) in the geriatric population as well as in the pregnant patient. An attempt to coordinate significant information from other chapters will follow and will focus on where we are today in the evaluation and treatment of GERD and airway disease. If you have read this book or selected chapters, you know that a large volume of information from multiple disciplines has been used to weave a tapestry of GERD-induced airway diseases. Starting with the embryo (Chap. 1) and progressing from infancy (Chap. 11) and childhood (Chap. 10) to the adult (Chaps. 4,5,6–8) and geriatric populations (Chap. 13), this volume attempts to follow the evolving relationships between the gastrointestinal tract and respiratory tract. It also follows the consequences of GERD from the mouth and dentition (Chap. 12) to the nasopharynx, larynx (Chaps. 4,5), and lungs (Chaps. 6–11). With the high prevalence of both GERD and airway disease in the population, a practicing physician usually sees at least one patient daily with these problems. The intent of this book is to awaken us to the concept that GERD, sometimes silent, can cause a variety of symptoms, and these relationships should always be considered in approaching the patient with airway disease. This is particularly important when the airway disease does not respond to a usually effective course of treatment. This concept helps us to better understand how GERD can contribute to the etiology of diseases and conditions previously considered idiopathic (see Chaps. 4,7,10–12).

I. GERD in the Geriatric Patient

The evaluation of GERD and airway disease in the geriatric population is especially complex. This complexity is due to the normal physiologic changes that occur with aging and the occurrence of additional diseases, which can complicate both diagnosis and treatment (1,2). The geriatric patient may have recent onset of GERD related to changes in weight, diet, or lifestyle, or he or she may have had longstanding GERD. Patients with many years of GERD may present with numerous complications or manifestations of this condition (see Chaps. 4,5,7,12). Figure 3 in Chapter 9 shows an outline for the progression of GERD from upright to supine and then bipositional reflux. The DeMeesters explain the changes based on tissue damage from bile salts in the refluxate causing further tissue damage. The older the patient with GERD and the longer he or she has had GERD, the greater are the chances that he or she will have these progressive changes.

As always, diagnosis starts with a good history. Unfortunately, a single question (Do you have heartburn?) is not likely to uncover this diagnosis, especially if the reflux is silent (no heartburn). After reviewing complex surveys for GERD (3), I have used the questionnaire shown in Table 1 for several years. This questionnaire has been easy to use and extremely helpful in obtaining clues to the presence of GERD and several of the supraesophageal manifestations of GERD. This questionnaire is most valuable in adults, since children often have problems communicating their symptoms. It helps to alert the clinician to a variety of possible otolaryngologic and lower respiratory problems, while relating symptoms to daily activities.

The geriatric patient, like younger patients, will often present with a variety of symptoms (e.g., cough, sore throat, episodic throat closing, and asthma), all of which may be due to GERD. Sometimes a questionnaire of this type will draw attention to this relationship. Often a patient of this type will be seen by multiple specialists, each of whom looks at only one aspect of the patient's problems without seeing the whole picture. This is a greater problem today with managed care, since the specialist may have a limited number of visits to arrive at a diagnosis and treatment plan. As explained in Chapter 4, the evaluation may differ based on the initial symptoms with supraesophageal symptoms, often requiring a dual pH probe study for correct diagnostic information, particularly in laryngeal diseases and with cough (see Chaps. 4,5) (4,5).

Evaluation of the geriatric patient with respiratory problems must be complete when suspecting GERD. The physical examination gives a few clues, including the dry rales of pulmonary fibrosis and the wet rales of a recent episode of aspiration. Extremely late findings include clubbing and increased anteroposterior chest diameter, which are often found with other types of lung disease. Pulmonary function testing is helpful in establishing the initial degree of restrictive and ob-

Table 1 Gastroesophageal Reflux Questionnaire for Patients with Cough, Sinusitis, Wheeze, or Voice Changes

Do you have	Yes	No	Not sure
1. Heartburn or indigestion? How often? _____			
2. Regurgitation of stomach contents (stomach contents coming into your mouth)? How often? _____			
3. Use of antacids (Rolaids, Tums, Maalox)? How often? _____			
4. Vomiting easily or frequently?			
5. Frequent burps or hiccups?			
6. Chronic cough worse after meals?			
7. Chronic cough worse after lying down?			
8. Chronic hoarseness or voice change?			
9. Chronic sinus disease?			
10. Chest pains?			
11. Stomach pain?			
12. Neck pain?			
13. Sore throat frequently?			
14. Feelings of throat closing or something stuck in throat?			
15. Adult-onset asthma?			
16. Asthma not relieved with usual treatments?			
17. Asthma worse after meals, alcohol, lying down, bending to tie shoes, or after onset of heartburn?			
18. Worse heartburn after theophylline?			
19. Anemia?			

structive changes and responsiveness to bronchodilators. Follow-up testing will gauge the additional responsiveness to inhaled or systemic steroids and treatment of GERD. A persistent residual restrictive component may suggest that aspiration has led to fibrosis. Nasopharyngoscopy with direct laryngoscopy has lead to a far greater appreciation of the types of tissue injury (see Chap. 4) resulting from GERD. The use of the fiberoptic instruments has greatly increased our ability to diagnose the posterior laryngitis of GERD.

With clues from the history and the questionnaire, physical examination, pulmonary functions, and direct laryngoscopy, the clinician is usually able to achieve a strong clinical impression that GERD is contributing to the patient's airway disease. This usually leads to a treatment plan that includes treatment for airway inflammation in addition to treatment of GERD. In the geriatric patient this association of GERD and airway disease is often missed. When this group of patients are seen, they are eager for some relief. In my experience, the best results are obtained with effective therapy of both the GERD and airway disease simultaneously. Caution is needed to avoid bronchodilators and other medications that may aggravate GERD (see Chap. 7). Relief of symptoms is more important to the patient than having full documentation of the extent of GERD. Once relief is achieved, the patient is generally more willing and able to cooperate with plans for further studies.

A. Pathophysiologic Changes with Advanced Age

Sensory Changes

As we age, many physiologic processes slowly, almost imperceptibly, change. Change occurs in many aspects of the swallowing process. The higher incidence of aspiration pneumonia in the elderly has been a stimulus for many of the studies that follow. Sensation in the upper airway decreases with age (6–10). While studying the increased incidence of aspiration pneumonia in the elderly, Aviv et al. studied sensory changes in the pharynx and supraglottic area. Using an air pulse pressure stimulus for testing the mucosa enervated by the superior laryngeal nerve (10,11), they demonstrated a decade-by-decade decrease in supraglottic and pharyngeal sensory discrimination threshold (8) (Table 2). Their study of two-point sensory discrimination in the mouth demonstrated an age-related decrease in the floor of the mouth and dorsal and ventral surface of the tongue, but not in the tip of the tongue (7). Calhoun et al. found that the lip had a decrease in tactile and vibratory sensation, the oral cavity had a slight decrease in proprioceptive and temperature sensation, and oral stereognostic ability declined for some shapes but not others (6). This change in stereognostic ability had been previously reported (9,11). These stereognostic skills are similar to those needed to estimate bolus size and may in part account for the larger bolus size swallowed by the elderly (11).

Anatomic Changes

Changes in the structure of nerves have been documented with aging. Electron-microscopic evaluation of age-related changes in postmortem human superior laryngeal nerve segments was performed by Mortelliti et al. (12). They compared tissue from young subjects (age 20–30 years) with tissue from old subjects (age 60–89, mean age of 76.2 years). There was a 31% decrease in number of myelinated nerve fiber counts in the older subjects, which was statistically significant ($p = 0.032$) (12). In addition, the small myelinated fiber group in the elderly

Table 2 Supraglottic and Pharyngeal Sensory Discrimination Thresholds by Decade

Age (yr)	Mean ± SD (mmHg)	N
20–30	2.06 ± 0.29	11
31–40	2.08 ± 0.12	17
41–50	2.08 ± 0.13	7
51–60	2.70 ± 0.48	2
Mean (20–60)	2.11 ± 0.24	
61–70	2.61 ± 0.49	8
71–80	2.49 ± 0.28	7
81–90	3.16 ± 1.15	4
Mean (61+)	2.68 ± 0.63*	
Total	2.30 ± 0.50	56

*$p < 0.001$.
Source: Ref. 8.

had decreased 67% ($p = 0.014$). These findings are important to the consideration of other changes of aging as it affects both GERD and its relationships to airway disease in the elderly. Most nerves supplying fibers to the gastrointestinal and respiratory tract have not been studied to this extent. However, it is reasonable to assume that similar changes occur in these nerves that account for some of the other findings to be described.

Reflex Changes And Aspiration

Reflex closure of the glottis was studied by Pontoppidan and Beecher in 1960 (13). Using the volume of 1.6% ammonia gas required to stimulate reflex glottic closure, they found that the threshold level increased sixfold from the second to the eighth or ninth decades of life (13). Changes in this glottic closure reflex coupled with decreased sensation make aspiration of even normal secretions more likely in the elderly. This is important, since aspiration of nasopharyngeal secretions occurs in normal individuals. This aspiration has been demonstrated in about 50% of normals, using radioisotopes instilled into the nasopharynx during sleep (14,15). Upper airway aspiration occurring in normal young subjects has significantly greater implications for the elderly. Those elderly at greatest risk for aspiration are those who have had a stroke. There is a 20% incidence of death from aspiration pneumonia in the first year after a stroke, with additional deaths from aspiration pneumonia each year thereafter (16). A careful assessment of the stroke patient is essential to find evidence of sensory or motor dysphagia, which could lead to aspiration and pneumonia. This is even more important in the patient with preexistent airway disease. With a stroke, questions arise about whether or not new respiratory symptoms are due to aspiration or an exacerbation of the preexistent disease. A new approach to this assessment includes a combined laryngopharyngeal sensory test and modified barium swallow. This combined approach appears to have a better ability to prognosticate the risks of aspiration, which leads to strategies to avoid the problem (17,18). Other investigators have demonstrated the usefulness of videofluoroscopy with or without the videoendoscopic swallow study in assessing dysphagia in the stroke patient (19,20). These same tools are at times helpful in evaluating the nonstroke patient with GERD and airway disease. Additional reflex changes are described in the next section.

Changes in Swallowing

Investigators have found a statistically significant increase in the threshold bolus volume of the pharyngeal swallow in the elderly (21–23). A delay in initiation of maximal hyolaryngeal excursion was the factor responsible for the significantly longer duration of oropharyngeal swallowing in patients over age 70 (24). Nondeglutitive lingual pressure is significantly lower in the elderly (25). Most studies have found that aging results in a significant decrease in resting upper esophageal sphincter (UES) pressure (21,25–27). The UES opening occurs earlier ($p = 0.01$), and the UES opening is significantly diminished ($p = 0.0001$) in the elderly (27,28). There is delayed UES relaxation and prolonged oral transit time (20,21). These factors result in increased hypopharyngeal intrabolus pressure (25,27,28). The net effect of these changes is that flow rates across the UES are unchanged with age. Although the compliance of the UES decreases with age, the increase in bolus pressure helps to compensate. It appears that these changes do not influence normal pharyngo-sphincteric coordination (27). The amplitude of the hypopharyngeal pressure wave varies in the elderly depending on what is swallowed. The amplitude is the same in the young and the elderly for mashed potato; however, with dry or water swallowing the amplitude was significantly greater in the elderly (25).

The term presbyesophagus evolved in the 1960s. It referred to certain patterns of esophageal dysfunction. Some of the early studies of patients in their eighth or ninth decades suggested that tertiary contractions, decreased primary peristalsis, decreased LES relaxation, delayed emptying of the esophagus, and dilatation of the esophagus were part of the normal aging process (29,30). More recent studies, using improved intraluminal manometry and better selection of patients to exclude other diseases (such as diabetes mellitus) that may effect esophageal motility, have changed our understanding of what is expected in the elderly. In one study there was a significant decrease in the amplitude of the peristaltic pressure wave in men over 80 years of age (31). Richter et al. found that the distal esophageal peristaltic wave amplitude was significantly higher with each increasing decade and peaked in the fifties (32). Severe motility disorders (presbyesophagus) in the elderly have not been found in recent studies. It is believed that the severe motility disturbances found at times in the elderly are caused by systemic diseases rather than the aging process (33,34).

Airway-Protective Mechanisms

There are two types of protective mechanisms: those preventing antegrade aspiration and those preventing retrograde aspiration. Retrograde transit includes gastroesophageal and esophagopharyngeal reflux, regurgitation, and vomiting. Airway-protective mechanisms for retrograde aspiration have been divided further into two subgroups (23,24). The first subgroup includes basal mechanisms that are active at all times. The second includes response mechanisms that become active with stimulation.

Of the basal mechanisms, the LES presents the first line of defense against GER. Many of the preceding authors have reviewed the problems that permit physiologic and pathologic reflux through the lower esophageal sphincter (LES). The UES provides a high-pressure zone separating the esophagus and pharynx; however, its resting pressure decreases during sleep and with aging (21). This may enhance risks for aspiration in the elderly, particularly during sleep.

Response mechanisms often include vagally mediated reflexes, such as the esophago-UES contractile reflex and esophagoglottal closure reflex. The esophagoglottal closure reflex is elicited when mechanical stretching of the esophagus occurs with abrupt distention from refluxate. The reflex results in adduction of the vocal cords. While this reflex is evoked with spontaneous reflux, it may be absent in about half of those over 70 years old (23,35).

Esophageal peristalsis is classified into primary, induced by swallowing, and secondary, initiated by local esophageal stimuli. Recent studies of the effect of aging on secondary peristalsis indicated that "in the healthy elderly volunteers, secondary peristalsis is either absent or its stimulation is inconsistent and significantly less frequent compared with young volunteers" (23).

For prevention of antegrade aspiration, swallowing is examined in more detail. The swallow is divided into the primary swallow, which is usually a voluntary act, and the secondary swallow, which involves a stimulus applied to the pharynx. The elderly, as mentioned before, require a significantly larger volume of liquid to trigger the secondary (pharyngeal) swallow (21-23). This could permit smaller volumes from the nasopharynx (14,15) or from gastric refluxate to be more easily aspirated. However, it has been suggested that the secondary swallow may help prevent aspiration by activating the swallow-induced glottal closure or at least clear the pharynx of refluxate (23). Injection of minute amounts of water into the pharynx stimulated the pharyngo-glottal adduction reflex with brief closure of the vocal cords (35,36). More recent evidence suggests that in the elderly a larger volume of liquid is needed to trigger this reflex (23,35). This implies that smaller volumes of liquid—antegrade or retrograde—would present a greater risk for aspiration.

Summary of Pathophysiologic Changes

With progressive aging there occurs loss of upper airway sensation, diminished protective reflexes, changes in swallowing, decreased airway protective mechanisms effecting laryngeal closure, and changes in voice (37). These changes are sometimes found to progress decade by decade, but some changes are only noticed in the seventh, eighth, and ninth decades. These changes appear to place the elderly at far greater risk for aspiration of fluids swallowed or refluxed. These changes of aging may then have serious implications in diagnosis and treatment of GERD and airway disease in the elderly, and they may explain why GERD and airway disease is more difficult to treat in this age group. While some have suggested that gastric acidity declines with age, Hurwitz et al. (38) indicate that 90% of elderly people were able to acidify gastric contents. This finding included the basal unstimulated state. Certainly this combination of findings increases the risk of aspiration pneumonia and other airway diseases (Chaps. 5–8, 12) in the elderly. One example of these differences, as seen in Figure 1 (39), is the fact the GERD moves from the third most common cause of chronic cough in patients of all ages (see Chap. 5) to the second most common cause in the elderly.

B. Evaluation of GERD in the Elderly

There are some unique aspects of evaluating GERD in the elderly. Sometimes the concomitant airway disease and/or additional medical problems (cardiac and orthopedic) prevent the clinician from obtaining the study he or she believes would be most helpful. Often the patient is not willing to go through invasive procedures. The evaluation of GERD has already been thoroughly reviewed (Chaps. 3, 4). Special evaluation techniques are sometimes needed in this group of patients, particularly when aspiration is suspected. Because of the pathophysiologic changes of aging and the possibility of other concomitant disorders (34) and occult stroke (17,18,40), videofluoroscopy carefully performed, using materials of differing consistencies, can be quite rewarding. It helps in identifying abnormal swallowing patterns and upper airway aspiration, as well as GERD with possible aspiration (19,41). The additional use of the laryngoscope can be invaluable in identifying changes of posterior laryngitis characteristic of GERD (Chap. 4) and assessing sensory function (9,17). The laryngoscope can also be used in combination with barium studies or videofluoroscopy to enhance accuracy (18,20,42). In the elderly you may diagnose GERD-associated airway disease, but if you have not considered the possibility of other disorders leading to aspira-

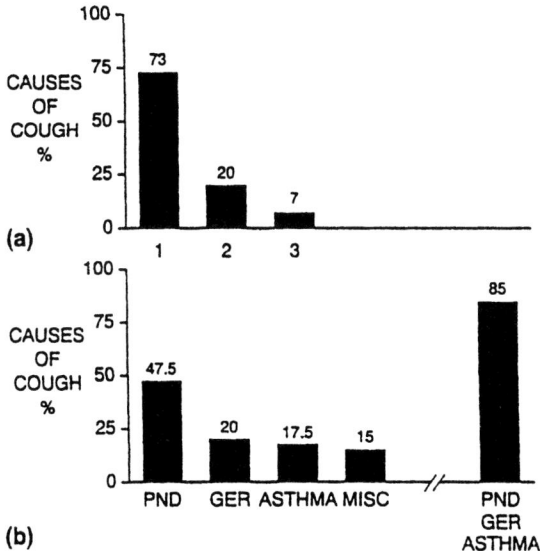

Figure 1 Causes of chronic cough in the elderly. (a) The cause was determined in 100% of patients; it was due to a single condition in 73% and multiple disorders in 27%. (b) The spectrum and frequency of the 40 causes. PND, postnasal drip syndrome; GER, gastroesophageal reflux; misc, miscellaneous.

tion, you may never achieve a successful treatment plan. When reflux symptoms have been present in this age group, it is extremely important to have an endoscopic exam to look for Barrett's esophagus (see Chaps. 3 and 6).

Studies of elderly patients suggest that they have more severe findings of GERD. Zhu et al. (43) studied 24 elderly patients with a mean age of 69 years (range 65–76) and compared them to 147 younger patients with a mean age of 45 years (range 21–64). Their studies using 24-hour pH monitoring and endoscopy demonstrated that the elderly patients had a higher incidence of pathologic reflux and reflux esophagitis (43). Their elderly patients had a pH < 4 for 32.5% of the time in 24 hours compared to 12.9% of the time in younger patients ($p < 0.05$). On endoscopy they found that the elderly had more severe esophageal lesions and a greater incidence of hiatal hernia ($p < 0.002$). The elderly had 20.8% incidence of grade III/IV esophagitis versus 3.4% in the younger patients (43). These are all findings that might be expected with the prolonged and progressive disease described in Chapter 9. Collen et al. (44) prospectively studied 228 consecutive symptomatic patients with GERD. Of these patients, 162 were less than 60 years old, and 66 patients were over 60 years old. All patients were evaluated for basal acid output and had endoscopic evaluations. There was a much higher incidence of mucosal disease (erosive esophagitis and Barrett's esophagus) in patients complaining of pyrosis who were elderly (81%) versus (47%) those who were younger ($p = 0.000002$, Fisher's exact test) (44). This difference in incidence of mucosal disease increased decade by decade from below 30 years to over 70 years, while there were no corresponding differences in basal acid outputs (38,44).

These studies taken together point to more severe mucosal disease in the elderly. They suggest there is an increase in acid-contact time and resultant damage to the mucosa. There may also be increased susceptibility to mucosal injury from decreased buffering of acid and decreased effective clearance of refluxate (23,25,43).

C. Treatment

Treatment programs for the elderly are similar, both medically (Chap. 8) and surgically (Chap. 9). The findings that the elderly have more severe disease (43,44) suggest the need for more aggressive therapy (44,45). One-third of the elderly patients studied by Collen et al. (44) required more than 600 mg of ranitidine per day for control of symptoms and healing of esophagitis. This finding and more severe disease in the elderly indicate that early use of proton pump inhibitors may be the most cost-effective therapeutic modality for initial treatment of this age group. As seen in other chapters (4,5,7,8), the proton pump inhibitors have been the most effective medical therapy for GERD and concomitant airway disease. It is not unusual with more severe disease to need combination therapy with a motility agent such as cisapride.

In the elderly there is an increase of coincident diseases or conditions that may limit the medications that can be used. This includes the increasing incidence of lactose intolerance with age, which leads to diarrhea with some products (omeprazole) (46). Sicca syndromes may also make the use of proton pump inhibitors more difficult to tolerate (47). The elderly are more prone to develop neurologic sequelae, especially movement disorders, from the use of metoclopramide. The elderly often have greater problems with side effects of medications and difficulties with multiple drug interactions. This is particularly important with the use of cisapride and the cytochrome p450 drug interactions (46). There is a significant list of drugs that can lead to torsade de pointes arrhythmias. Once an effective treatment plan is established, the patient will have questions about cost, safety, and duration of therapy. Cost can be a major factor in all age groups, but elderly patients are often living on fixed incomes and may not have insurance with prescription coverage. Table 3 shows the recent average retail costs of medications, including generics (when available), in one local market. It is apparent that GERD is an expensive disease (47,48). When combined with medications to treat airway

Table 3 Daily Cost of Therapy

Drug	Dose	Average cost per day
Cimetidine	800 mg bid	$5.48
generic	800 mg bid	$2.04
Ranitidine	150 mg bid	$2.98
generic	150 mg bid	$1.87
Famotidine	20 mg bid	$3.08
Nizatidine	150 mg bid	$3.10
Omeprazole	20 mg daily	$3.44
Lansoprazole	30 mg daily	$3.28
Cisapride	20 mg bid	$2.87
Sucralfate	1 g qid	$2.89
generic	1 g qid	$2.05

Cost calculations are based on the average retail price of 100 tablets in the Palm Beach County area, December 1997.

disease, the combined cost can be overwhelming. It may force some patients into health maintenance organization insurance coverage just to obtain coverage for the cost of medications.

Failure of medical treatment to control either GERD or GERD-induced respiratory disease is a reason for surgical intervention. Some patients will not follow lifestyle changes (particularly weight loss) and/or the long-term costs of medical therapy are unacceptable. These factors can also lead to a rational choice regarding surgical intervention. With newer laparoscopic approaches (see Chap. 9), patients who would not have been considered surgical candidates in the past are now acceptable for surgery. Just as the adjustment of the medication program for GERD can be difficult, so the decision for surgery and type of procedure can be difficult. The clinician must have a surgeon with appropriate skills for fundoplication. Sometimes this means referral to a surgeon out of the immediate area.

One of the biggest mistakes in the elderly patient can be procrastination about the decision for surgery. If the patient is suffering from severe respiratory problems because of GERD, appropriate medical and surgical therapy will be needed. Aspiration from GERD will cause progressive fibrosis. Waiting until the patient requires continuous oxygen is a mistake. Sometimes the patient is responsible for the delay in treatment; the physician who has read this far should realize the appropriate time and place for surgical intervention. With the population in this country living longer, we must constantly reassess the question: How old is too old for surgery for GERD?

II. GERD and Airway Disease During Pregnancy

Pregnancy is frequently accompanied by heartburn. Baron et al. (50) thoroughly reviewed the literature on GERD in pregnancy. While heartburn is present in 30–80% of pregnancies, it is usually most troublesome during the third trimester (50). The same precipitating factors will be problems in pregnancy as they are in other patients with GERD (see Chap. 8). Smoking and alcohol intake should be avoided during pregnancy for the benefit of the fetus as well as to avoid precipitating GERD.

Therapy for GERD during pregnancy is approached with caution because of concerns about teratogenicity of any drug used. Consequently, in this group of patients lifestyle changes are an extremely important first step (see Chap. 8). Antacids have been used by 35% of patients in some populations during third trimester pregnancies (57). Antacids (other than sodium bicarbonate) or alginic acid are usually the drugs of first choice. Sucralfate has been described as apparently safe and has proven effective in a randomized controlled study during pregnancy (50). For the more difficult-to-control GERD of pregnancy, it appears that ranitidine (51) at a dose of 150 mg twice daily is effective. An additional study found no adverse side effects of this class of drugs taken at any time during pregnancy (52). The H_2-blockers are listed as pregnancy category B drugs, while cisapride and omeprazole are category C (46). Lansoprazole is a pregnancy category B drug, but studies of its use in pregnancy have yet to be published. The benefits and risks of therapy are always most closely weighed during pregnancy, and the safest, most effective drug is always preferred. Clearly this is a subject requiring future research.

III. State of the Art

While the first descriptions of GERD and airway disease date back to the twelfth century (see Chap. 6), it has taken a long time to gather enough scientific evidence to have this relationship enter the mainstream of medical education. In 1996, the First Multi-Disciplinary International Symposium on Supraesophageal Complications of Reflux Disease was held in Tucson, Arizona. The proceedings of this symposium were published in December 1997 (53). It was also a milestone when in 1997 a textbook was published on asthma with passages dedicated to the relationships between GERD and asthma (54). Unfortunately, in that large textbook no chapter was devoted to GERD and asthma. Still, this was a major advance in the recognition that GERD does influence airway disease, and seven authors in the textbook at least devoted space to point out these relationships.

A. Evolution of the Human Larynx

Going beyond the embryological development of our aerodigestive system (Chap. 1), comparative and developmental anatomy studies of primates have shown the evolution of the human aerodigestive system (55,56). The descent of the larynx into the neck has resulted in the ability to speak, while losing the more complete separation of the respiratory and digestive systems seen in our closest relatives, nonhuman primates (57). As the human embryo and infant develop, we witness the evolution of this descent of the larynx into the neck (see Chaps. 1,11).

B. GERD and Inflammation

In Chapter 2, we have an excellent detailed review of inflammation in asthma. It details the role of the vagus nerve and both the cholinergic and nonadrenergic, noncholinergic nerves in providing reflex changes and inflammation as explanations for part of the mechanism by which GERD causes airway disease. Sanico et al. (58) demonstrated capsaicin-sensitive nerves stimulating neurogenic inflammation in the human upper airway of patients with allergic rhinitis. It is anticipated that reflex nasal inflammation of this type may play a role in some types of rhinitis (59) and sinusitis associated with GERD (Chaps. 4,10,11). Rolla et al. (60) noted that patients with sinusitis have pharyngeal biopsies demonstrating a thinning of the epithelium and increase in density of submucosal nerve fibers. Their study suggests that in nonasthmatics with sinusitis, pharyngeal mucosal changes lead to increased access of irritants to submucosal nerve endings. These changes in the pharyngeal mucosa are associated with an increase in extrathoracic airway responsiveness to histamine and, in some cases, activation of a pharyngobronchial reflex with wheezing. The investigators infer that the mucosal changes are due to chronic postnasal drip of mediators and inflammatory cells from the affected sinuses. Their study did not look for evidence of GERD. It would be easy to infer that this mucosal injury could be a result of reflux into the upper airway. There appears to be evidence for a subgroup of patients with severe sinusitis (61) in whom treatment of GERD can significantly improve the sinusitis, thereby avoiding the need for surgery (62,63). This is an area in need of additional research since confirmation of such a relationship could lead to a major change in the approach to treating severe chronic sinus disease.

C. Diagnostic Approaches to GERD and Airway Diseases

The approaches to diagnosis of GERD were reviewed in detail in Chapter 3. However, in Chapter 4, evidence was discussed that patients with reflux laryngitis differ in their findings from patients with symptomatic esophagitis. It appears that studies directed at diagnosing esophagitis (endoscopy and biopsy) and use of a single pH probe in the lower esophagus may mislead the investigator. The importance of using a dual pH probe is stressed, as well as the fact that proximal reflux may not show up on a single study. It may be intermittent but frequent enough to cause persistent damage to the sensitive tissues of the upper airway, which are not able to protect against the damage from acid and pepsin. The specificity of the proximal pH probe is excellent (91%), but the sensitivity and reproducibility is only 55% (64,65). This suggests that a single negative test does not exclude proximal reflux as a cause of upper or lower airway disease. Some studies have suggested very high rates of positive proximal pH studies (Chap. 4) (66). Other investigators have suggested a more invasive approach using simultaneous tracheal and esophageal pH probes as a means of detecting microaspiration (67). Ruth et al. (68) are the latest to find a role for scintigraphic detection of aspiration in patients with GERD. This technique has met with mixed results in other studies (see Chap. 7), but some modifications may make it helpful in the pediatric population (69). The patient's age and state of health will often dictate which diagnostic approach is most appropriate (Chaps. 3–13).

D. Prevalence of GERD in Airway Disease and Airway Disease in GERD

In spite of the high prevalence of GERD in asthmatics (60–80% in adults and 50–60% in children) (Chap. 6), one of the most important deficiencies of studies reported to date has been small numbers of patients studied (Chaps. 6,8,10). While we would all like to see a large prospective study, this would be very expensive and take many years to complete. An interesting study appeared in 1997, with a large retrospective review of the comorbid occurrence of laryngeal or pulmonary disease with esophagitis (70). This research starts with patients who have severe esophagitis or stricture and looks at the prevalence of airway diseases. In 1970, the hospital records of 172 Veterans Affairs (VA) hospitals became computerized. These files are managed by the VA Central Automation Center. Since 1981, the ICD 9 coding has been used for discharge diagnoses. The study group included all patients discharged between 1981 and 1994 who had a primary or secondary diagnosis of GERD-related esophagitis (ICD 9 code 530.1) or esophageal stricture (ICD 9 code 530.3). This group consisted of 101,366 patients. They were compared to an identical number of unmatched control patients selected randomly from the remaining files. These populations were then compared looking at associated medical conditions considered to be extraesophageal manifestations of GERD. There was a significant difference in comorbity for sinusitis, pharyngitis, laryngeal stenosis, chronic bronchitis, bronchial asthma, chronic obstructive pulmonary disease, pulmonary fibrosis, bronchiectasis, pulmonary collapse, and pneumonia ($p < 0.0001$) (70). Sinusitis was the most frequent upper airway problem. Odds ratios showed a strong association between laryngitis and laryngeal stenosis and esophagitis (70). Asthma and pulmonary fibrosis had the highest odds ratios for association with esophagitis or stricture (70). This study shows an increased risk or a variety of extraesophageal manifestations of GERD in the study population. Because of the severity of GERD required to be in the study, it may underestimate the risk for extraesophageal manifestations of GERD. Certainly this study will have its critics, but it is unlikely that another study of this size will appear. It helps to point out the clinical significance between GERD and a variety of airway diseases.

E. An Office Approach to GERD and Airway Disease

It is important to have a good clinical approach to the diagnosis of GERD (Chaps. 3,4) and a high level of suspicion for the diagnosis of GERD-associated airway diseases (3–12). Keeping in mind that some conditions like cough, reflux laryngitis, and asthma may have silent GERD, the use of a questionnaire, as seen in Table 1, may provide the clinician with a tool to raise levels of suspicion. Beyond a good history, the routine physical exam offers only a few clues (abnormal breath sounds) most of the time. The extension of the examination to include direct fiberoptic laryngoscopy, as described in Chapter 4, is often most rewarding. Pulmonary function testing will help detect obstructive and restrictive components of airway disease. The addition of a flow volume loop will help find those cases of extrathoracic obstruction. This finding helps identify those patients with vocal cord dysfunction syndrome (71,72), a condition that has been associated with GERD (73). Two additional cases, evaluated at the National Jewish Center for Immunology and Respiratory Medicine, are followed in my practice; both have responded well to treatment of GERD and speech therapy. Failure to diagnose vocal cord dysfunction syndrome can have serious consequences for the patient (71), who is frequently treated with high-dose steroids for suspected asthma.

Therapeutic trials of therapy for GERD can often be helpful in leading to the diagnosis, but this therapeutic trial must involve sufficient amounts of proton pump inhibitors and an adequate period of treatment, which differs significantly for conditions such as asthma (see Chaps. 7,8) or laryngitis (see Chap. 4). This choice of drugs for therapeutic trial is also affected by age (see Chaps. 10,11) and pregnancy. It is important for each clinician to have confidence in his ability to refer this patient to an appropriate gastroenterologist or otolaryngologist for further evaluation of the underlying GERD-induced problem, especially one familiar with the importance of the dual pH probe study. The next most important decision is when to consider the surgical option. This is an extremely important decision in all age groups (see Chaps. 8–11 and 13). Multiple factors must be considered here, including severity of respiratory disease, rate of progression of respiratory disease, occupation, costs of long-term medical therapy, adequacy of relief of symptoms with maximum medical therapy, availability of a surgeon skilled in laparoscopic fundoplication, and whether the patient has an esophageal motility disorder (see Chap. 9). Consideration should also be given to the stages of the progressive damage to the esophagus from bile salts, as described in Chapter 9. So far, long-term studies have suggested that surgery is superior to medical therapy (see Chaps. 7–9). This is another area where we await further research comparing long-term use of high-dose proton pump inhibitors versus long-term follow-up of (laparoscopic or open) fundoplications.

IV. Conclusions

Since this book was written for clinicians, it did not cover the large amount of information available on the normal physiology of swallowing (e.g., the complex interactions of the tongue, pharynx, hypopharynx, UES, esophagus, and LES). This information has been addressed in a recent publication (74), and additional information was presented at the First Multi-Disciplinary International Symposium on Supraesophageal Complications of Reflux Disease, November 21–23, 1996. These proceedings were published in 1997 (62).

In this book, each contributing author has attempted to present the latest information to help the clinician understand the complex relationships between GERD and airway disease, including approaches to diagnosis and treatment. The large amount of published material referenced and the number of articles in various stages of preparation for print attest to the importance of these relationships in various fields of medical research. It is anticipated that research will continue to confirm additional relationships between GERD and both upper and lower airway diseases (63,75). The development of a new assay for human pepsin may open some new avenues for evaluating the distribution of supraesophageal refluxate (J. A. Koufman, personal communication). There are studies in progress further evaluating the use of cisapride alone in treatment of GERD-induced asthma. Additional proton pump inhibitors and motility agents are in various states of research or near final approval for release in this country. Early evidence suggests that new therapeutic agents may be available to modulate some mediators of neurogenic inflamation (76). The future looks bright for the progressive increase in our armamentarium of treatment modalities and expansion of our knowledge of the relationships between GERD and airway diseases (77).

References

1. Jones B, Ravich WJ, Donner MW. Dysphagia in systemic disease. Dysphagia 1993; 8:368–383.
2. Smyrnios NA, Irwin RS. Wheeze and cough in the elderly. In: Mahler DA, ed. Pul-

monary Disease in the Elderly Patient. New York: Marcel Dekker, Inc., 1993:113–157.
3. Locke GR, Talley NJ, Weaver AL, Zinsmeister AR. A new questionnaire for gastroesophageal reflux disease. Mayo Clin Proc 1994; 69:539–547.
4. Vaezi MF, Richter JE. Twenty-four-hour ambulatory esophageal pH monitoring in the diagnosis of acid reflux-related chronic cough. South Med J 1997; 90:305–311.
5. Shaker R, Milbrath M, Ren J, Toohill R, Hogan WJ, Li Q, Hofmann CL. Esophagopharyngeal distribution of refluxed acid in patients with reflux laryngitis. Gastroenterology 1995; 109:1575–1582.
6. Calhoun KH, Gibson B, Hartley L, Minton J, Hokanson JA. Age-related changes in oral sensation. Laryngoscopy 1992; 102:109–116.
7. Aviv JE, Hecht C, Weinberg H, Dalton JF. Surface sensibility of the floor of the mouth and tongue in healthy controls and in radiated patients. Otolaryngol Head Neck Surg 1992; 107:418–423.
8. Aviv JE, Martin JH, Jones ME, Wee TA, Diamond B, Keen MS, Blitzer A. Age-related changes in pharyngeal and supraglottic sensation. Ann Otol Rhinol Laryngol 1994; 103:749–752.
9. Aviv JE, Martin JH, Keen M, Debell M, Blitzer A. Air pulse quantification of supraglottic and pharyngeal sensation: a new technique. Ann Otol Rhinol Laryngol 1993; 102:777–780.
10. Aviv JE. Effects of aging on sensitivity of the pharyngeal and supraglottic areas. Am J Med 1997; 103 (5A):74S–76S.
11. Williams WN, LaPointe LL. Intra-oral recognition of geometric forms by normal subjects. Percept Mot Skills 1971; 32:419–426.
12. Mortelliti AJ, Malmgren LT, Gacek RR. Ultrastructural changes with age in the human superior laryngeal nerve. Arch Otolaryngol Head Neck 1990, 116:1062–1069.
13. Pontoppidan H, Beecher HK. Progressive loss of protective reflexes in the airway with the advance of age. JAMA 1960; 174:2209–2213.
14. Huxley FJ, Viroslav J, Gray WR, Pierce AK. Pharyngeal aspiration in normal adults and patients with depressed consciousness. Am J Med 1978; 64:564–568.
15. Gleeson K, Eggli DF, Maxwell SL. Quantitative aspiration during sleep in normal subjects. Chest 1997; 111:1266–1272.
16. Schmidt EV, Smirnov VE, Ryabova VS. Results of the seven year prospective study of stroke patients. Stroke 1988; 19:1942–1949.
17. Aviv JE, Martin JH, Sacco RL, Zagar D, Diamond B, Keen MS, Blitzer A. Supraglottic and pharyngeal sensory abnormalities in stroke patients with dysphagia. Ann Otol Rhinol Laryngol 1996; 105:92–97.
18. Aviv JE, Sacco RL, Mohr JP, Thompson JLP, Levin B, Sunshine S, Thompson J, Close LG. Laryngopharyngeal sensory testing with modified barium swallow as predictors of aspiration pneumonia after stroke. Laryngoscope 1997; 107:1254–1260.
19. Feinberg MJ, Ekberg O. Videofluoroscopy in elderly patients with aspiration: importance of evaluating both oral and pharyngeal stages of deglutition. Am J Roentgenol 1991; 156:293–296.
20. Bastian RW. The videoendoscopic swallowing study: an alternative and partner to the videofluoroscopic swallow study. Dysphagia 1993; 8:359–367.

21. Shaker R, Ren J, Podvrsan B, Dodds WJ, Hogan WJ, Kern M, Hoffman R, Hintz J. Effect of aging and bolus variables on pharyngeal and upper esophageal sphincter motor function. Am J Physiol 1993; 264 (Gastrointest Liver Physiol 27):G427–G432.
22. Shaker R, Ren J, Sarna A, Liu J, Sui Z. Effect of aging, position, and temperature on the threshold volume triggering pharyngeal swallows. Gastroenterology 1994; 107:396–402.
23. Shaker R. Airway protective mechanisms: current concepts. Dysphagia 1995; 10: 216–227.
24. Robbins J, Hamilton JW, Lof GL, Kempster GB. Oropharyngeal swallowing in normal adults of different ages. Gastroenterology 1992; 103:823–829.
25. Shaker R, Lang IM. Effect of aging on the deglutitive oral, pharyngeal, and esophageal motor function. Dysphagia 1994; 9:221–228.
26. Fulp SR, Dalton CB, Castell MS, Castell DO. Aging-related alterations in human upper esophageal sphincter function. Am J Gastroenterol 1990; 85:1569–1572.
27. Shaw DW, Cook IJ, Gabb M, Holloway RH, Simula ME, Panagopoulos V, Dent J. Influence of normal aging on oral-pharyngeal and upper esophageal sphincter function during swallowing. Am J Physiol 1995; 268 (Gastrointest Liver Physiol 31): G389–G396.
28. Tracy JF, Logemann JA, Kahrilas PJ, Jacob P, Kobara M, Krugler C. Preliminary observations on the effects of age on oropharyngeal deglutition. Dysphagia 1989; 4:90–94.
29. Soergel KH, Zboralske FF, Amberg JR. Presbyesophagus: esophageal motility in nonagenarians. J Clin Invest 1964; 43:1472–1479.
30. Zboralske FF, Amberg JR, Soergel KH. Presbyesophagus: cineradiologic manifestations. Radiology 1964; 82:463–467.
31. Hollis JB, Castell DO. Esophageal function in elderly men—a new look at "presbyesophagus." Ann Intern Med 1974; 80:371–374.
32. Richter JE, Wu WC, Johns DN, Blackwell JN, Nelson JL, Castell JA, Castell DO. Esophageal manometry in 95 healthy adult volunteers. Dig Dis Sci 1987; 32:583–592.
33. Richter JE. Motility disorders of the esophagus. In: Yamada T, Alpers DH, Powell DW, Owyang C, Silverstein FE, eds. Textbook of Gastroenterology. Philadelphia: J.B. Lippincott Company, 1995:1174–1213.
34. Ren J, Shaker R, Kusano M, Podvran B, Metwally N, Dua KS, Sui Z. Effect of aging on the secondary esophageal peristalsis: presbyesophagus revisited. Am J Physiol 1995; 268 (Gastrointest Liver Physiol 31):G772–G779.
35. Shaker R, Lang IM. Reflex mediated airway protective mechanisms against retrograde aspiration. Am J Med 1997; 103(5A):64S–73S.
36. Ren J, Shaker R, Dua K, Trifan A, Podvrsan B, Sui Z. Glottal adduction response to pharyngeal water stimulation: evidence for a pharyngoglottal closure reflex. Gastroenterology 1994; 106:A558.
37. Ward PH, Colton R, McConnell F, Malmgren L, Kashima H, Woodson G. Aging of the voice and swallowing. Otolaryngol Head Neck Surg 1989; 100:283–286.
38. Hurwitz A, Brady DA, Schaal SE, Samloff IM, Dedon J, Ruhl CE. Gastric acidity in older adults. JAMA 1997; 278:659–662.
39. Smyrnios NA, Irwin RS. Wheeze and cough in the elderly. In: Mahler DA, ed. Pul-

monary Disease in the Elderly Patient. New York: Marcel Dekker, Inc., 1993:113–157.

40. Hamdy S, Aziz Q, Rothwell JC, Hughes D, Tallis RC, Thompson DG. Explaining oropharyngeal dysphagia after unilateral hemispheric stroke. Lancet 1997; 350:686–692.

41. Feinberg MJ. Radiographic techniques and interpretation of abnormal swallowing in adult and elderly patients. Dysphagia 1993; 8:356–358.

42. Kaye GM, Zorowitz RD, Baredes S. Role of flexible laryngoscopy in evaluating aspiration. Ann Otol Rhinol Laryngol 1997; 106:705–709.

43. Zhu H, Pace F, Sangaletti O, Bianchi Porro G. Features of symptomatic gastroesophageal reflux in elderly patients. Scand J Gastroenterol 1993; 28:235–238.

44. Collen MJ, Abdulian JD, Chen YK. Gastroesophageal reflux in the elderly: more severe disease that requires aggressive therapy. Am J Gastroenterol 1995; 90:1053–1057.

45. Waring JP. Management of gastroesophageal reflux disease in the elderly: more aggressive or more appropriate? Am J Gastroenterol 1995; 90:1037.

46. Physicians' Desk Reference. Montvale, NJ: Medical Economics Publications, 1997.

47. Teare JP, Spedding C, Whitehead MW, Greenfield SM, Challacombe SJ, Thompson RPH. Omeprazole and dry mouth. Scand J Gastroenterol 1995; 30:216–218.

48. Pope CE II. Acid-reflux disorders. N Engl J Med 1994; 331:656–660.

49. Harding SM, Richter JE. The role of gastroesophageal reflux in chronic cough and asthma. Chest 1997; 111:1389–1402.

50. Baron TH, Richter JE. Gastroesophageal reflux disease in pregnancy. Gastroenterol Clin North Am 1992; 21:777–791.

51. Larson JD, Patatanian E, Miner PB, Rayburn WF, Robinson MG. Double-blind, placebo-controlled study of ranitidine for gastroesophageal reflux symptoms during pregnancy. Obstet Gynecol 1997; 90:83–87.

52. Magee LA, Inocencion G, Kamboj L, Rosetti F, Koren G. Safety of first trimester exposure to histamine H_2 blockers. A prospective cohort study. Dig Dis Sci 1996; 4:1145–1149.

53. Shaker R, ed. First multi-disciplinary international symposium on supraesophageal complications of reflux disease. Am J Med 1997; 103(5A):1S–150S.

54. Barnes PJ, Grunstein MM, Leff AR, Woolcock AJ, eds. Asthma. Philadelphia: Lippincott-Raven, 1997.

55. Laitman JT, Reidenberg JS. Specialization of the human upper respiratory and upper digestive systems as seen through comparative and developmental anatomy. Dysphagia 1993; 8:318–325.

56. Laitman JT, Reidenberg JS. The human aerodigestive tract and gastroesophageal reflux: and evolutionary perspective. Am J Med 1977; 103(5A):2S–8S.

57. Sasaki CT, Weaver EM. Physiology of the larynx. Am J Med 1997; 103(5A):95–185.

58. Sanico AM, Atsuta S, Proud D, Togias. Dose-dependent effects of capsaicin nasal challenge: in vivo evidence of human airway neurogenic inflammation. J Allergy Clin Immunol 1997; 100:632–641.

59. Contencin P, Narcy P. Nasopharyngeal pH monitoring in infants and children with chronic rhinopharyngitis. Int J Pediatr Otorhinolaryngol 1991; 22:249–256.

60. Rolla G, Colagrande P, Scappaticci E, Bottomicca F, Magnano M, Brussino L, Dutto L, Bucca C. Damage of the pharyngeal mucosa and hyperresponsiveness of airway in sinusitis. J Allergy Clin Immunol 1997; 100:52–57.
61. Hogan WJ. Spectrum of supraesophageal complications of gastroesophageal reflux disease. Am J Med 1997; 103(5A):77S–83S.
62. Yellon RF. The spectrum of reflux-associated otolaryngologic problems in infants and children. Am J Med 1997; 103(5A):125S–129S.
63. Bothwell MR, Parsons DS, Talbot A, Barbero GJ, Wilder B. Outcome of reflux therapy on pediatric sinusitis. Otolaryngol Head Neck Surg 1999; 121:255–262.
64. Vaezi MF, Schroeder PL, Richter JE. Reproducibility of proximal probe pH parameters in 24-hour ambulatory esophageal pH monitoring. Am J Gastroenterol 1997; 92:825–829.
65. Richter JE. Ambulatory esophageal pH monitoring. Am J Med 1997; 103(5A):130S–134S.
66. Loughlin CJ, Koufman JA. Paroxysmal laryngospasm secondary to gastroesophageal reflux. Laryngoscope 1996; 106:1502–1505.
67. Jack CIA, Calverley PMA, Donnelly RJ, Tran J, Russel G, Hind CRK, Evans CC. Simultaneous tracheal and esophageal pH measurements in asthmatic patients with gastroesophageal reflux. Thorax 1995; 50:201–204.
68. Ruth M, Carlsson S, Mansson I, Bengtsson U, Sandberg N. Scintigraphic detection of gastro-pulmonary aspiration in patients with respiratory disorders. Clin Physiol 1993; 13:19–33.
69. Collier BD. Detection of aspiration: scintigraphic techniques. Am J Med 1997; 103(5A):135S–137S.
70. El-Serag HB, Sonnenberg A. Comorbid occurrence of laryngeal or pulmonary disease with esophagitis in United States military veterans. Gastroenterology 1997; 113:755–760.
71. Butani L, O'Connell EJ. Functional respiratory disorders. Ann Allergy Asthma Immunol 1997; 79:91–101.
72. Reisner C, Nelson HS. Vocal cord dysfunction with nocturnal awakening. J Allergy Clin Immunol 1997; 99:843–846.
73. Gutierrez M, Nelson HS, Weber R. Gastroesophageal reflux disease–induced vocal cord dysfunction masquerading as asthma. Presented in abstract at the American College of Allergy, Asthma, and Immunology 1996 annual meeting, Boston.
74. Castell DO, ed. The Esophagus. Boston: Little, Brown and Co. 1995.
75. Halstead LA. Role of gastroesophageal reflux in pediatric upper airway disorders. Otolaryngol Head Neck Surg 1999; 120:208–214.
76. Shinoda M, Watanabe N, Suko T, Mogi G, Takeyama M. Effects of anti-allergic drugs on substance P(SP) and vasoactive intestinal peptide (VIP) in nasal secretions. Am J Rhinol 1997; 11:237–241.
77. Second Multi-Disciplinary International Symposium on Supraesophageal Complications of Gastroesophageal Reflux Disease. Seattle, Washington, August 6–8, 1998.

AUTHOR INDEX

Italic numbers give the page on which the complete reference is cited.

A

Abbott, WO, 69, *87*
Abdulian, JD, 311, 312, *321*
Abelli, L, 37, *51*
Abrahamsson, H, 274, *282*
Abrams, JS, 21, *43*
Abramson, SJ, 276, *284*
Abucan, A, 255, *266*
Ackroyd, R, 214, *234*
Adami, B, 187, *205*
Adams, GK, 23, *43*
Adams, PF, 246, *263*
Adcock, IM, 31, *48*
Addis, A, 187, *205*
Adeleine, P, 20, 24, *41*, 170, 171, 172, 173, *178*, 196, 198, *207*
Advenier, C, 30, 31, 33, *47*, *48*, *49*
Agee, J, 26, *45*
Ahlstedt, S, 20, 21, *42*
Ahmad, M, 180, 181, *203*
Akers, S, 89, 90, 103, *107*
Alam, R, 19, 23, *40*
Albanese, C, 279, *284*
Albertucci, M, 99, *111*, 225, 227, 228, 230, *236*
Alexander, RW, 20, *41*, 104, *112*, 146, 147, 148, 157, 158, 170, 172, *174*, *178*, 250, 256, 257, *265*
Alger, L, 28, *46*
Alland, S, 243, *263*
Allen, CJ, 90, 95, 96, 99, 103, 104, 105, 106, *107*, *110*
Allen, F, 274, *282*
Allen, FW, 247, *263*
Allen, ML, 103, *112*
Allen, TGJ, 37, *52*
Aloe, L, 33, *49*
Altemus, JB, 37, 38, *51*
Altorki, NK, 161, *175*
Altschuler, SM, 95, 105, *110*, 274, *282*
Amberg, JR, 308, *320*
Ambrecht, U, 255, *266*
Amemiya, T, 33, *49*, 90, *107*
Ament, ME, 60, *67*, 90, 92, 99, *108*, 129, 130, *138*, 244, 247, 259, *263*, *267*, 274, 279, *281*, *284*
Amodio, JB, 276, *284*
Amoury, RA, 276, *284*
Amyot, R, 168, *177*, 183, *205*
Andersen, C, 33, *49*
Andersen, LI, 20, *41*, 95, *109*, 143, 158, *173*
Anderson, JA, 20, *41*

323

Anderson, P, 28, 31, 39, *46*
Andersson, KE, 131, *138*, 165, 167, *177*
Ando, MI, 28, 29, *46*
Andreotti, MR, 275, *283*
Andze, GO, 129, 130, *138*
Angelides, A, 272, *281*
Angelucci, F, 33, *49*
Anggard, A, 37, *51*
Ansaldi, N, 285, *300*
Arakawa, M, 90, 93, *108*
Arana, J, 105, *113*
Arciniega-Oliver, RM, 104, *112*
Arenberg, B, 77, *87*
Arguelles-Martin, F, 251, 258, *265*, 267
Arndorfer, R, 244, *263*, 270, *280*
Aronow, E, 272, *281*
Ashcraft, E, 244, *263*
Ashcraft, KW, 276, *284*
Asher, MI, 244, *263*
Ashraf, MM, 152, *174*
Assoufi, B, 20, 21, 24, *42*, *44*
Atsuta, S, 315, *321*
Aubert, A, 224, 228, 230, *235*, 260, *267*
Aubier, M, 247, *263*, 265
Auricchio, S, 270, *280*
Austin, J, 168, *177*, 183, *204*, 274, *282*
Averill, DB, 77, *87*
Avert, ME, 253, *266*
Aviv, JE, 306, 308, 310, *319*
Avner, D, 189, 192, *206*
Aye, R, 225, *236*
Ayers, JG, 179, 197, *203*
Aziz, Q, 310, *321*
Azizkhan, RG, 258, *267*
Azzar, D, 20, 24, *41*, 170, 171, 172, 173, *178*, 196, 198, *207*

B

Badalamenti, S, 105, *113*, 185, *205*
Badier, M, 105, *113*, 125, 126, *137*
Bafrett, J, 65, *68*
Bagley, CJ, 19, 23, *40*
Bai, TR, 31, *48*

Bailey, B, 187, *205*
Bain, WM, 70, 78, *85*, 241, 242, 243, *262*
Baker, DG, 38, *52*
Baker, J, 28, *46*
Baker, LA, 99, *111*
Bakewell, M, 270, *279*
Balaban, DH, 161, 162, 163, 164, 169, *175*, 247, *263*
Ballantine, T, 275, 279, *283*, *284*
Ballard, RD, 144, 158, *174*, 248, *265*
Balocco, P, 285, *300*
Balson, B, 251, 252, 256, 257, *265*
Baltazan, MH, 257, *267*
Baluk, P, 26, 28, 31, 39, *45*, *46*
Bannister, WK, 152, *174*
Baraniuk, JN, 30, 33, 34, *48*, *49*
Barbara, L, 254, *266*
Barbero, GJ, 318, *322*
Bardelli, E, 94, 95, *109*
Bardham, KD, 56, 60, *67*
Baredes, S, 310, *321*
Barkans, J, 21, 24, *43*, *44*
Barneon, G, 20, 21, *41*
Barnert, J, 168, *177*
Barnes, BE, 270, *280*
Barnes, P, 248, *265*
Barnes, PJ, 20, 22, 25, 26, 28, 30, 31, 33, 34, 37, 38, 39, *41*, *42*, *46*, *47*, *48*, *49*, *51*, *52*, 314, *321*
Barnett, C, 271, *280*
Baron, TH, 314, *321*
Barradell, LB, 189, 192, *206*
Barrison, GM, 275, *283*
Bartelsman, JF, 104, *112*, 192, 194, *206*, 257, *267*
Barter, CE, 161, 162, 169, *176*
Barthlow, HG, 22, 28, 31, 39, *43*
Bartolotti, M, 270, *280*
Bartter, T, 89, 90, 103, *107*
Barudi, C, 129, 130, *138*, 184, *205*
Barundi, C, 240, *261*
Bastian, RW, 308, 310, *319*
Batch, AJ, 90, *108*
Battaglia, G, 105, *113*

Author Index

Bauer, FE, 37, *52*
Bauman, N, 274, *282*
Bauman, NM, 77, *87*
Baumgarten, CR, 23, 31, *42*
Beasley, CRW, 20, 21, *41*
Beatty, TW, 70, 78, *86*
Beaudy, PH, 244, *263*
Becker, DJ, 103, *112*, 183, 184, *204*, *205*
Beckett, HA, 285, *300*
Beecher, HK, 307, *319*
Behar, J, 105, *113*, 189, 192, *206*
Bel, A, 90, *107*, 123, 124, *137*
Beland, J, 37, *51*
Belenky, WM, 240, *262*
Bellamy, JF, 30, 31, *47*
Belmont, JR, 240, 241, *261*, 275, *283*
Belsey, R, 117, *136*, 224, 228, 230, *235*
Belvisi, M, 37, 38, *51*, *52*
Bendig, DW, 275, *283*
Bengtsson, U, 155, *175*, 316, *322*
Benini, S, 94, 95, *109*
Benjamin, SB, 83, *88*, 92, 93, *108*, *109*, 241, 242, *262*, 270, *279*
Bennett, FM, 20, *41*, 90, 92, 93, 94, 95, 96, 97, 98, 99, 100, 101, 103, *107*
Bennett, JR, 103, *112*, 180, 184, *203*, *205*, 260, *267*
Bensoussan, AL, 224, 228, 230, *235*
Bentley, AM, 20, 21, 24, *42*, *43*, *44*
Berant, M, 273, *281*
Berdon, WE, 276, *284*
Berenberg, W, 69, 80, *87*
Berenguer, J, 180, 197, *203*
Berenson, NN, 189, 192, *206*
Berger, K, 183, *204*
Berghammer, G, 272, *281*
Bergren, A, 186, 188, *205*
Berkowtiz, D, 273, *281*
Berkson, J, 123, *137*
Bermejo, J, 214, *234*
Berni Canani, J, 243, *263*
Berni Canani, R, 243, *263*
Bernsford, RG, 215, *234*
Bernstein, A, 24, *44*, 186, 188, *205*

Bernstein, J, 241, *262*
Bernstein, LM, 99, *111*
Berquist, WE, 24, *44*, 119, 129, 130, 131, *136*, *138*, 165, *177*, 183, *204*, 247, *263*, 274, *281*, *282*
Berrisford, RG, 156, 157, *175*
Berstad, A, 192, *206*
Bertrand, C, 28, 31, *46*
Bervoets, D, 292, *301*
Beste, DJ, 99, *111*
Bettagha, G, 185, *205*
Bettex, M, 276, *284*
Beumont, PJV, 286, *300*
Bevenius, J, 287, *300*
Beveridge, BR, 214, *234*
Biancani, P, 105, *113*
Bianchi Porro, G, 311, 313, *321*
Bierman, CW, 239, *261*
Bittinger, M, 168, *177*
Bjornsdottir, US, 20, 22, 23, *42*
Bjornsson, E, 285, *300*
Blackburn, KS, 93, *109*
Blackshaw, LA, 163, *176*
Blackwell, JN, 309, *320*
Blalock, PD, 70, 71, 76, *86*
Blane, Ce, 279, *284*
Blaser, K, 24, *44*
Blitzer, A, 306, 308, 310, *319*
Block, SM, 93, *109*
Bloom, BS, 83, *88*, 182, *204*
Bloom, SR, 37, *52*
Bluestone, CD, 242, *262*
Blum, AL, 187, *205*
Blum, AM, 23, *42*
Blum, D, 274, 275, *282*
Bochner, BS, 20, 21, 22, 23, *42*
Bochnowitz, S, 38, *53*
Bocus, P, 254, *266*
Bode, E, 24, *44*
Boer, L, 24, *44*
Bogdasarian, RS, 70, 71, 78, *86*
Boichot, E, 33, *49*
Boileau, R, 37, 38, *51*
Boisen, RJ, 103, *112*, 183, *204*
Bolio, A, 253, *266*

Bolser, DC, 31, *48*
Boman, G, 285, *300*
Bonavina, L, 105, *113*, 125, 126, *137*, 170, 171, *178*, 197, *207*, 217, 225, 227, 228, 230, 232, *235*, *236*
Bondy, GP, 31, *48*
Bonini, S, 33, *49*
Book, LS, 273, 274, *281*
Bordeaux, EA, 73, *87*
Borish, L, 21, *43*
Bornhofen, B, 255, *266*
Bothwell, MR, 318, *322*
Bottomicca, F, 315, *322*
Boushey, HA, 33, *49*, 180, *203*
Bousquet, J, 20, 21, *41*
Bouzo, MH, 187, *205*
Bovo, P, 94, 95, *109*
Bowden, JJ, 26, 37, 38, *46*, *52*, *53*
Boyle, JT, 95, 105, *109*, *110*, 152, 153, 154, 155, 158, 160, *175*, 274, *282*
Bradding, P, 21, 22, *42*
Bradley, B, 24, *44*
Bradley, LA, 20, *41*, 104, *112*, 145, 146, 147, 148, 157, 158, 170, 172, *174*, *178*, 250, 256, 257, *265*
Brady, DA, 310, 312, *320*
Brady, JM, 289, *301*
Brady, JP, 287, *300*
Braillon, G, 20, 24, *41*, 119, *137*, 170, 171, 172, 173, *178*, 196, 198, *207*
Braman, SS, 89, *106*
Brand, L, 24, *44*, 123, 124, 125, 126, 128, 129, *137*, 163, 168, 170, *176*, 180, 196, 197, 199, 200, *203*, *207*
Brandstatter, G, 187, *205*
Brandt, ML, 129, 130, *138*
Brant, R, 124, *137*, 160, 169, 170, *175*, 180, *203*, 285, *300*
Braunstein, G, 30, *47*
Bray, GW, 116, *136*
Bray, PF, 273, 274, *281*
Bredt, DS, 37, 39, *51*
Bremner, CG, 196, 199, *207*, 211, 212, 215, 224, 228, 230, *234*, *235*, 258, *267*
Bremner, RM, 215, 222, 226, *234*, 235

Brenic, S, 104, *112*
Breslin, ABX, 90, 92, 93, 94, 95, 96, 98, 99, *107*, *109*, 243, *263*
Bret, P, 90, *108*
Bretza, J, 119, *137*
Brewer, JP, 21, *43*
Britton, WJ, 21, *43*
Broaddus, VC, 24, 25, *45*
Brodin, E, 34, *50*
Brooks, LS, 60, *68*
Brown, CM, 286, *300*
Brown, CR, 31, *48*
Brown, M, 248, *265*
Brown, MA, 244, *263*
Brown, P, 125, 126, *137*, 186, 188, *205*
Bruce, AN, 20, 25, 26, 31, *41*
Brummer, RJ, 144, 158, *174*, 248, *265*
Brussino, L, 315, *322*
Bruyns, J, 260, *267*
Bryant, GH, 161, *175*
Bryne, WJ, 253, *266*
Brzana, RJ, 98, 101, *110*
Bucca, C, 315, *322*
Buckner, CK, 22, 28, 31, 39, *43*
Bulluck, GR, 23, *42*
Bundgaard, A, 20, *41*, 95, *109*, 143, 158, *173*
Bunnett, NW, 26, *46*
Burden, DT, 38, *53*
Burghard, G, 93, 97, 98, *109*, 142, 148, 157, 158, *173*, 180, *203*
Burke, AJ, 70, 78, *86*
Burne, WJ, 60, *67*
Burnstock, G, 37, *52*
Burrows, B, 21, *43*
Busse, WW, 20, 22, 23, *42*
Butani, L, 317, *322*
Butland, RJ, 104, *112*, 192, 193, 194, *206*
Buts, JP, 129, 130, *138*, 184, *205*, 240, *261*
Buttery, LDK, 37, *51*
Button, B, 274, *282*
Byrne, WJ, 90, 92, 99, *108*, 129, 130, *138*, 244, 253, *263*, *266*

C

Cabezas, GA, 38, *53*
Cadiere, GB, 260, *267*
Cadieux, A, 37, *52*
Cadman, D, 244, *263*
Cahill, JL, 276, *284*
Caletti, GC, 254, *266*
Calhoun, J, 257, *267*
Calhoun, KH, 306, *319*
Calhoun, WJ, 21, *43*
Calus, D, 129, 130, *138*
Calverley, PMA, 156, 157, 158, *175*, 316, *322*
Cameron, AJ, 90, *108*
Campbell, AM, 161, 162, 169, *176*
Campbell, BH, 70, 78, *86*
Campbell, M, 244, *263*
Campfield, J, 272, *281*
Canning, BJ, 22, 28, 30, 31, 34, 35, 37, 38, 39, *42*, *47*, *50*, *52*
Carceller-Blanchard, A, 224, 228, 230, *235*
Carling, L, 192, *206*
Carlsson, S, 155, *175*, 316, *322*
Carrasco, E, 20, 24, *41*, 56, *67*, 125, 126, *137*, 170, 171, 172, *178*, 186, 188, 196, 197, *205*, 260, *267*, 279, *284*
Carre, IJ, 272, *281*
Carstairs, JR, 30, *48*
Casale, TB, 25, 38, 39, *45*
Casimir, G, 243, *263*
Castell, DO, 56, 59, 61, 62, 65, 66, *67*, *68*, 78, *87*, 90, 93, 94, 96, 98, 99, 103, *107*, *110*, *111*, *112*, 125, *138*, 152, 155, 156, 170, 171, 172, *174*, *175*, *178*, 182, 183, 184, 185, 192, *204*, *205*, *206*, 216, *235*, 255, 256, *266*, *267*, 308, 309, 318, *320*, *322*
Castell, JA, 63, 65, *68*, 90, 94, 99, *107*, 156, 170, 171, 172, *175*, *178*, 184, *205*, 309, *320*
Castell, MS, 308, *320*
Cattau, EL, 93, *109*

Catto-Smith, A, 274, *282*
Caughey, G, 38, *53*
Cavallini, G, 94, 95, *109*
Cervero, F, 25, 31, *45*
Challacombe, SJ, 298, *302*, 312, *321*
Chan, B, 26, *45*
Chandler, JP, 122, *137*
Chanez, P, 20, 21, *41*
Chang, MH, 275, *283*
Chapman, RW, 23, *43*
Charette, L, 247, 248, 249, *263*
Charpin, D, 105, *113*, 125, 126, *137*
Chastang, JF, 78, *88*
Cheadle, WG, 78, *88*, 183, *204*
Chejfec, B, 196, 197, 199, 200, *207*
Chejfec, G, 20, 24, *40*, *44*, 125, 126, 128, 129, *137*, 163, 168, 170, *176*, 180, 196, 198, *203*, *207*
Chen, MY, 242, *262*
Chen, PH, 275, *283*
Chen, XR, 33, *49*
Chen, YK, 311, 312, *321*
Cherian, P, 56, 60, *67*
Chernow, B, 90, 93, *107*, 125, *138*, 155, 156, *175*
Cherry, J, 69, 70, 71, *86*, 117, *136*
Chesrown, SE, 37, 38, *51*
Cheung, A, 37, *52*
Chinchilli, VM, 180, *203*
Chintam, R, 20, *40*, 196, 198, *207*
Chobanian, SJ, 56, 57, 60, 64, *67*
Christensen, J, 167, *177*
Christian, EP, 26, *46*
Christie, DL, 129, 130, *138*, 247, *263*, 276, *284*
Christofides, ND, 37, *52*
Chudry, N, 33, *50*
Chung, KF, 28, *46*
Church, MK, 21, 22, *42*, *43*
Ciarleglio, C, 93, *109*
Cirillo, B, 243, *263*
Clarke, DD, 270, *279*
Claus, D, 240, *261*
Close, LG, 308, 310, *319*
Cloutier, MM, 90, *107*, 243, *263*
Coben, RM, 93, *109*

Cobos, A, 272, 274, *280*
Coburn, RF, 37, 38, *51*
Cochran, W, 75, *87*, 241, *262*
Coffman, RL, 21, *43*
Coghlan, HC, 147, 148, 150, 162, 169, *174*
Cognon, C, 31, *48*
Cohen, D, 93, *109*
Cohen, S, 95, 105, *109*, *110*, 131, *138*, 152, 153, 154, 155, 158, 160, 167, *175*, *177*, 182, *204*, 247, *263*, 274, *282*
Colagrande, P, 315, *322*
Colasurdo, GN, 38, *53*
Colebatch, HJH, 152, *174*
Coleman, RA, 37, *51*
Coleridge, HM, 26, 34, 35, 37, *45*, *50*, 92, *108*
Coleridge, JCG, 26, 34, 35, 37, *45*, *50*, 92, *108*
Collen, MJ, 311, 312, *321*
Collier, BD, 316, *322*
Collins, KA, 93, *109*
Colon, AR, 270, *279*
Colton, R, 310, *320*
Colton, T, 121, *137*
Colturi, T, 69, 70, 71, 72, 79, *86*
Conley, SF, 99, *111*
Constantini, M, 222, 226, *235*
Contencin, P, 70, 75, 80, *86*, 239, 240, 241, 253, *261*, 315, *321*
Cook, I, 270, *280*
Cook, IJ, 308, *320*
Cooke, HJ, 38, *53*
Cooper, DN, 24, *44*, 186, 188, *205*
Cooper, JB, 66, *68*, 69, 71, 72, *87*, 96, *110*, 156, *175*
Coran, AG, 244, 259, *263*, *267*, 276, *279*, *284*
Corey, M, 275, *283*
Cornu, G, 129, 130, *138*, 240, *261*
Corrales, R, 97, *110*
Corrao, WM, 56, *67*, 89, 90, *106*, 243, *263*
Corrigan, CJ, 20, 21, 23, 24, *42*, *43*, *44*

Corsello, BF, 20, *41*, 143, 145, 148, 157, 158, *173*
Corwin, RW, 155, *175*
Costa, DL, 26, *46*
Coumaros, D, 93, 97, 98, *109*, 125, 126, *137*, 142, 148, 157, 158, *173*, 180, *203*
Courtney, JV, 105, *113*, 125, 126, *137*, 170, 171, *178*, 197, *207*, 217, 232, *235*
Cowan, RJ, 81, *88*
Cowie, RL, 124, *137*, 160, 169, 170, *175*, 180, *203*, 285, *300*
Crausaz, FM, 155, *175*
Craven, MA, 90, 95, 99, 103, 104, 105, 106, *107*, *110*
Crookes, PF, 222, 226, *235*
Cucchiara, S, 270, 275, *280*, *283*
Cuello, C, 26, 30, 39, *45*
Cui, YY, 33, *49*
Culebras, A, 162, *176*
Cummins, MM, 69, 70, 72, 76, 78, 84, *85*
Cunha, FQ, 33, *49*
Cunningham, ET, 140, 141, *173*
Curley, FJ, 20, *41*, 89, 90, 91, 92, 93, 94, 95, 96, 97, 98, 99, 100, 101, 102, 103, *106*, *107*, *108*, 170, 171, 172, *178*, 180, *203*, 243, *262*
Curran, J, 93, *109*
Cuschieri, A, 183, *204*, 259, *267*

D

D'Esopo, W, 244, *263*
Dab, I, 105, *113*, 275, *283*
daCosta, FAM, 37, *51*
Dahlqvist, A, 37, *52*
Dale, HH, 34, *50*
Dalton, CB, 56, 62, 63, *67*, *68*, 99, *111*, 184, *205*, 308, *320*
Dalton, JF, 306, *319*
Damme, JV, 24, *44*
Daneman, A, 275, *283*

Daouli, S, 31, 33, *48*, *49*
Davi, G, 105, *113*, 185, *205*
Davidson, A, 275, *284*
Davidson, GP, 270, *279*, *280*
Davis, MV, 119, *137*
Davis, P, 272, *281*
Davis, PB, 161, *176*
Davis, PM, 255, *266*
Davis, RS, 119, *136*, 143, 144, 148, 157, *173*, 248, 249, *265*, 273, *281*
Dawson, D, 56, 60, *67*
de Blieck-Hogervorst, JMA, 292, *301*
de Caestecker, JS, 96, *110*
de la Bellacasa, JP, 272, 274, *280*
de Ritis, G, 275, *283*
Debell, M, 306, 310, *319*
deBlic, Y, 247, 248, *265*
DeBruijne, JW, 192, *206*
Dechner, WK, 241, 242, *262*
Dedon, J, 310, 312, *320*
Dees, SC, 248, *265*
DeGennaro, FC, 31, *48*
Dekkers, CP, 192, *206*
DeKruyff, RH, 21, *44*
Delagado-Munoz, MD, 239, *261*
Delahunty, JE, 70, 71, *85*
Delattre, JF, 163, *176*
Della Roandi, GM, 243, *263*
dellaRocca, A, 270, *280*
Delpierre, S, 38, *52*
DeLuca, G, 270, *280*
DeMeester, TR, 62, *68*, 96, 99, 103, 105, *110*, *111*, *112*, *113*, 125, 126, *137*, 161, 162, 170, 171, *175*, *176*, *178*, 183, 196, 197, 199, *204*, *207*, 211, 212, 214, 215, 217, 222, 223, 224, 225, 226, 227, 228, 229, 230, 232, *234*, *235*, *236*, 258, *267*, 270, *280*, 291, *301*
Denault, L, 270, *280*
Denis, P, 20, *40*, 196, 198, *207*
Denjean, A, 20, 33, *41*, 95, *109*, 150, 151, 158, *174*, 248, *265*
Dennish, DW, 78, *87*
Dennish, GW, 183, *204*

Denoyelle, F, 77, *87*
Dent, J, 61, *68*, 104, *112*, 163, *176*, 214, *234*, 238, *260*, 270, *280*, 308, *320*
Depla, AC, 104, *112*, 192, 194, *206*, 257, *267*
Derkx, HHF, 253, *266*
deRoy, C, 188, *205*
Desai, MC, 28, *46*
Deschner, WK, 93, 97, 98, *109*
Deshazo, RD, 20, 21, 23, *42*
DeVault, KR, 61, *68*, 99, 103, *111*, 182, 185, *204*, *205*
DeVita, C, 243, *263*
Dey, RD, 30, 35, 37, 38, *47*, *51*, *52*
Deynoyelle, F, 70, 80, *86*
Di Mario, F, 105, *113*
Di Simone, MB, 254, *266*
Diamond, B, 306, 308, 310, *319*
Diamond, L, 37, 38, *51*
Dillard, VL, 271, *280*
Dillon, PW, 276, *284*
DiLorenzo, C, 270, *280*
DiMarino, AJ, 131, *138*, 167, *177*, 247, *263*, 274, *282*
DiMario, F, 185, *205*
DiMartino, AJ, 93, *109*
DiPalma, J, 270, *279*
Djukanovic, R, 20, 21, 31, *41*, *48*
Do Vale, J, 69, *87*
Dobhan, R, 62, *68*, 216, *235*
Dodds, WJ, 73, 79, *87*, 156, *175*, 238, 244, *260*, *263*, 270, *280*, 291, *301*, 308, 309, *320*
Doerschuk, CM, 28, *46*
Dollery, C, 248, *265*
Domeij, S, 37, *52*
Don, H, 38, *52*
Donnelly, RJ, 156, 157, *175*, 215, *234*, 316, *322*
Donner, MW, 140, 141, *173*, 242, *262*, 304, *319*
Dordal, MT, 257, *267*
Dowdeswell, R, 162, *176*
Downing, SE, 273, 274, *281*

Drane, WE, 93, *109*
Dray, A, 28, 32, *47, 48*
Drazen, JM, 31, 37, 38, 39, *48, 51, 53,* 180, *203*
Dua, KS, 309, 310, *320*
Dubois, J, 89, 90, 103, *107*
Ducasse, A, 163, *176*
Ducolone, A, 93, 97, 98, *109*, 125, 126, *137*, 142, 148, 157, 158, *173*, 180, *203*
Dunbar, J, 271, *280*
Dunnill, MS, 20, *41*
Dupin, B, 105, *113*, 125, 126, *137*
Duranceau, A, 168, *177*, 183, *205*
Durham, SR, 20, 21, 24, *42, 43, 44*
Durie, P, 275, *283*
Duroux, P, 20, 33, *41*, 95, *109*, 150, 151, 158, *174*, 248, *265*
DuSouich, P, 168, *177*, 183, *205*
Dutto, L, 315, *322*

E

Eappon, S, 28, *46*
Earis, JE, 24, *44*, 186, 188, *205*
Eccles, JD, 288, 290, 292, *301*
Edmonds-Alt, X, 31, 33, *48, 49*
Egan, RW, 23, *43*
Eggli, DF, 307, 309, *319*
Eizaguirre, I, 105, *113*
Ekberg, O, 308, 310, *319*
Ekstrom, F, 248, *265*
Ekstrom, P, 192, *206*
Ekstrom, T, 95, *109*, 144, 158, 162, 165, 166, 170, 171, 172, *174, 176, 177, 178*, 186, 187, 188, *205*
El-Serag, HB, 316, *322*
Elbon, CL, 39, *54*
Ellis, JL, 22, 28, 31, 39, *43, 47*
Elta, G, 69, 70, 71, 72, 79, *86*
Emonds-Alt, X, 30, 31, *47*
Enander, I, 20, 21, *41*
Ercolini, P, 275, *283*
Erzurum, SC, 180, 181, *203*
Euler, AR, 60, *67*, 90, 92, 99, *108*, 129, 130, *138*, 244, 253, *263, 266*, 279, *284*
Evans, CC, 156, 157, 158, *175*, 215, 216, *234, 235*, 316, *322*
Evans, S, 272, *280*
Everett, SL, 270, *279*

F

Fahrenkrug, J, 37, *51*
Fajac, I, 30, *47*
Fame, TM, 38, *53*
Farmer, SG, 22, 33, *43*
Farrar, JF, 247, *263*, 274, *282*
Faulds, D, 189, 192, *206*
Favez, G, 155, *175*
Federman, Q, 79, *88*
Feigelson, J, 275, *283*
Fein, M, 211, 228, *234*
Feinberg, MJ, 308, 310, *319, 321*
Feinstein, AR, 122, *137*
Feldman, M, 271, *280*
Feldman, W, 244, *263*
Fendrick, M, 83, *88*, 182, *204*
Fenton, BH, 81, *88*
Fernandez, X, 23, *43*
Ferrari, A, 254, *266*
Ferrari, M, 94, 95, *109*
Ferriera, SH, 33, *49*
Ferriero, J, 241, *262*
Ferry, GD, 275, *283*
Festen, HP, 192, *206*
Festen, HPM, 83, *88*
Fett, SL, 56, *67*, 180, 197, *203*
Field, SK, 124, *137*, 160, 169, 170, *175*, 180, *203*, 285, *300*
Filipi, CJ, 223, 229, *235*
Filler, SJ, 98, *111*, 286, 288, 291, 292, *300, 301*
Fischer, A, 26, 30, 33, 34, 35, 37, 38, 39, *45, 47, 49, 50, 51, 52, 53*
Fish, JE, 180, *203*
Fitzgerald, G, 248, *265*
FItzgerald, JM, 90, 99, 103, 104, 106, *107*

Fitzgerald, S, 26, *46*
Flament, JB, 163, *176*
Flanagan, TL, 26, *45*
Flannery, EM, 21, *43*
Flores, AF, 273, *281*
Foda, HD, 37, *52*
Foglia, RP, 105, *113*
Folkesson, HG, 24, 25, *45*
Follette, D, 279, *284*
Fong, T, 31, *48*
Fonkalsrud, EW, 24, *44*, 90, 92, 99, 105, *108*, *113*, 244, 259, *263*, *267*, 276, 279, *284*
Fontana, R, 189, *206*, 257, *267*
Foran, SK, 23, *43*
Forbes, DA, 257, *267*
Ford, GA, 104, *112*, 192, 193, 194, *206*
Forge, P, 90, *108*
Forget, PP, 105, *112*, 189, *206*, 247, *263*
Forichon, J, 20, 24, *41*, 170, 171, 172, 173, *178*, 196, 198, *207*
Fornes, MF, 56, *67*
Forsgren, S, 37, *52*
Foster, AC, 275, *283*
Foster, LJ, 165, 167, *177*
Foster, PS, 23, *43*
Fowler, AA, 24, *44*
Fox, AJ, 28, *47*
Fox, WW, 274, *282*
Franco, P, 274, 275, *282*
Franconi, G, 38, *53*
Franssila, S, 289, *301*
Fraser, R, 270, *279*
Frazer, A, 247, *263*
Freeman, JK, 270, *280*
Freeman, SR, 170, 172, *177*, 192, 193, 194, *206*
Freije, JE, 70, 78, *86*
French, CL, 20, *41*, 89, 90, 91, 92, 93, 94, 95, 96, 97, 98, 99, 100, 101, 102, 103, *106*, *107*, *108*, 170, 171, 172, *178*, 180, *203*
Freston, JW, 99, *111*, 182, *204*
Friedland, GW, 129, 130, *138*
Frieling, T, 38, *53*

Frisken, K, 286, *300*
Frossard, N, 30, *47*
Fryer, AD, 22, 39, *42*, 53, *54*
Fuchs, KH, 99, *111*
Fuentes, P, 105, *113*, 125, 126, *137*
Fuji, K, 28, 29, *46*
Fujimori, K, 90, 93, *108*
Fujimura, M, 33, *49*, 90, *107*
Fukuchi, Y, 24, *45*
Fukumura, D, 33, *50*
Fuller, RW, 30, *48*, 103, *112*
Fulp, SR, 308, *320*
Fumagalli, J, 187, *205*
Furkert, J, 23, 31, *42*

G

Gabb, M, 308, *320*
Gacek, RR, 306, *319*
Gadmundsson, K, 239, *261*
Gall, DG, 257, *267*, 275, *283*
Gallant, SP, 93, *108*, 155, *175*
Galleano, E, 285, *300*
Galleguillos, F, 20, 24, *41*, 56, *67*, 125, 126, *137*, 170, 171, 172, *178*, 186, 188, 196, 197, *205*, 260, *267*, 279, *284*
Galmiche, JP, 187, *205*
Gambone, LM, 39, *54*
Garabedian, EN, 77, *87*
Garay, J, 105, *113*
Gardiner, DG, 38, *53*
Garland, A, 28, *46*
Gastal, OL, 156, *175*
Gaston, B, 37, 39, *51*
Gaudric, M, 167, *177*, 183, *204*
Geisinger, KR, 93, *109*
Gelder, C, 31, *48*
Gelfand, DW, 59, *67*, 81, *88*
Gentles, MG, 258, *267*
Geppetti, P, 28, 31, *46*
Gergen, PJ, 246, *263*
Gerhardt, DC, 73, *87*
Germain, N, 33, *49*
German, VG, 97, *110*

Germonpre, PR, 23, 30, *42*, *47*
Gervaise, E, 270, *279*
Geubelle, F, 90, *108*
Ghaed, N, 155, *175*
Ghanekar, SV, 22, 28, 31, 39, *43*
Ghavanian, N, 20, 21, *41*
Ghillebert, G, 98, 99, 101, *110*, *111*
Giachetti, A, 26, *45*
Gibbins, IL, 35, 37, 38, *50*, *52*, *53*
Gibbs, CP, 24, *44*
Gibson, B, 306, *319*
Gibson, GG, 214, *234*
Gibson, WS, 75, *87*, 241, *262*
Gideon, RM, 90, *107*
Gilmour, AG, 285, *300*
Girault, F, 275, *283*
Giudicelli, R, 105, *113*, 125, 126, *137*
Glab, N, 95, *109*, 140, 142, 148, 157, *173*, 273, *281*
Glanz, H, 70, 71, 78, *86*
Gleeson, K, 307, 309, *319*
Gleich, GJ, 21, *43*
Glicklich, M, 244, *263*
Glock, MS, 70, 80, *86*
Godard, P, 20, 21, *42*
Gold, WM, 37, 38, *51*
Goldberg, AB, 21, *43*
Goldberg, H, 79, *88*
Goldie, RG, 22, 33, *43*
Goldman, AL, 165, 167, *177*
Goldman, G, 24, *44*, *45*
Goldman, JM, 180, *203*, 260, *267*
Goldstein, BD, 32, *48*
Goldsworthy, W, 270, *279*
Gomes, H, 253, *266*
Gonzalez-Fernandez, F, 251, 258, *265*, *267*
Good, JT, 24, *44*
Goodall, RJ, 24, *44*, 186, 188, *205*
Goodwin, C, 276, *284*
Gooszen, HG, 224, 228, 230, *235*
Gormand, F, 20, 24, *41*, 119, *137*, 170, 171, 172, 173, *178*, 196, 198, *207*
Gourley, GR, 259, *267*
Gower, VC, 240, *262*
Gozetti, G, 254, *266*

Grad, R, 240, *262*
Graf, PD, 38, *53*
Grand, RJ, 256, *266*, 275, *283*
Grant, AK, 214, *234*
Grant, JA, 24, *44*
Graves, J, 38, *53*
Gray, WR, 97, *110*, 307, 309, *319*
Greenfield, SM, 298, *302*, 312, *321*
Greenlee, G, 196, 197, 199, 200, *207*
Greenlee, H, 20, 24, *40*, *44*, 125, 126, 128, 129, *137*, 163, 168, 170, *176*, 180, 196, 198, *203*, *207*
Gremillion, DE, 142, 148, 157, 158, *173*
Grette, K, 98, 99, *111*
Greyson, ND, 155, *175*
Grob, JC, 93, 97, 98, *109*, 125, 126, *137*, 142, 148, 157, 158, *173*, 180, *203*
Gross, NJ, 33, 34, *49*
Grundfast, K, 240, 241, *261*, 275, *283*
Grunstein, MM, 119, 129, 130, *136*, *138*, 143, 144, 148, 157, *173*, 248, 249, *265*, 273, *281*, 314, *321*
Gudmundsson, K, 291, 292, *301*
Guenel, P, 78, *88*
Guerre, J, 167, *177*, 183, *204*
Guiffre, RM, 275, *283*
Guivarch, M, 224, 228, 230, *235*, 260, *267*
Gunasekaren, TS, 256, 258, *267*
Gunther, T, 69, *87*
Gupta, RR, 103, *112*, 183, *204*
Gustafsson, PM, 129, 130, *138*, 247, 256, 258, *263*, *267*
Gutierrez, M, 317, *322*
Guzzo, MR, 20, *41*, 56, 60, *67*, 104, *112*, 146, 147, 148, 150, 157, 158, 162, 169, 170, 172, *174*, *178*, 250, 256, 257, *265*

H

Haber, M, 189, 192, *206*
Haberberger, R, 37, *52*

Hagen, JA, 196, 199, *207*, 211, 212, 222, 226, 228, 230, *234*, *235*, *236*
Haile, JM, 145, 146, 148, 157, 158, *174*
Hall, AE, 31, *48*
Hall, AW, 291, *301*
Hall, WJ, 90, 103, *107*
Halpern, L, 274, *283*
Halstead, LA, 318, *322*
Ham, H, 260, *267*
Hamamoto, J, 28, 29, *46*
Hamdy, S, 310, *321*
Hameister, HH, 95, *109*, 140, 142, 148, 157, *173*, 273, *281* Hamid, Q, 20, 21, *42*, *43*
Hamilton, JW, 103, *112*, 183, *204*, 308, 309, *320*
Hamman, RF, 24, *44*
Hammer, B, 96, *110*
Hamosh, M, 270, *279*
Hanaway, PJ, 243, *263*
Hand, CRK, 156, 157, 158, *175*
Handy, D, 275, *284*
Hansel, TT, 24, *44*
Hanson, DG, 70, 71, 72, 78, 81, 83, *86*, *87*, 88, 104, *112*, 240, *261*
Harder, RV, 90, 103, *107*
Harding, SM, 19, 20, 24, *40*, *41*, 56, 60, 63, *67*, *68*, 104, *112*, 145, 146, 147, 148, 150, 157, 158, 162, 169, 170, 172, *174*, *178*, *179*, 192, 194, 197, *203*, *206*, 250, 256, 257, *265*, 313, *321*
Hardy, KA, 246, *263*
Harmon, JW, 94, *109*
Harned, HS, 241, *262*
Harper, PC, 186, 188, *205*
Harrington, JW, 70, 78, *85*, 241, 242, 243, *262*
Hartley, L, 306, *319*
Haslam, R, 270, *279*
Hassall, CJS, 37, *52*
Hassall, EG, 256, 258, *267*, 275, *284*
Hathaway, T, 26, *45*
Hatlebakk, JG, 192, *206*
Hautmann, G, 30, *47*
Havu, N, 192, *206*

Hawroth, SG, 37, *51*
Hay, DWP, 22, 30, 31, 33, *43*, *48*, *49*
Hayashi, S, 31, *48*
Hazinski, TA, 244, *263*
Heading, RC, 96, *110*
Hebbeln, H, 187, *205*
Heberden, W, 116, *136*
Hebert, CA, 24, 25, *45*
Hecht, C, 306, *319*
Hechtman, HB, 24, *44*, *45*
Hegele, R, 31, *48*
Heimbucher, J, 224, 230, *235*, 258, *267*
Heine, R, 274, *282*
Heinrich, C, 96, *110*, 167, *177*, 183, *204*, 247, *263*
Heldt, GP, 240, 244, 245, 246, *262*, 275, *283*
Helm, JF, 73, 79, *87*, 291, *301*
Henry, RL, 241, *262*, 275, *283*
Hentschel, E, 187, *205*
Herbison, GP, 21, *43*
Herbst, JJ, 60, *68*, 237, 239, 255, *260*, *261*, 273, 274, 276, *281*, *284*
Hernandez, C, 28, *46*
Herve, P, 20, 33, *41*, 95, *109*, 150, 151, 158, *174*
Hervonen, A, 37, *51*
Herz, R, 255, *266*
Hetzel, D, 61, *68*
Hetzel, DJ, 104, *112*, 214, *234*
Hetzel, DP, 292, *301*
Heudebert, GR, 83, *88*
Hevre, P, 248, *265*
Hewitt, CJ, 21, *43*
Hewson, EG, 56, *67*
Hey, JA, 31, *48*
Heym, C, 26, 38, *45*
Higenbottom, T, 26, *45*
Hill, LD, 225, *235*, *236*
Hillman, AL, 83, *88*, 182, *204*
Hilman, BC, 237, 255, *260*
Himpens, J, 260, *267*
Hind, CRK, 216, *235*, 316, *322*
Hinder, RA, 223, 229, *235*
Hine, MK, 294, *301*
Hintz, J, 308, 309, *320*

Hirata, N, 28, 29, *46*
Hirayama, Y, 23, 31, *42*
Hirsch, B, 272, *281*
Hirsch, W, 254, *266*
Hirschowitz, BI, 81, *88*, 189, 192, *206*
Hislop, AA, 37, *51*
Hiss, J, 77, *87*
Hobson, CE, 26, *45*
Hodgson, TA, 246, *263*
Hoeffel, JC, 260, *267*
Hoeft, SF, 222, 226, *235*
Hoffer, DK, 243, *263*
Hoffman, B, 37, 38, *51*
Hoffman, CL, 240, *261*
Hoffman, PJ, 20, *41*, 92, 93, 94, 95, 96, 97, 99, 102, 103, *108*
Hoffman, R, 308, 309, *320*
Hoffpauir, J, 37, *52*
Hoffstein, V, 90, 103, *106*
Hofman, CL, 100, 102, *111*
Hofmann, CL, 304, *319*
Hogan, NJ, 240, *261*
Hogan, SP, 23, *43*
Hogan, WJ, 100, 102, *111*, 156, *175*, 244, *263*, 270, *280*, 291, *301*, 304, 308, 309, 315, *319*, *320*, *322*
Hokanson, JA, 306, *319*
Hokfelt, T, 26, 30, 37, 39, *45*, *51*
Holbrook, WP, 239, *261*, 291, 292, *301*
Holdaway, MD, 21, *43*
Holder, TM, 276, *284*
Holgate, ST, 20, 21, 22, 31, *41*, *42*, *48*
Holinger, LD, 90, 103, *107*, 243, *262*
Hollender, L, 93, 97, 98, *109*, 142, 148, 157, 158, *173*, 180, *203*
Hollis, JB, 309, *320*
Holloway, RH, 163, *176*, 183, *204*, 308, *320*
Hollwarth, ME, 255, *266*
Holmes, PW, 161, 162, 169, *176*
Holt, S, 81, *88*, 189, 192, *206*
Holtzman, MA, 33, *49*
Holzer, P, 20, 25, 26, *41*
Hongo, M, 183, *204*
Hood, CI, 24, *44*, 216, 228, *235*
Horback, JMLM, 224, 228, 230, *235*

Horowitz, RI, 122, *137*
Horton, PF, 61, *68*
Hosie, KB, 214, *234*
Hotz, P, 289, *301*
Howarth, PH, 20, 21, 31, *41*, *48*
Howden, CW, 182, *204*
Howden, GF, 285, *300*
Hoyoux, C, 90, *108*
Hrabovsky, EE, 272, *281*
Hsu, SO, 275, *283*
Hubbard, W, 33, *49*
Huber, HL, 20, *41*
Huber, RM, 167, *177*, 183, *204*, 247, *263*
Hubert, D, 167, *177*, 183, *204*
Hughes, D, 310, *321*
Hughes, DM, 95, 105, *110*, 119, *136*
Hughes, DMN, 247, 249, *263*
Humbert, M, 24, *44*
Hunter, J, 259, *267*
Hureau, J, 163, *176*
Hurwitz, A, 310, 312, *320*
Huttemann, W, 187, *205*
Huxley, EJ, 97, *110*, 307, 309, *319*
Hyams, JS, 255, *266*, 272, *281*
Hyman, PE, 270, *279*, *280*
Hyvarinen, H, 286, 290, *300*

I

Iascone, C, 105, *113*, 125, 126, *137*, 170, 171, *178*, 197, *207*, 217, 232, *235*
Ichinose, M, 23, 31, 38, *42*, *52*, *53*
Idrissi, MSS, 224, 228, 230, *235*
Ikeda, H, 33, *49*
Imaeda, H, 33, *50*
Ing, AJ, 90, 92, 93, 94, 95, 96, 97, 98, 99, *107*, *108*, *109*, 243, *263*
Ingelfinger, FJ, 69, *87*
Inocencion, G, 185, *205*, 314, *321*
Inoue, H, 38, *52*, *53*
International Asthma Project, 19, *40*
Ireland, AP, 211, 212, 224, 228, 230, *234*, *235*, 258, *267*

Irvin, CG, 37, 38, *51*
Irwin, RI, 90, 99, 103, *107*
Irwin, RS, 20, *41*, 56, *67*, 89, 90, 91, 92, 93, 94, 95, 96, 97, 98, 99, 100, 101, 102, 103, *106*, *107*, *108*, *110*, 155, 170, 171, 172, *175*, *178*, 180, *203*, 243, 262, 304, 310, *318*, *320*
Ismail-Beigi, F, 61, *68*
Isolauri, E, 229, *236*
Isolauri, J, 229, *236*
Israel, D, 275, *284*
Israel, E, 180, *204*
Israel, RH, 90, 103, *107*
Iwagoe, H, 28, 29, *46*

J

Jack, CIA, 156, 157, 158, *175*, 215, 216, *234*, *235*, 316, *322*
Jackson, C, 69, *87*
Jackson, M, 28, *46*
Jacob, P, 308, *320*
Jacobs, F, 33, *48*
Jacobson, KW, 165, 166, *177*, 247, *263*, 274, *282*
Jacoby, DB, 22, 39, *42*, *54*
Jain, NK, 163, *176*
Jammes, Y, 38, *52*
Jancso, N, 26, 38, *45*
Jancso-Gabor, A, 26, 38, *45*
Janowitz, WR, 90, 93, *107*, 155, 156, *175*
Jansen, HM, 104, *112*, 192, 194, *206*, 257, *267*
Jansen, JB, 192, *206*
Jansen, JBMJ, 83, *88*
Janson, C, 285, *300*
Janssens, J, 98, 99, 101, *110*, *111*
Jarvinen, V, 286, 290, 295, *300*, *301*
Jarvis, D, 31, *48*
Jeffery, PK, 24, *44*
Jenkins, GN, 298, *302*
Jenkins, WG, 288, 290, 292, *301*
Jian, R, 20, 33, *41*, 95, *109*, 150, 151, 158, *174*, 248, *265*

Jiminez-Isabel, MA, 239, *261*
Jindal, JR, 70, *86*
Joelsson, B, 131, *138*, 165, 167, *177*
Johannesson, N, 131, *138*, 165, 167, *177*
Johns, DN, 309, *320*
Johnson, D, 274, *283*
Johnson, DA, 93, *109*
Johnson, DG, 252, 258, 259, *266*, *267*, 276, *284*
Johnson, L, 270, *280*
Johnson, LF, 62, *68*, 94, 96, 103, *109*, *110*, *112*, 155, 156, 162, *175*, *176*, 183, *204*, 217, *235*, 291, *301*
Johnson, WE, 196, 199, *207*, 232, *236*
Johnston, BT, 90, *107*
Jolley, SG, 274, 276, *283*, *284*
Jones, B, 140, 141, *173*, 242, 262, 304, *318*
Jones, ME, 306, *319*
Joos, GF, 23, 30, *42*, *47*
Joseph, GJ, 291, *301*
Jouin, H, 93, 97, 98, *109*, 125, 126, *137*
Jovin, H, 142, 148, 157, 158, *173*, 180, *203*
Juodis, E, 275, *283*
Just, R, 192, *206*

K

Kadakia, SC, 183, *204*
Kadden, M, 24, *44*, 165, *177*, 183, *204*, 247, *263*, 274, *281*
Kahn, A, 274, 275, *282*
Kahrilas, PJ, 65, *68*, 71, 72, 81, 83, *87*, *88*, 103, 104, *112*, 161, *176*, 183, *204*, 237, 238, 240, 242, 243, 250, *260*, *261*, 285, *300*, 308, *320*
Kalia, M, 34, *50*
Kaliner, MA, 33, *49*, 161, *176*
Kallay, MC, 90, 103, *107*
Kallenback, JC, 162, *176*
Kamada, SK, 180, *203*
Kambie, V, 239, *261*
Kamboj, L, 185, *205*, 314, *321*

Kamel, P, 104, *112*
Kamel, PL, 71, 72, 81, 83, *87*, *88*, 240, *261*
Kangas, M, 298, *301*
Kanno, T, 39, *53*
Karakousis, PC, 30, 35, 38, *47*
Karl, S, 279, *284*
Karlsson, JA, 92, *108*, 140, 160, *173*
Karvonen, A, 229, *236*
Kashima, H, 310, *320*
Katayama, H, 24, *45*
Katsumata, U, 38, *53*
Katz, AJ, 273, *281*
Katz, PO, 62, 63, 65, *68*, 83, *88*, 99, *111*, 216, *235*
Katz, RM, 24, *44*, 90, 92, 99, *108*, 165, *177*, 244, 247, *263*, 274, *281*, *282*
Katzka, DA, 192, *206*, 256, *267*
Kauer, WKH, 196, 199, *207*, 211, 212, 224, 230, *234*, *235*, *236*, 258, *267*
Kaufman, JA, 56, *67*
Kaul, B, 98, 99, *111*
Kavuru, MS, 180, 181, *203*
Kawahara, H, 270, *280*
Kawano, O, 28, 29, *46*
Kay, AB, 20, 21, 23, 24, *42*, *43*, *44*
Kaye, GM, 310, *321*
Kaye, MD, 186, 188, *205*
Kays, JS, 22, 28, 31, 39, *43*
Kedan, R, 254, *266*
Keen, MS, 306, 308, 310, *319*
Keens, T, 275, *283*
Keir, R, 33, *49*
Keith, IM, 37, *51*
Kempster, GB, 308, 309, *320*
Kennedy, JH, 117, *136*
Kern, M, 308, 309, *320*
Kerr, GD, 125, 126, *137*, 186, 188, *205*
Kerr, P, 162, *176*
Keyrilainen, O, 229, *236*
Khan, A, 93, *109*
Khandelwal, S, 24, *44*, 56, 60, 63, *67*, *68*, 125, 126, 128, 129, 131, 134, *137*, *138*, 150, 160, 163, 168, 169, 170, *174*, *175*, *176*, 180, 196, 197, 199, 200, *203*, *207*, 211, 214, 217, *234*, *235*, 247, *263*
Kianmanesh, R, 224, 228, 230, *235*, 260, *267*
Kikendall, JW, 183, *204*
Kimmitt, P, 24, *44*
Kimura, K, 38, *53*
Kingsnorth, AN, 214, *234*
Kinsbourne, M, 251, *265*
Kirk, CL, 270, *279*
Kirubakaran, C, 270, *280*
Kita, H, 21, *43*
Kitchin, LI, 182, *204*
Kjellen, G, 143, 148, 157, *173*, 184, *205*
Kjellman, NIM, 129, 130, *138*, 247, *263*
Kjellman, WIM, 256, 258, *267*
Klauser, A, 272, *281*
Klauser, AG, 99, *111*
Klein, M, 244, *263*
Kleinsasser, O, 70, 71, 78, *86*
Klemetti, E, 239, *261*, 286, 289, 291, *300*
Klinkenberg-Knol, EC, 81, 83, *88*, 192, *206*
Knoblich, R, 244, *263*
Knuff, TE, 83, *88*
Kobara, M, 308, *320*
Kobzik, L, 24, 30, 37, *44*, *45*, *51*
Koch, A, 276, *284*
Koch, KL, 98, 101, *110*
Kocoshis, SA, 241, *262*, 275, *283*
Koessler, KK, 20, *41*
Kofman, J, 123, 124, *137*
Kohrogi, H, 28, 29, *46*
Kohut, RI, 70, 73, 78, *86*
Kokonos, M, 95, *109*, 152, 153, 154, 155, 158, 160, *175*
Kolut, RI, 242, *262*
Konig, A, 96, *110*
Koren, G, 185, *205*, 314, *321*
Korpas, J, 92, *108*
Koufman, JA, 62, *68*, 69, 70, 71, 72, 73, 74, 75, 76, 77, 78, 79, 80, 81, 82, 83, 84, *85*, *86*, *87*, *88*, 98, 99,

Author Index

111, 156, *175*, 239, 242, 243, 245, 261, 262, 316, *322*
Kozarek, RA, 225, *236*
Kraemer, SJM, 225, *236*
Krause, JE, 32, *48*
Kravitz, E, 251, 252, 256, 257, *265*
Krekel, J, 37, *52*
Kreutner, W, 23, *43*
Kristleifsson, G, 239, *261*, 291, 292, *301*
Kron, IL, 26, *45*
Kronborg, IJ, 152, *174*, 192, 194, 196, *206*
Kroon, L, 289, *301*
Krugler, C, 308, *320*
Kryger, MH, 162, *176*
Kuck, EJ, 24, *44*
Kuhns, L, 257, *267*
Kuittnen, T, 298, *301*
Kummer, W, 26, 28, 30, 31, 33, 34, 35, 37, 38, 39, *45*, *47*, *49*, *52*, *53*
Kunkel, G, 23, 31, *42*
Kuo, B, 66, *68*, 152, *174*
Kurkowski, R, 26, 38, *45*
Kurose, I, 33, *50*
Kurucar, C, 123, 124, 129, *137*
Kurup, VP, 21, *43*
Kusano, M, 309, *320*

L

L'Estrange, PL, 287, *300*
Labarre, JF, 90, *107*
Lacey, SR, 258, *267*
Lacoste, JY, 20, 21, *41*
Lacronique, J, 30, *47*
Lagente, V, 33, *49*
Lahdenuso, A, 90, *107*
Laitinen, LA, 37, *51*
Laitman, JT, 271, *280*, 315, *321*
Lama, A, 38, *52*
Lambert, J, 256, *266*
Lambiase, A, 33, *49*
Lambrechts, L, 90, *108*
Lamers, CB, 192, *206*, 224, 228, 230, *235*
Lami, CA, 189, *206*, 257, *267*
Lander, M, 272, 273, *280*, *281*
Lang, IM, 308, 309, 310, *320*
Lange, RC, 163, *176*
Langley, JN, 35, *50*
Langman, J, 163, *176*
Langou, RA, 122, *137*
Langtry, HD, 81, *88*
Lanza, F, 189, 192, *206*
Lapicque, JC, 105, *113*, 125, 126, *137*
LaPointe, LL, 306, *319*
Larrain, A, 20, 24, *41*, 56, 60, *67*, 125, 126, *137*, 170, 171, 172, *178*, 186, 188, 196, 197, *205*, 260, *267*, 279, *284*
Larsen, GL, 38, *53*, 119, 129, 130, *136*, *138*, 143, 144, 148, 157, *173*, 248, 249, *265*, 273, *281*
Larson, JD, 314, *321*
Larsson, O, 37, *51*
Laughlin, GM, 245, *263*
Laukka, MA, 90, *108*
Laurence, BH, 214, *234*
Law, SKY, 230, *236*
Lawrence, LF, 90, 93, *107*
Lazarchik, DA, 98, *111*, 286, 288, 291, 292, *300*, *301*
Lazarus, S, 38, *53*
Lazarus, SC, 180, *204*
Leandro, G, 105, *113*, 185, *205*
Lebenthal, E, 270, *279*
Lecocguic, Y, 247, *265*
Ledbetter, MS, 242, *262*
Leduc, T, 168, *177*, 183, *205*
Lee, A, 187, *205*
Lee, JC, 273, 274, *281*
Lee, P, 33, *49*, 270, *279*
Lefevre, PM, 26, *46*
Leff, AR, 314, *321*
Leite, L, 256, *267*
Lemanske, RF, 180, *204*
Lemen, RJ, 244, *263*

Lemper, JC, 260, *267*
Leport, J, 224, 228, 230, *235*, 260, *267*
Lerner, E, 244, *263*
Lester, LA, 275, *283*
Levi-Schafer, F, 21, *43*
Levin, B, 308, 310, *319*
Levison, H, 95, 105, *110*, 119, *136*, 247, 249, *263*, 275, *283*
Levy, BM, 294, *301*
Levy, GP, 37, *51*
Lew, C, 275, *283*
Lewis, J, 279, *284*
Lewis, T, 20, 25, 26, 31, *41*
Li, BUK, 259, *267*
Li, Q, 100, 102, *111*, 240, *261*, 304, *319*
Lichtenstein, LM, 20, 21, 22, 23, *42*
Liew, VP, 286, *300*
Lilly, CM, 31, *48*
Lindahl, H, 276, *284*
Lindgren, BR, 170, 171, 172, *178*, 186, 187, 188, *205*
Lindsey, JR, 26, *46*
Liron, R, 214, *234*
Little, AG, 161, *175*
Little, FB, 70, 73, 78, *86*, 242, *262*
Little, JP, 70, 80, *86*
Litwin, D, 180, 181, *203*
Liu, J, 308, 309, *320*
Liu, YC, 155, *175*
Llyod, DA, 162, *176*
Lo Cascio, V, 94, 95, *109*
Loader, JE, 38, *53*
Locke, GR, 56, *67*, 180, 197, *203*, 304, *319*
Lockhart, A, 167, *177*, 183, *204*
Lodi, U, 147, 148, 150, 162, 169, *174*
Lof, GL, 308, 309, *320*
Loftor, DW, 257, *267*
Logemann, JA, 308, *320*
Lomansey, TL, 105, *113*
Lombard-Platet, R, 20, 24, *41*, 170, 171, 172, 173, *178*, 196, 198, *207*
Lomena, F, 272, 274, *280*
Londong, W, 272, *281*

Lopez, AF, 19, 23, *40*
Lorenzetti, BB, 33, *49*
Lotti, T, 30, *47*
Loughlin, CJ, 70, 76, 77, 81, *86*, *87*, 316, *322*
Loughlin, GM, 90, *107*, 243, 274, *263*, *282*
Louhimo, I, 276, *284*
Low, DE, 225, *235*
Lowenstein, CJ, 37, 39, *51*
Lowry, R, 26, *45*
Luce, D, 78, *88*
Luckers, A, 192, *206*
Luckmann, K, 252, *266*
Ludviksdottir, D, 285, *300*
Lundberg, JM, 26, 28, 30, 31, 34, 37, 38, 39, *45*, *46*, *50*, *51*, *52*
Luostarinen, M, 229, *236*, 259, *267*
Lussi, A, 289, *301*
Lutz, J, 270, *280*
Lyrenas, E, 274, *282*

M

MacGlashan, DW, 24, *44*
Machida, HM, 257, *267*
MacIagan, J, 39, *53*
Mackinnon, M, 104, *112*
Mackinnon, WD, 214, *234*
Macklem, PT, 37, 38, *51*, 165, 169, *177*, 247, *263*
Macklin, CC, 25, *45*
Maclagan, J, 28, 31, 39, *47*
Madgy, DM, 240, *262*
Magee, LA, 185, *205*, 314, *321*
Maggi, CA, 25, 26, *45*
Maggi, JC, 93, *108*, 155, *175*
Magrini, L, 33, *49*
Maher, J, 274, *282*
Maimonides, M, 116, *136*
Maisels, M, 275, 279, *283*, *284*
Malagelada, JR, 99, *111*
Maldonado, J, 95, *109*
Malfroot, A, 105, *113*, 275, *283*

Malmagyi, DFJ, 152, *174*
Malmgren, LT, 306, 310, *319*, 320
Mandel, ID, 292, *301*
Mangano, M, 315, *322*
Mannerberg, F, 292, *301*
Manni, L, 33, *49*
Mansfield, LE, 20, *40*, *41*, 92, 93, 95, *108*, *109*, 140, 142, 148, 157, 158, 165, 166, 167, *173*, *177*, 248, *265*, 273, 274, *281*, *282*
Mansfield, TE, 247, *263*
Mansson, I, 155, *175*, 316, *322*
Maples, RV, 147, 148, 158, *174*
Marano, MA, 246, *263*
Marcinkiewicz, M, 298, *302*
Marco, V, 95, *109*, 180, 197, *203*
Margulies, SI, 69, 70, 71, *86*, 117, *136*
Marinkovich, VA, 129, 130, *138*
Marino, W, 274, *282*
Markewitz, BA, 22, 33, *43*
Marks, R, 83, *88*
Marmon, L, 275, *283*
Marques, L, 257, *267*
Marsac, J, 167, *177*, 183, *204*
Marshall, RB, 242, *262*
Martin, JH, 306, 308, 310, *319*
Martin, ME, 129, 130, *138*
Martin, RJ, 144, 158, *174*, 180, *203*, 248, *265*
Martin, RR, 37, 38, *51*
Martin, TR, 21, *43*
Martinez de Haro, LF, 214, *234*
Martling, CR, 26, 28, 30, 31, 37, 39, *45*, *46*, *51*
Masclee, AAM, 224, 228, 230, *235*
Massarella, GR, 20, *41*
Mathay, MA, 24, 25, *45*
Mathews, JK, 38, *53*
Mathis, R, 93, *108*, 155, *175*
Matlak, ME, 276, *284*
Maton, PN, 189, *206*
Matran, R, 35, 37, *51*
Matsuda, T, 33, *49*, 90, *107*
Matsumoto, S, 39, *53*
Matsuse, T, 24, 33, *45*, *49*

Matsushima, K, 33, *49*
Matthaei, KI, 23, *43*
Matthews, BL, 70, 80, *86*
Mattoli, S, 254, *266*
Mattox, HE, 96, 99, *110*
Matute-Cardenas, JA, 239, *261*
Mauser, PJ, 23, *43*
Maxwell, SL, 307, 309, *319*
Maydonovitch, C, 183, *204*
Mayer, B, 37, 38, *51*, *53*
Mays, EE, 125, 128, *138*, 161, 163, *176*, 180, 197, *203*
McCallum, RW, 99, *111*, 163, *176*, 183, *204*, 292, 298, *301*, *302*
McCarson, KE, 32, *48*
McCarthy, JH, 214, *234*
McCloy, RF, 99, *111*
McCombs, A, 276, *284*
McConnell, F, 310, *320*
McCourtie, DR, 162, *176*
McDonald, DM, 22, 26, 28, 31, 39, *42*, *45*, *46*, *47*
McDonnell, JT, 165, 166, *177*, 247, *263*, 274, *282*
McGeady, SJ, 250, 251, 252, 256, 257, *265*
McGregor, GP, 33, *49*
McKay, K, 31, *48*
McLeod, RL, 31, *48*
McMahan, J, 104, *112*
McNally, EF, 103, *112*
McNally, PR, 170, 172, *177*, 192, 193, 194, *206*
McTavish, D, 189, 192, *206*
Mehlhop, PD, 21, *43*
Meier, JH, 170, 172, *177*, 192, 193, 194, *206*
Mela, GS, 185, *205*
Meli, A, 25, 26, *45*
Mellis, CM, 241, *262*, 275, *283*
Mello, CJ, 90, 92, 96, 97, 98, 99, 101, 103, *106*, *110*, 243, *262*
Mellow, MH, 103, *112*
Melton, LJ, 56, *67*, 180, 197, *203*
Meltzer, SJ, 69, *87*

Menanteau, B, 253, *266*
Menchausky, B, 180, *203*
Meng, Q, 24, *44*
Menon, AP, 274, *282*
Menz, G, 24, *44*
Meraud, P, 90, *108*
Mertz, H, 270, *280*
Mesulam, MM, 34, *50*
Methlin, G, 14, 93, 97, 98, *109*, 148, 157, 158, *173*, 180, *203*
Metwally, N, 309, *320*
Meunier, L, 38, *53*
Meurman, JH, 286, 289, 290, 291, 295, 298, *300*, *301*
Meuwissen, SG, 81, *88*, 192, *206*
Meyer, C, 93, 97, 98, *109*, 125, 126, *137*, 142, 148, 157, 158, *173*, 180, *203*
Meyer, E, 270, *280*
Meyers, WF, 252, *266*
Michael, JR, 22, 33, *43*
Michel, FB, 20, 21, *42*
Michel, ME, 183, *204*
Michoud, MC, 168, *177*, 183, *205*
Mickey, MR, 165, *177*, 247, *263*, 274, *281*
Mickflikier, AB, 162, *176*
Miki, K, 270, *279*
Milbrath, MM, 70, *86*, 100, 102, *111*, 240, *261*, 304, *319*
Miles, JF, 179, 197, *203*
Millar, NSC, 162, *176*
Millar, T, 162, *176*
Miller, FA, 69, *87*
Miller, SA, 20, *41*, 143, 145, 148, 157, 158, *173*
Miller, SJ, 123, 124, 129, *137*
Miller, T, 24, *44*, 56, *67*, 122, 123, 124, 125, 126, 128, 129, 131, 134, *137*, *138*, 160, 163, 168, 169, 170, *175*, *176*, 180, 196, 197, 199, 200, *203*, *207*, 211, 214, *234*, 247, *263*
Mills, SE, 26, *45*
Milner, AD, 274, *282*
Minella, R, 270, 275, *280*, *283*

Miner, PB, 314, *321*
Minton, J, 306, *319*
Minton, SD, 60, *68*, 273, 274, *281*
Miralbes, M, 180, 197, *203*
Mitchell, B, 214, *234*
Mitchell, I, 275, *283*
Mittal, R, 161, 162, 163, 164, 169, *175*, *176*, 247, *263*
Miura, M, 23, 31, 38, *42*, *52*, *53*
Miura, S, 33, *50*
Mizuguchi, M, 33, *49*, 90, *107*
Mobassaleh, M, 256, *266*
Modell, JH, 24, *44*
Moffatt, JD, 34, 35, *50*
Mogi, G, 318, *322*
Mohr, JP, 308, 310, *319*
Molimard, M, 30, 31, *47*
Molina, J, 214, *234*
Moore, DJ, 253, *266*
Moote, DW, 162, *176*
Morabito, A, 285, *300*
Morales, G, 214, *234*
Morgan, TM, 96, *110*
Morley, J, 33, 34, *49*
Morris, BA, 244, *263*
Morris, JL, 35, *50*
Morrison, MD, 70, 78, *86*
Mortelliti, AJ, 306, *319*
Mosher, HP, 69, *87*
Mosmann, TR, 21, *43*
Mosnier, H, 224, 228, 230, *235*, 260, *267*
Moulin, D, 129, 130, *138*, 240, *261*
Muller-Lissner, SA, 99, *111*, 167, *177*, 183, *204*, 247, *263*, 272, *281*
Mullett, MD, 272, *281*
Muls, V, 260, *267*
Munciano, D, 247, *265*
Murat, BW, 96, 99, *110*
Murphy, DW, 103, *112*
Murphy, SA, 275, *283*
Murtomaa, H, 286, 290, *300*
Myers, AC, 22, 28, 29, 30, 31, 33, 39, *43*, *46*, *47*, *48*, *54*
Myracle, J, 241, *262*
Myrvold, HE, 98, 99, *111*

N

N'Duwlmana, M, 274, 275, *282*
Nadel, JA, 26, 28, 31, 33, 38, 39, *45, 46, 47, 48, 49, 53*, 97, *110*, 248, 265
Nagase, T, 24, *45*
Nagata, H, 33, *50*
Nagayama, T, 39, *53*
Nagel, RA, 125, 126, *137*, 186, 188, 205
Naik, DR, 253, *266*
Nakajima, N, 23, 31, *42*
Naline, E, 30, 31, *47*
Namiot, Z, 292, *301*
Narcy, P, 70, 75, 80, *86*, 239, 240, 241, 253, *261*, 315, *321*
Nardi, R, 99, *111*
Narielvala, RM, 104, *112*, 214, *234*
Nash, M, 93, *109*
National Heart, Lung and Blood Institute, 19, *40*
Naveh, Y, 273, *281*
Neary, P, 223, 229, *235*
Nebel, OT, 56, *67*
Nelis, F, 192, *206*
Nelson, HS, 165, 166, *177*, 247, 252, 255, *263, 266*, 274, *282*, 317, *322*
Nelson, JL, 309, *320*
Nemchausky, B, 20, 24, *40, 44*, 125, 126, 129, 131, 134, *137, 138*, 160, 169, 170, *175*, 196, 198, *207*, 211, 214, *234*, 247, *263*
Nemchausky, T, 196, 197, 199, 200, *207*
Netzer, P, 96, *110*
Neuhauser, EBD, 69, 80, *87*
Neurna, JH, 239, *261*
Newhouse, MT, 90, 95, 99, 103, 104, 105, 106, *107, 110*
Ngu, MC, 90, 92, 93, 94, 95, 96, 97, 98, 99, *107, 109*, 243, *263*
Nieber, K, 23, 31, *42*
Nielson, DW, 240, 244, 245, 246, *262*, 275, *283*
Nihoul-Fekete, C, 260, *267*
Nishi, K, 33, *49*, 90, *107*
Nixon, TE, 95, 105, *110*, 274, *282*
Nogami, H, 38, *52*
Nohr, D, 37, *52*
Nomura, M, 33, *49*
Noordzij, P, 70, 79, *86*
Nouvet, G, 20, *40*
Nouvet, TG, 196, 198, *207*
Novak, LB, 38, *53*
Novembre, E, 189, *206*, 257, *267*
Novey, HS, 119, *137*
Nowak, L, 71, *87*
Nussbaum, E, 93, *108*, 155, *175*
Nutinen, P, 239, *261*
Nuutinen, P, 286, 289, 291, *300*

O

O'Connell, EJ, 317, *322*
O'Connell, F, 103, *112*
O'Connell, S, 20, 24, *40, 44*, 56, 60, 63, *67, 68*, 123, 124, 125, 126, 128, 129, 131, 134, *137, 138*, 150, 160, 163, 168, 169, 170, *174, 175, 176*, 180, 196, 197, 198, 199, 200, *203, 207*, 211, 214, 217, *234, 235*, 247, *263*
O'Donnell, M, 37, 38, *51*
O'Neal, M, 275, *283*
O'Reilly, S, 31, *48*
Oakley, GD, 56, 60, *67*
Obach, S, 33, *49*
Oehme, P, 23, 31, *42*
Oestreich, A, 271, *280*
Oettgen, HC, 21, *43*
Oggero, V, 275, *283*
Ohga, E, 24, *45*
Ohka, T, 33, *49*
Okubo, T, 33, *49*
Oldham, KT, 259, *267*, 279, *284*
Olinksy, A, 274, *282*
Oliver, PS, 104, *112*, 192, 193, 194, *206*

Oliviera, H, 37, *51*
Olivieri, M, 94, 95, *109*
Ollerenshaw, SL, 31, *48*
O'Loughlin, EV, 275, *283*
Olson, NR, 70, 71, 73, 78, *86*
Omari, T, 270, *279*
Once, J, 180, 197, *203*
Ong, TH, 272, 273, *280*, *281*
Ooka, T, 90, *107*
Opdenakker, G, 24, *44*
Orenstein, DM, 238, 241, 257, *260*, *262*, *267*, 272, 275, *280*, *283*
Orenstein, S, 98, 99, *111*, 238, 239, 240, 241, 244, 245, 246, 251, 252, 253, 255, 256, 257, 259, *260*, *261*, *262*, *263*, *266*, *267*, 270, 272, 273, 275, 278, *280*, 281, *283*, *284*
Oritz, A, 214, *234*
Orlando, RC, 96, 98, 99, 103, 105, *110*, 182, *204*
Orr, WC, 99, 103, *111*, *112*
Orringer, MB, 224, 225, 228, 230, *235*, *236*
Osborn, RR, 38, *53*
Osler, WB, 116, *136*, 139, 140, *173*, 246, *263*
Ossakow, DJ, 69, 70, 71, 72, 79, *86*
Ote, JB, 184, *205*
Otis, RD, 152, *174*
Otsuka, M, 26, 30, *45*
Ott, DJ, 59, *67*, 81, *88*, 242, 252, *262*, *266*
Otte, JB, 129, 130, *138*, 240, *261*
Overholt, RH, 119, *136*, 152, *174*

P

Pace, F, 311, 313, *321*
Pack, AI, 95, 105, *109*, *110*, 144, 152, 153, 154, 155, 158, 160, *174*, *175*
Page, C, 19, *40*
Palmer, ED, 65, *68*
Palombini, B, 37, 38, *51*
Palot, JP, 163, *176*

Panagopoulos, V, 308, *320*
Panconesi, E, 30, *47*
Pandey, R, 144, 158, *174*
Panetti, M, 71, *87*
Pantalena, M, 105, *113*, 185, *205*
Paoletti, V, 256, *267*
Pariente, R, 247, *265*
Parker, AF, 276, *284*
Parkes, MW, 38, *53*
Parrilla, P, 214, *234*
Parsons, DS, 318, *322*
Partanen, M, 37, *51*
Pasquis, P, 20, *40*, 196, 198, *207*
Passot, E, 90, *107*
Pastma, GN, 71, *87*
Patacchini, R, 26, *45*
Patatanian, E, 314, *321*
Patel, B, 78, *88*, 183, *204*
Paterson, WG, 96, 99, *110*
Pathial, K, 156, *175*
Patterson, D, 33, *49*
Patterson, JE, 214, *234*
Paulson, DL, 117, *136*
Pauwels, RA, 23, 30, *42*, *47*
Pearlman, DS, 239, *261*
Peat, JK, 21, *43*
Pecau, Y, 275, *283*
Pecova, R, 91, *108*
Pedersen, KE, 22, *42*
Peghini, P, 65, *68*
Pellegrini, CA, 162, *176*, 217, *235*
Pellett, JR, 259, *267*
Pellicer, C, 95, *109*
Pelto-Huikko, M, 37, *51*
Pelttari, A, 289, *301*
Pen, J, 240, *261*
Penagini, R, 163, *176*
Perdikis, G, 223, 229, *235*
Perin, P, 250, *265*
Perks, WH, 125, 126, *137*, 186, 188, *205*
Perlman, LV, 244, *263*
Permutt, S, 38, *53*
Perpina, M, 95, *109*, 180, 197, *203*
Perrault, S, 168, *177*, 183, *205*

Perrin-Fayolle, M, 20, 24, *41*, 119, 123, 124, *137*, 170, 171, 172, 173, *178*, 196, 198, *207*, 246, *263*
Perry, M, 170, 172, *177*, 192, 193, 194, *206*
Persson, CGA, 131, *138*, 165, 167, *177*
Pesendorfer, P, 255, *266*
Peters, JH, 196, 197, 199, *207*, 211, 212, 214, 222, 224, 226, 228, 230, *234*, *235*, 258, *267*
Peters, M, 31, *48*
Petersen, H, 98, 99, *111*
Pfister, R, 24, *44*
Phelan, P, 274, *282*
Philbrick, JT, 122, *137*
Philip, G, 30, *47*
Philippin, B, 33, *49*
Phillips, AM, 89, *107*
Phillips, RW, 89, *107*
Piascik, R, 292, *301*
Piedimonte, G, 28, *46*
Pien, L, 180, 181, *203*
Piepsz, A, 105, *113*
Pierce, AK, 97, *110*, 307, 309, *319*
Pieretti, R, 276, *284*
Pilotto, A, 105, *113*, 185, *205*
Pindborg, JJ, 287, *300*
Piper, DW, 81, *88*
Pitchumoni, C, 274, *282*
Pitman, AM, 23, *43*
Plaschkes, J, 276, *284*
Plaxico, D, 274, *282*
Plebani, M, 105, *113*, 185, *205*
Podvran, B, 308, 309, 310, *320*
Poe, RH, 90, 103, *107*
Pohl, J, 255, *266*
Polak, JM, 31, 37, *48*, *51*, *52*
Pollmann, H, 255, *266*
Polonovski, JM, 240, *261*
Ponce, J, 95, *109*
Ponce-Castro, H, 104, *112*
Pondez, R, 248, *265*
Pontoppidan, H, 307, *319*
Poole, S, 33, *49*
Pope, CE, 20, 24, *41*, 61, *68*, 99, *111*, 125, 126, *137*, 163, 170, 171, 172, *176*, *178*, 182, 186, 188, 196, 197, *204*, *205*, 248, 250, 260, *265*, *267*, 279, *284*, 285, *300*, 312, *321*
Posavac, EJ, 122, *137*
Postma, GN, 84, *88*
Pratter, MR, 56, *67*, 89, 90, 103, *106*, *107*
Preiss, U, 254, *266*
Prescott, CA, 239, *261*
Pride, NB, 103, *112*
Prince, R, 247, *263*, 274, *282*
Prinsen, J, 275, *284*
Prior, JS, 104, *112*, 192, 193, 194, *206*
Proud, D, 33, *49*, 315, *321*
Proujansky, R, 241, *262*, 275, *283*
Proulx, F, 168, *177*, 183, *205*
Puetz, TR, 106, *113*
Pulijoki, H, 90, *107*
Punja, M, 170, 172, *177*, 192, 193, 194, *206*
Putnam, PE, 98, 99, *111*, 240, 252, *261*, *262*, 273, *281*

Q

Quan, SF, 20, 22, 23, *42*

R

Rachelefsky, GS, 24, *44*, 90, 92, 99, *108*, 165, *177*, 183, *204*, 244, 247, *263*, 274, *281*, *282*
Rademaker, AW, 65, *68*
Radsel, Z, 239, *261*
Rajan, A, 260, *267*
Ramirez, B, 98, *111*, 286, 291, 292, *300*, *301*
Ramphal, R, 216, 228, *235*
Ramsay, AJ, 23, *43*
Ransohoff, DF, 122, *137*
Rathsack, R, 23, 31, *42*

Ravich, WJ, 140, 141, *173*, 242, *262*, 304, *318*
Ray, DW, 28, *46*
Rayburn, WF, 314, *321*
Reboud, E, 105, *113*, 125, 126, *137*
Rebuffat, E, 274, 275, *282*
Reed, WD, 61, *68*, 104, *112*, 214, *234*, 286, *300*
Regoli, D, 30, 31, *47*
Rehm, D, 270, *280*
Reichelderfer, M, 103, *112*
Reid, RH, 155, *175*
Reid, S, 123, 124, 129, *137*
Reidenberg, J, 271, *280*
Reinach, SG, 162, *176*
Reisner, C, 317, *322*
Ren, J, 304, 308, 309, *319*, *320*
Resti, M, 189, *206*, 257, *267*
Reulbach, TR, 84, *88*
Revillon, Y, 247, 248, *265*
Reyes, C, 276, *284*
Riccio, MM, 29, 33, *47*, *49*
Richards, J, 244, *263*
Richardson, CA, 38, *52*
Richardson, J, 37, *51*
Richter, JE, 19, 20, 24, *40*, *41*, 56, 59, 60, 62, 63, 66, *67*, *68*, 80, *88*, 96, 98, 99, 100, 101, 104, *110*, *111*, *112*, 145, 146, 147, 148, 156, 157, 158, 170, 172, *174*, *175*, *178*, 179, 185, 192, 194, 197, *203*, *205*, *206*, *207*, 210, *234*, 239, 250, 251, 255, 256, 257, *261*, *265*, *266*, 286, 291, 292, *300*, *301*, 304, 309, 313, 314, 316, *319*, *320*, *321*, *322*
Ricker, DH, 240, 252, *262*, 273, *281*
Ricks, P, 252, *266*
Riedel, DR, 73, 79, *87*
Riedenberg, JS, 315, *321*
Riera, C, 272, 274, *280*
Rintala, R, 276, *284*
Rio-Navarro, BE, 104, *112*
Ritter, MP, 196, 199, *207*, 211, 228, *234*
Rivein, J, 247, 249, *263*
Rivlin, J, 95, 105, *110*, 119, *136*

Robb, ND, 285, *300*
Robbins, J, 308, 309, *320*
Roberts, CC, 252, *266*, 276, *284*
Roberts, MW, 285, *300*
Robinson, DS, 20, 21, 24, *42*, *43*, *44*
Robinson, MG, 99, 103, *111*, *112*, 182, 189, 192, *204*, *206*, 314, *321*
Robinson, P, 152, *174*, 192, 194, 196, *206*
Roca, I, 257, *267*
Roche, WR, 20, 21, *41*
Rochester, DF, 163, *176*
Rodd, A, 37, 38, *51*
Rodrigues-Roisin, R, 272, 274, *280*
Rodriguez-Villarrel, H, 125, 126, 128, *138*
Rodriquez de Quesada, B, 251, *265*
Roessle, R, 270, *280*
Roger, G, 70, 77, 80, *86*, *87*
Rogers, DF, 28, 31, 35, 37, *47*
Rohr, S, 276, *284*
Rohwedder, JJ, 168, *177*, 183, *204*, 274, *282*
Rolla, G, 315, *322*
Ron, J, 100, 102, *111*
Roos, CM, 104, *112*, 192, 194, *206*, 257, *267*
Ros, E, 272, 274, *280*
Rosemeyer, D, 255, *266*
Rosen, SN, 99, *111*
Rosenwasser, L, 21, *43*
Rosetti, F, 185, *205*, 314, *321*
Rosman, AS, 79, *88*
Ross, A, 279, *284*
Ross, JA, 70, 79, *86*
Rothberg, RM, 275, *283*
Rothwell, JC, 310, *321*
Roulet, F, 270, *280*
Rourk, RM, 292, *301*
Roussos, C, 165, 169, *177*
Roussos, E, 247, *263*
Rovero, P, 26, *45*
Rowshan, N, 274, *282*
Rubin, S, 275, *283*
Ruggins, NR, 274, *282*
Ruhl, CE, 310, 312, *320*

Russell, G, 156, 157, 158, *175*, 316, *322*
Ruth, M, 155, *175*, 316, *322*
Ruzkowski, CJ, 168, *177*, 183, *204*, 274, *282*
Ryabova, VS, 307, 309, *319*
Ryan, P, 273, *281*
Rytomaa, I, 286, 289, 290, 295, *300*, *301*

S

Sacco, RL, 308, 310, *319*
Sackner, MA, 98, *107*
Sacre, L, 188, *205*
Sacre-Smits, L, 270, *280*
Sadek, SA, 183, *204*
Sagar, PM, 214, *234*
Said, SI, 37, 38, *51*, *52*
Saito, H, 33, *49*
Sakamoto, T, 28, *46*
Salari, H, 33, *49*
Salem, H, 248, *265*
Salome, CM, 21, *43*
Salter, HH, 25, 31, *45*
Samloff, IM, 310, 312, *320*
Sampson, AP, 21, 22, *42*
Sampson, M, 247, *263*
Sand, C, 274, *282*
Sandberg, N, 155, *175*, 316, *322*
Sanders, AD, 77, *87*, 90, 103, *107*, 243, *262*
Sandler, A, 274, *282*
Sandro Mela, G, 105, *113*
Sangaletti, O, 311, 313, *321*
Sanico, AM, 30, *47*, 315, *321*
Sann, H, 37, *52*
Sanowski, RA, 168, *177*, 183, *204*, 274, *282*
Sant'Ambrogio, G, 92, *108*, 140, 160, *173*
Santamaria, F, 275, *283*
Sarahan, TM, 244, *263*
Saria, A, 26, 28, 30, 31, 33, 34, 39, *45*, *46*, *49*, *50*

Sarna, A, 308, 309, *320*
Sarosiek, J, 292, 298, *301*, *302*
Sasagawa, M, 90, *108*
Sasaki, CT, 315, *321*
Sataloff, RT, 69, 72, 81, 82, 83, *86*
Satch, M, 90, *108*
Sattilaro, AJ, 152, *174*
Saubier, E, 90, *108*
Savarino, V, 105, *113*, 185, *205*
Saye, Z, 105, *112*, 189, *206*
Sbai-Idrassi, MS, 260, *267*
Scappaticci, E, 315, *322*
Schaal, SE, 310, 312, *320*
Schaffner, M, 289, *301*
Schaible, HG, 32, *48*
Schalling, M, 37, *51*
Schan, CA, 20, *41*, 104, *112*, 145, 146, 147, 148, 157, 158, 170, 172, *174*, *178*, 250, 256, 257, *265*
Schefft, GL, 274, *282*
Schei, AJ, 90, *108*
Schellenberg, RR, 33, *49*
Schemann, M, 37, *52*
Scheurich, CJ, 298, *302*
Schidlow, DV, 246, *264*, 275, *283*
Schindlbeck, NE, 96, 99, *110*, *111*, 167, *177*, 183, *204*, 247, *263*, 272, *281*
Schleimer, RP, 21, 24, *43*
Schmidt, A, 20, *41*, 95, *109*, 143, 158, *173*
Schmidt, C, 77, *87*, 274, *282*
Schmidt, EV, 307, 309, *319*
Schmidt, RF, 32, *48*
Schmitt, M, 260, *267*
Schnatz, PF, 63, *68*, 90, 94, 99, *107*, 170, 171, 172, *178*, 216, *235*
Schnell, TG, 20, 24, 40, *44*, 56, *67*, 125, 126, 128, 129, 131, 134, *137*, *138*, 160, 163, 168, 169, 170, *175*, *176*, 180, 196, 197, 198, 199, 200, *203*, *207*, 211, 214, *234*, 247, *263*
Schoeb, TR, 26, *46*
Schroeder, JT, 24, *44*
Schroeder, PL, 98, *111*, 286, 291, 292, *300*, *301*, 316, *322*
Schuck, TJ, 73, *87*

Schultz, E, 187, *205*
Schultz, HD, 26, 34, *45*
Schwartz, DJ, 24, *44*
Schwartz, J, 95, *109*, 152, 153, 154, 155, 158, 160, *175*
Schwartz, LB, 21, 22, 23, *42, 43*
Schwartz, S, 182, *204*
Schwiebert, LM, 21, 24, *43*
Scott, RB, 257, *267*, 275, *283*
Searl, JP, 81, *88*
Sears, MR, 19, 21, *40, 43*
Sedgwick, JB, 21, *43*
Seheinmann, P, 247, 248, *265*
Seibert, J, 244, *263*
Seidel, UJ, 24, *44*, 125, 126, 128, 129, *137*, 163, 168, 170, *176*
Seidel, WJ, 180, *203*
Seilheimer, DK, 275, *283*
Sekizuka, E, 33, *50*
Sellner, JC, 142, 148, 157, 158, *173*, 273, *281*
Sembenini, C, 94, 95, *109*
Sepulveda, R, 20, 24, *41*, 125, 126, *137*, 170, 171, 172, *178*, 186, 188, 196, 197, *205*, 260, *267*, 279, *284*
Serizawa, H, 33, *50*
Serlovsky, R, 24, *44*, 125, 126, 129, 131, 134, *137, 138*, 160, 169, 170, *175*, 180, *203*, 211, 214, *234*
Serra-Battles, J, 272, 274, *280*
Shafer, SG, 294, *301*
Shah, B, 272, *281*
Shaker, R, 69, 70, 72, *86*, 93, 100, 102, *108, 111*, 156, *175*, 240, *261*, 304, 308, 309, 310, 312, 314, *319, 320, 321*
Shalaby, T, 270, *280*
Shandling, B, 276, *284*
Shannon, WA, 37, *51*
Shapiro, GG, 129, 130, *138*, 247, *263*
Shatz, A, 77, *87*
Shaw, DW, 308, *320*
Shaw, GY, 81, *88*
Sheahan, GG, 105, *113*
Shearman, DJC, 104, *112*, 214, *234*

Shelhamer, JH, 161, *176*
Sheller, JR, 33, *49*
Shepherd, P, 273, *281*
Shepherd, RW, 272, *280*
Shepro, D, 24, *44, 45*
Sherloosky, R, 247, *263*
Shimizu, T, 39, *53*
Shimizu, Y, 22, 23, *42*
Shimosegawa, T, 37, *52*
Shinoda, M, 318, *322*
Shiozaki, H, 33, *50*
Shirasaki, H, 31, *48*
Shirato, K, 23, 31, *42*
Shoenut, JP, 162, *176*
Shore, SA, 31, *48*
Shou-Hua, L, 285, *300*
Siegel, SC, 24, *44*, 90, 92, 99, *108*, 165, *177*, 244, 247, *263*, 274, *281, 282*
Sienra-Monge, JJ, 104, *112*
Sigmund, CJ, 103, *112*
Silver, PB, 33, *49*
Silverberg, M, 272, *281*
Silverman, M, 33, *50*
Silverman, W, 247, 248, 249, *263*
Simonneau, G, 20, 33, *41*, 95, *109*, 150, 151, 158, *174*, 248, *265*
Simonsson, B, 33, *48*
Simony-Lafontaine, J, 20, 21, *42*
Simpson, WG, 20, *41*, 182, *204*, 285, *300*
Simula, ME, 308, *320*
Sinclair, J, 103, *112*, 183, 184, *204, 205*
Sinclair, JW, 56, *67*, 96, *110*
Sindel, B, 275, 279, *283, 284*
Singh, V, 163, *176*
Siu, Z, 308, 309, *320*
Skinner, DB, 105, *113*, 125, 126, *137*, 161, 162, 170, 171, *175, 176, 178*, 197, *207*, 217, 224, 228, 230, 232, *235*, 291, *301*
Skloot, G, 38, *53*
Sloan, S, 65, *68*, 161, *176*
Smart, SJ, 25, 38, 39, *45*
Smirnov, VE, 307, 309, *319*
Smith, BGN, 285, *300*

Smith, DL, 20, 21, 23, *42*
Smith, H, 275, *284*
Smith, LF, 56, 60, *67*
Smith, LJ, 161, *176*
Smith, N, 273, *281*
Smith, NJ, 95, *109*, 140, 142, 148, 157, *173*
Smith, R, 274, *282*
Smith, S, 279, *284*
Smyrnios, NA, 89, 90, 92, 97, 98, 99, 103, *107*, 304, 310, *318*, *320*
Snel, P, 192, *206*
Snider, RM, 28, *46*
Soergel, KH, 308, *320*
Sognnaes, RF, 289, *301*
Solcia, E, 104, *112*
Soll, AH, 73, *87*
Solway, J, 28, *46*
Sondheimer, JM, 244, *263*, 270, *279*
Sonnenberg, A, 316, *322*
Sontag, SJ, 20, 24, *40*, *44*, 56, 60, 63, *67*, *68*, 81, *88*, 123, 124, 125, 126, 128, 129, 131, 134, *137*, *138*, 150, 160, 163, 168, 169, 170, *174*, *175*, *176*, 180, 189, 192, 196, 197, 198, 199, 200, *203*, *206*, *207*, 211, 214, 217, *234*, *235*, 247, 250, *263*, *265*
Sorvari, R, 289, *301*
Spannhake, EW, 30, *48*
Spaulding, HS, 95, *109*, 140, 142, 148, 157, 158, 170, 172, *173*, *177*, 192, 193, 194, *206*, 273, *281*
Spechler, SJ, 62, *68*, 105, *113*, 229, *236*
Spedding, C, 298, *302*, 312, *321*
Spier, S, 95, 105, *110*, 119, *136*, 247, 249, *263*
Spitzer, AR, 95, *109*, 152, 153, 154, 155, 158, 160, *175*, 274, *282*
Sprigg, A, 275, *283*
Springall, DR, 31, 37, *48*, *51*, *52*
Spurling, TJ, 56, 57, 60, 64, *67*
St Vil, D, 129, 130, *138*
Staiano, A, 270, *280*
Stamler, JS, 37, 39, *51*
Stanciu, C, 103, *112*, 184, *205*

Stealman, CR, 253, *266*
Steens, RD, 162, *176*
Stein, MR, 20, *41*, 92, 93, *108*, 131, *138*, 142, 148, 155, 157, 158, 165, 166, 167, *173*, *175*, *177*, 247, 248, 254, *263*, *265*, *266*, 273, 274, *281*, *282*
Stellato, C, 21, 24, *43*
Stephens, CA, 276, *284*
Sterling, C, 274, *283*
Stocker, N, 170, 172, *177*, 192, 193, 194, *206*
Stoddard, CJ, 214, *234*
Stolar, CJ, 276, *284*
Storz, C, 24, *44*
Stow, RB, 26, *46*
Stringer, D, 275, *283*
Strobel, CF, 244, 253, *263*, *266*
Strobel, CT, 90, 92, 99, *108*
Stulbarg, M, 90, *107*
Sudduth, RH, 170, 172, *177*, 192, 193, 194, *206*
Sudo, E, 24, *45*
Suematsu, M, 33, *50*
Sugarbaker, D, 37, 39, *51*
Sui, Z, 309, 310, *320*
Suko, T, 318, *322*
Sullivan, CE, 31, *48*
Sunshine, S, 308, 310, *319*
Surpas, P, 105, *113*, 125, 126, *137*
Suter, P, 289, *301*
Sutphen, JL, 271, *280*
Suzuki, E, 90, 93, *108*
Svedberg, LE, 192, *206*
Szefler, SJ, 180, *203*
Szentivanyi, A, 25, *45*
Szolcsanyi, J, 26, 38, *45*

T

Taborda-Barata, L, 24, *44*
Tadjkarimi, S, 37, *51*
Takahashi, T, 38, *53*
Takeyama, M, 318, *322*

Takishima, T, 38, *52*, *53*
Talbot, A, 318, *322*
Talerico, SD, 26, *46*
Talley, NJ, 56, *67*, 180, 197, *203*, 304, *319*
Tallis, Rc, 310, *321*
Taminiau, JA, 253, *266*
Tamplin, B, 248, *265*
Tan, WC, 144, 158, *174*, 248, *265*
Tardif, C, 196, 198, *207*
Tardiff, C, 20, *40*
Tashiro, H, 33, *50*
Tatar, M, 91, *108*
Tatemoto, K, 37, *51*
Taussig, LM, 240, *262*
Taylor, LA, 258, *267*
Teague, WG, 26, *45*
Teare, JP, 298, *302*, 312, *321*
Teichtahl, H, 152, *174*, 192, 194, 196, *206*
Temple, JG, 24, *44*
ten Velde, GPM, 144, 158, *174*, 248, *265*
Tepper, JS, 26, *46*
Termini, R, 105, *113*, 185, *205*
Thach, BT, 274, *282*
Theodors, A, 239, *261*, 291, 292, *301*
Thivolle, P, 90, *107*
Thomas, D, 275, *283*
Thomas, LE, 70, 78, *85*
Thomas, M, 275, *284*
Thomas, P, 155, *175*
Thomas, PE, 241, 242, 243, *262*
Thomas, VE, 103, *112*
Thompson, DG, 310, *321*
Thompson, JL, 89, *107*
Thompson, JLP, 308, 310, *319*
Thompson, RPH, 298, *302*, 312, *321*
Thompson, SWN, 32, *48*
Thomson, AH, 247, 248, 249, *263*
Thomson, HG, 90, *108*
Thomson, RJ, 33, *49*
Thorpe, J, 56, 60, *67*
Thurston, G, 26, *46*
Tibbling, L, 95, *109*, 129, 130, *138*, 143, 144, 148, 157, 158, 162, 165, 166, 170, 171, 172, *173*, *174*, *176*, *177*, *178*, 184, 186, 187, 188, *205*, 247, 248, 256, 258, *263*, *265*, *267*
Tileson, W, 69, *87*
Tinsdale, RS, 122, *137*
Toews, GB, 21, 22, *43*
Togias, A, 30, 38, *47*, *53*
Tokiwa, Y, 248, *265*
Tolia, V, 257, *267*
Tomaki, M, 23, 31, *42*
Tombelaine, R, 20, *40*, 196, 198, *207*
Tomita, T, 37, *51*
Tomori, Z, 92, *108*, 152, *174*
Toohill, R, 69, 72, 81, 82, 83, *86*, 100, 102, *111*, 240, *261*, 304, *319*
Tooley, WH, 240, 244, 245, 246, *262*, 275, *283*
Torres, A, 272, 274, *280*
Toscano, MS, 291, *301*
Toskala, J, 239, *261*, 286, 289, 291, *300*
Touyz, SW, 286, *300*
Tovar, JA, 105, *113*
Towbin, R, 279, *284*
Towner, TG, 131, *138*, 165, 166, *177*, 247, *263*, 274, *282*
Tracy, JF, 308, *320*
Tran, JA, 156, 157, 158, *175*, 215, 216, *234*, *235*, 316, *322*
Treem, WR, 255, *266*, 272, *281*
Tremblay, J, 37, 38, *51*
Tribble, CG, 26, *45*
Trifan, A, 309, 310, *320*
Triglia, JM, 70, 80, *86*
Trudeau, WL, 165, 167, *177*
Tseng, P, 286, *300*
Tsicopoulos, A, 21, *43*
Tsuchiya, M, 33, *50*
Tsujiura, M, 33, *49*
Tsukiji, J, 33, *49*
Tucci, F, 189, *206*
Tucci, J, 257, *267*
Tuchman, DN, 95, 105, *109*, *110*, 152, 153, 154, 155, 158, 160, *175*, 274, *282*
Tuisku, T, 298, *301*
Tunnell, W, 274, *283*

Turnage, RH, 259, *267*, 279, *284*
Turner, CR, 26, 33, *46*, *49*
Turner, CW, 122, *137*
Twentyman, OP, 20, 21, *41*
Tytgat, GN, 104, *112*, 192, 194, *206*, 257, *267*

U

Uejima, Y, 24, *45*
Ueki, IF, 97, *110*
Ulman, I, 279, *284*
Umeno, E, 28, 31, *46*, *47*
Umetsu, DT, 21, *44*
Undem, BJ, 20, 21, 22, 23, 28, 29, 30, 31, 32, 33, 34, 35, 37, 38, 39, *42*, *43*, *46*, *47*, *48*, *49*, *50*, *53*, *54*
Undem, FJ, 30, *48*
Underwood, DC, 38, *53*
Underwood, M, 124, *137*, 160, 169, 170, *175*, 180, *203*, 285, *300*
Unge, P, 192, *206*
Uray, E, 255, *266*
Urbain, D, 260, *267*
Urban, L, 28, 32, *47*, *48*
Urschel, HC, 117, *136*
Utell, MJ, 90, 103, *107*

V

Vadas, MA, 19, 23, *40*
Vaezi, MF, 98, 100, 101, *111*, 286, 291, 292, *300*, *301*, 304, 316, *319*, *322*
Vakil, N, 106, *113*
Valeri, CR, 24, *44*, *45*
Van de Rijn, M, 21, *43*
Van Drunen, M, 20, *40*, 196, 198, *207*
Vandenplas, Y, 105, *113*, 188, *205*, 270, *280*
Vandevenne, A, 93, 97, 98, *109*, 125, 126, *137*, 142, 148, 157, 158, *173*, 180, *203*
Vantini, I, 94, 95, *109*
Vantrappen, G, 98, 99, 101, *110*, *111*

Varkey, B, 156, *175*
Varry, M, 95, 105, *110*
Velvisi, MG, 30, 34, *48*
Venge, P, 20, 21, *41*
Venlloch, E, 180, 197, *203*
Venter, JC, 161, *176*
Venugopalan, CS, 37, 38, *51*
Verlinden, M, 105, *113*
Viala, P, 240, *261*
Vierucci, A, 189, *206*, 257, *267*
Vignal, J, 20, 24, *41*, 170, 171, 172, 173, *178*, 196, 198, *207*
Vigneri, S, 105, *113*, 185, *205*
Viljakka, M, 229, *236*
Vingerling, P, 292, *301*
Vinocur, CD, 275, *283*
Virchow, JC, 24, *44*
Viroslav, J, 97, *110*, 307, 309, *319*
Vitale, GC, 78, *88*, 183, *204*
Voderholzer, WA, 99, *111*
von Rosenstein, NR, 116, *136*
Voorhees, RJ, 119, *136*
Vos, M, 211, 228, *234*
Voyles, JB, 275, *283*

W

Wagner, JI, 103, *112*
Wagner, JL, 183, *204*
Wagner, ML, 275, *283*
Wagner, PH, 93, *109*
Waki, EY, 240, *262*
Walker, B, 31, *48*
Walker, C, 24, *44*
Walker, LH, 147, 148, 150, 162, 169, *174*
Wallwork, J, 26, *45*
Walner, DL, 243, *262*
Walshaw, MJ, 216, *235*
Wanner, J, 20, *40*, 196, 198, *207*
Ward, JK, 37, *51*
Ward, PH, 70, 78, *86*, 310, *320*
Waring, JP, 168, *177*, 183, *204*, 274, *282*, 312, *321*
Washburn, LK, 93, *109*

Wastwood, TF, 183, *204*
Watanabe, N, 318, *322*
Waterfall, WE, 95, 96, 105, *110*
Watson, J, 33, *49*
Watson, N, 28, 31, 39, *47*
Weaver, AL, 304, *319*
Weaver, EM, 315, *321*
Weber, E, 37, *52*
Weber, R, 274, *282*, 317, *322*
Weber, RW, 131, *138*, 165, 166, *177*, 247, *263*
Webster, T, 162, *176*
Wee, Ta, 306, *319*
Weihe, E, 37, *52*
Weinbech, M, 168, *177*
Weinberg, H, 306, *319*
Weinberger, M, 247, *265*
Weiner, GJ, 56, 66, *67*, *68*, 96, *110*, 156, *175*
Weiner, T, 258, *267*
Weinreich, D, 32, 33, 38, 39, *48*, *49*, *53*, *54*
Weinstock, JV, 23, *42*
Weintraub, A, 93, *109*
Weintraub, WH, 275, *283*
Weir, T, 31, *48*
Weiss, KB, 246, *263*
Welbourn, R, 24, *44*, *45*
Welch, M, 274, *282*
Welch, RW, 252, *266*
Wells, GA, 162, *176*
Werlin, SL, 99, *111*, 244, *263*, 270, *280*
Wernly, JA, 161, *175*
Wesley, JR, 244, 259, *263*, *267*, 276, *284*
Wesseling, G, 144, 158, *174*
Wessling, G, 248, *265*
Westra, SJ, 253, *266*
Wetmore, RF, 77, *87*
Wetscher, G, 223, 229, *235*
Wheatley, MJ, 259, *267*, 276, *284*
White, SJ, 244, *263*
Whitehead, MW, 298, *302*, 312, *321*
Whittington, PF, 98, *111*, 241, *262*, 272, 275, *280*, *283*

Widdicombe, JG, 89, 92, *106*, *108*, 140, 152, 160, *173*, *174*
Wiebecke, B, 99, *111*
Wiener, CJ, 69, 70, 72, 84, *85*
Wiener, GJ, 69, 70, 71, 72, 80, *87*, 98, 99, *111*
Wilcox, CM, 83, *88*
Wilde, MI, 81, *88*
Wilder, B, 318, *322*
Wilkinson, SP, 104, *112*, 192, 193, 194, *206*
Williams, H, 286, *300*
Williams, JC, 26, *46*
Williams, WN, 306, *319*
Willing, J, 270, *280*
Wills-Karp, M, 38, *53*
Wilson, JW, 20, 21, 31, *41*, *48*
Wilson, NM, 33, *50*, 247, 248, 249, *263*
Wilson, RS, 186, 188, *205*, 242, *262*
Wilson, RSE, 125, 126, *137*
Winkelstein, A, 69, 71, *87*
Winter, CS, 62, *68*
Winters, C, 56, 57, 60, 64, *67*
Wohl, MEBG, 246, *263*
Wolcott, RB, 289, *301*
Wolfe, B, 253, 259, *266*, *267*
Wolfe, MM, 73, *87*
Wolgtens, JHM, 292, *301*
Wong, L, 275, *284*
Woo, P, 70, 79, *86*
Wood, JD, 38, *53*
Wood, RD, 289, *301*
Woodson, G, 310, *320*
Woolcock, AJ, 19, 21, 31, *40*, *43*, *48*, 314, *321*
Working Group of the European Society of Gastroenterology and Nutrition, 252, *266*
Wouters, EFM, 144, 158, *174*, 248, *265*
Wrannge, B, 143, 148, 157, *173*, 184, *205*
Wren, J, 272, *280*
Wright, RA, 20, *41*, 143, 145, 148, 157, 158, *173*
Wu, WC, 56, 59, *67*, 69, 70, 71, 72, 80,

84, *85*, *87*, 96, 98, 99, 103, *110*, *111*, *112*, 156, *175*, 183, *204*, 309, *320*
Wynne, JW, 24, *44*, 216, 228, *235*

X

Xhonga, FA, 289, *301*

Y

Yacoub, MH, 37, *51*
Yafuso, N, 38, *52*
Yamamoto, DT, 103, *112*, 183, *204*
Yamasaki, M, 39, *53*
Yamate, M, 129, 130, *138*
Yamauchi, H, 23, 31, *42*
Yamawaki, I, 28, *46*
Yanaihara, N, 37, *52*
Yarkony, KA, 39, *54*
Yazbeck, S, 224, 228, 230, *235*
Yellon, RF, 318, *322*
Yeomans, ND, 104, *112*, 152, *174*, 192, 194, 196, *206*
Ying, S, 20, 21, 24, *42*, *43*, *44*

Yip, P, 37, 38, *51*
Yoshioka, K, 26, 30, *45*
Young, IG, 23, *43*
Young, JL, 81, *88*
Yu, XY, 30, *48*

Z

Zaeri, W, 246, *263*
Zagar, D, 308, 310, *319*
Zannoli, R, 254, *266*
Zawacki, JK, 20, *41*, 90, 92, 93, 94, 95, 96, 97, 98, 99, 100, 101, 102, 103, *107*, *108*
Zboralske, FF, 308, *320*
Zfass, A, 274, *282*
Zhou, D, 31, *48*
Zhu, H, 311, 313, *321*
Zhu, W, 37, *52*
Zillessen, E, 255, *266*
Zinsmeister, AR, 56, *67*, 180, 197, *203*, 304, *319*
Zorowitz, RD, 310, *321*
Zuccali, V, 94, 95, *109*
Zwi, S, 162, *176*

SUBJECT INDEX

A

Acid,
  aspiration, 135
    see also Aspiration
  basal output, 311
  citric, 28
  contact time, 72, 160 (see also pH monitoring)
  hydrochloric, 29, 285, 289
  hypersecretion, 197
  laryngeal, 248
  pepsin, 73
  suppression, 64, 66, 67, 72, 170, 297
  tracheal, 152–154, 160
Albuterol (see Pharmaceuticals)
Alginic acid (see Pharmaceuticals)
Alpha-adrenergic agonists (see Pharmaceuticals)
Aminophylline (see Pharmaceuticals)
Animal model, 21, 24–26, 28, 33–35, 37–39, 73, 74, 77, 91, 95, 97, 140, 152, 241, 243
  acid-pepsin, 73, 74, 241
Angiotensin-converting enzyme inhibitors (see Pharmaceuticals)
Anorexia nervosa, 285, 286
Anticholinergic agents (see Pharmaceuticals)
Aspiration, 197, 215, 216, 234, 244, 273, 276, 305, 316
  acid, 135 (see also Acid)
  antegrade, 309, 310
  gastric, 20, 24, 28, 33
  gross, 93
  macrophage, lipid laden, 93, 154, 155, 276
  microaspiration, 93, 139, 140, 145, 148, 152, 155–158, 160, 246, 273
  nasopharyngeal, 307
  nocturnal, 93
  pneumonia, 56, 57, 215, 244, 276, 306–308, 310
  retrograde, 93, 309
  stroke, 307, 308, 310
  tracheal, 157, 216 (see also Acid)
Asthma,
  acute attack, 31, 162
  adult, 60, 118, 119, 129, 130, 305
  airway hyperresponsiveness, 21, 32–34, 36, 38, 135, 144, 150, 152, 158, 160, 162, 180, 187, 217, 246, 248–250

353

[Asthma]
  airway responses, 35, 39, 273
  atopic, 21, 24, 33, 39
  bronchoconstriction (spasm), 20, 28–30, 32, 33, 36, 148, 248, 273
  childhood (*see* Children and adolescents)
  cough variant, 243
  nocturnal, 172, 248
  prevalence of association with GERD (*see* Prevalence)
  severe, 246, 305
  stimulus (*see* Stimulus, for asthma)
  symptom scores, 194, 195
Atropine (*see* Pharmaceuticals)
Attapulgite (*see* Pharmaceuticals)
Autonomic function testing, 147

B

Barrett's esophagus, 56, 57, 60–62, 67, 81, 125, 170, 197, 211, 212, 214, 259, 260, 311
Benzocaine (*see* Pharmaceuticals)
Bernstein Acid-Perfusion Test, 94, 95, 99, 142, 144–148, 249, 253, 276
Beta-adrenergic agonists (*see* Pharmaceuticals)
Benzocaine (*see* Pharmaceuticals)
Benzodiazepams (*see* Pharmaceuticals)
Bethanecol (*see* Pharmaceuticals)
Bile salts, 211–213
  bilirubin, esophageal, 211
Bronchial,
  airway, infantile, 271
  biopsy, 2, 21, 31, 93
  bronchitis, 57, 91, 244, 245
  lavage, 20, 21
Bronchiectasis, 91, 215, 234, 244, 245
Bronchiolitis obliterans, 244, 246
Bronchodilators (*see* Pharmaceuticals)
Bronchopulmonary dysplasia, 244, 269, 272
Bulimia, 285–287, 296

C

Calcium channel blockers (*see* Pharmaceuticals)
Capsaicin (*see* Pharmaceuticals)
Central nervous system,
  brainstem nuclei, 34, 92
    nucleus ambiguus, 92, 140
    nucleus retroambiguus, 92
    nucleus of the salivary tract, 140
    nucleus of the vagal nerve, dorsal, 161
  developmental delay, 244
  hindbrain, fish, 4
  injury, neurologic, 244
  level of consciousness, depressed, 244
  medulla, ventrolateral, 140, 144
  stroke, 307, 308, 310
    aspiration pneumonia (*see* Aspiration)
    dysphasia (*see* Gastroesophageal reflux disease)
    occult, 310
Children and adolescents, 237–268
  asthma, 60, 118, 119, 129–130, 237
  croup, 239, 240
  infants, 269–284
    GERD, 272–279
    nasal breathing, 271
    physiology, 269–272
    premature, 272
    therapy, 277–279
Cimetidine (*see* Pharmaceuticals)
Cisapride (*see* Pharmaceuticals)
Congenital anomalies,
  atresia, esophageal, 244, 269
  atresia, tracheal, 15
  diverticulum, of trachea, 15
  eventration of the diaphragm, 16
  fistula, tracheoesophageal, 15, 16
  hernia, diaphragmatic, 16, 269
  stenosis, tracheal, 15
  tracheal lobe, 16
  web, laryngeal, 15

Corticosteroids (*see* Pharmaceuticals)
Cough, chronic, 56, 58, 61, 63, 64, 70, 72, 74–76, 89–113, 189, 214, 239, 243, 305, 311
  asthma (*see* Asthma)
  awake, 97
  bronchiectasis (*see* Bronchiectasis)
  bronchitis (*see* Bronchial)
  gastroesophageal reflux (*see* Gastroesophageal reflux)
  multiple, 91, 92
  postnasal drip (*see* Allergic rhinitis)
  duration, 97
  nocturnal, 92
  relationship to reflux, temporal, 96
  sputum, 97
  threshold, 94
  upright, 97
Cystic fibrosis, 79, 269
Cytochrome p450 (*see* Pharmaceuticals)

D

Dental erosions, 56, 98, 285–302
  acid-induced, 285 (*see also* Acid)
    dietary, 288
    industrial, 288
  classification, 287, 288, 290
  diagnosis, differential, 292–296
  enamel, 291
  etiology, 288, 289
    reflux, gastric acid (*see* Acid)
    vomiting, chronic, 289
  hypersensitivity, dentinal, 286, 287
  prevention, 297–298
    mouth guard, 298
  treatment, 298, 299
    dental restoration, 299
Diagnostic evaluation of GERD, 55–88, 121–125, 250, 315
  barium studies, 57–60, 66, 74, 79–81, 92, 93, 98, 252, 308
    bolus, solid, 60
    hiatal hernia (*see* Hiatal hernia)

[Diagnostic evaluation of GERD]
    rings, 59, 81
    webs, 59
  Bernstein test (*see* Bernstein acid-perfusion test)
  biopsy, esophageal, 58, 61, 62, 74, 92, 253, 277, 291, 316
  bronchoscopy, 275, 276
  endoscopy, 57, 58, 61, 62, 66, 67, 69, 72–81, 92, 93, 99, 120, 201, 312
  history, 250
  laryngoscopy, 61, 66, 70–81, 251, 275, 305, 310, 317
  manometry, esophageal, 57, 58, 62, 65, 73, 74, 78, 79, 92, 95, 96, 139, 160–169, 171, 201, 217–222, 232–234, 252, 308, 309
    preoperative, 65, 217–222, 232–234
    sphincter, lower (LES), 57, 62, 65, 73, 78, 82, 139, 160, 161, 163, 165–169, 183, 187, 197, 209, 211–213, 247, 270, 309
    sphincter upper (UES), 73, 74, 79, 238, 270, 308, 309
  methylene blue, 276
  nasopharyngoscopy (*see* rhinopharyngoscopy)
  pH monitoring, 57, 58, 61–64, 66, 67, 71, 92, 97, 99, 100, 145–160, 166, 167, 181, 186–188, 192, 196, 201, 215, 217, 218, 240, 243, 249, 252, 253, 257, 275, 276, 304, 311, 316, 317
    ambulatory, 62, 99
    distal, 63, 64, 172
    dual, 64, 66, 80, 81, 84, 94, 99, 145–156, 171, 172, 216, 233, 252, 291, 304, 316, 317
    hypopharyngeal, 63, 80, 81
    intragastric, 63
    nasopharyngeal, 241
    proximal, 63, 64, 156, 172, 173, 196, 216

[Diagnostic evaluation of GERD]
   tracheal, 154–157 (*see also* Aspiration)
   values, normal, 63
   rhinopharyngoscopy, 251, 305
   scintigraphy, 93, 154, 155, 251, 252, 275, 316
   Tuttle test, 253
   ultrasonography, 253, 254
   x-ray, chest, 90
Diaphragm, 10–12
   central tendon, 12
   crural, 139, 163–165
   eventration (*see* Congenital anomalies)
   hernia (*see* Congenital anomalies)
Diazepam (*see* Pharmaceuticals)
Diphenhydramine (*see* Pharmaceuticals)
Domperidone (*see* Pharmaceuticals)
Dopamine (*see* Pharmaceuticals)
Dyclonine (*see* Pharmaceuticals)

E

Epiglottis, 5–7
Epinepherine (*see* Pharmaceuticals)
Esophageal acid clearance, 58, 73, 74, 79, 80, 95, 96, 147, 189, 210, 214
   factors,
      activity, motor, 210
      anchoring of distal esophagus, 210
      gravity, 210
      salivation, 210 (*see also* Saliva)
   ineffective, 210
Esophagus, 4, 7, 13, 14
   distention, 95, 142
   epithelial glands, 14
   esophagitis, 57, 60, 61, 72, 73, 93, 125, 148, 153, 170–172, 181, 185–189, 193, 194, 211–215, 248, 311, 316
   infantile, 270
   injury, progressive, 211
   length, 161, 197, 219

[Esophagus]
   malignancy, 57, 62, 81, 99, 214
   presbyesophagus, 308, 309
   short, 209, 220, 224, 238
   stricture, peptic, 56, 57, 59, 79, 81, 98, 197, 211, 214, 220, 260, 316
   ulceration, 57, 98, 125

F

Famotidine (*see* Pharmaceuticals)
Fenoterol (*see* Pharmaceuticals)
Fish, 2–4
   lung fish, 4, 7
   swim bladder, 3
Foregut,
   embryonic, 2, 13, 15

G

Ganglionic blocker (*see* Pharmaceuticals)
Gastroesophageal reflux disease (GERD), 25, 55, 90–92, 213, 309
   asthma, as a cause, 247, 248
   complications, 56
      bleeding, 56
      esophagitis, 57, 60, 61, 72, 73, 93
      stricture, 56, 57, 59, 79, 81
      ulceration, 57, 98, 125
   diagnosis (*see* Diagnostic evaluation of GERD)
   medical therapy, 179–207
   occult, 97, 181, 202, 215, 238, 304
   physical findings,
      erythema, pharyngeal, 251
      headcocking (*see* Sandifer's syndrome)
   reflux,
      acid (*see* Acid)
      alkaline, 95
      bipositional, 212, 213, 304
      daytime, 72, 73

[Gastroesophageal reflux disease (GERD)]
  duodenal, 211
  duration, 96
  frequency, 64
  gastroduodenal, 212
  laryngitis, 58, 59, 70, 74, 81, 84, 100, 215, 239, 240, 305, 310
  nasal, 269, 274
  nocturnal, 73, 80, 183
  number of episodes, 96
  pathologic, 73, 96, 311
  pharyngeal, 74, 238, 243, 270, 274, 285, 309
  physiologic, 73, 96, 237
  postprandial, 96
  provoked by treatment, 274
  response to therapy, 66
  supine, 64, 72–74, 80, 83, 212, 213, 304
  symptom score, 172
  trypsin, 95
  upright, 64, 72–74, 80, 83, 96, 212, 213, 304
  voluntary, 285
  risk factors, 211
  silent, 97, 181, 202, 215, 238, 304
  spectrum, 55–57
  symptoms, 56, 238
    anemia, 61, 260, 305
    apnea, infantile, 215, 269, 271, 272, 274, 275
    aspiration pneumonia (see Aspiration)
    asthma (see Asthma)
    belching, 251, 305
    bleeding, 61, 260
    bronchitis (see Bronchial)
    cervical pain, 305
    chest pain 56, 61, 63, 98, 214, 305
    choking, 72, 214
    cough, chronic (see Cough)
    crying, intractable in infant, 273
    drip, postnasal, 70
    dysparunia, 56
    dyspepsia, 56

[Gastroesophageal reflux disease (GERD)]
    dysphagia, 59, 61, 70, 75, 76, 79, 84, 160, 251, 308
    dysphonia, 70, 75, 76, 84
    erosion, dental (see Dental erosions)
    globus, 56, 70, 72, 74–76, 79, 84, 98, 239, 242
    heartburn, 55, 57–60, 74, 97, 117, 145, 179, 181, 187, 251, 260, 305
    hiccups, 36, 305
    hoarseness, 56, 57, 61, 72, 74, 98, 215, 239, 240, 305
    mouth burning, 286, 298
    mouth dry, 286
    mucous, excessive throat, 70
    night sweats, 56
    odynophagia, 61
    otalgia, 56, 241
    postural worsening, 117
    questionnaire, 304, 317
    regurgitation, 55–57, 97, 145, 160, 172, 173, 179, 181, 187, 196, 214, 305
    sore throat, 72, 79, 98, 242, 305
    stridor, 98, 240, 269, 272, 275
    taste, sour, 98
    teeth, sensitive (see Dental erosions)
    throat clearing, chronic, 70, 72, 75, 76, 84, 214, 239, 242
    tongue, sensitive, 286
    ulcers, oral, 56, 286, 298
    voice fatigue, 70
    waterbrash, 97, 251
    weight loss, 61
  Geriatric, 304–313
    anatomic, 306, 307
    lactose intolerance, 312
    reflex changes (see Reflex, geriatric changes)
    sicca syndrome, 312
    sensory changes, 306
      airways, upper, 306

[Geriatric]
   lip, 306
   pharynx, 306, 307
   proprioceptive, 306
   stereognostic, 306
   supraglottic, 306, 307
   temperature, 306
   tongue, 306
   two point, 306
Glottis, 5

H

hexamethonium (*see* Pharmaceuticals)
H$_2$-receptor antagonists (*see* Pharmaceuticals)
Hiatal hernia, 59, 98, 117, 125, 127–130, 161, 197, 210, 220, 253, 274, 311
   incidence, 163
   large, 65
   paraesophageal, 220
   sliding, 220
Histamine challenge (*see* Asthma, airway hyperresponsiveness)

I

Immunoglobulin E, 246
Inflammation, 19–54, 89, 180, 306, 315
   cells,
      basophils, 21–24
      endothelial, 33
      eosinophils, 20–23
      epithelial, 20, 22, 23, 26, 33
      hyperalgesia, 31, 32
      macrophages, 21, 22 (*see also* Aspiration)
      mast cells, 21, 22, 24, 33
      mononuclear, 20
      neutrophil, 24
   mediators (*see* Mediators of inflammation)
   mucosal edema, 20

[Inflammation]
   neurogenic, 24–54, 158, 160
   neuronal activation, 25
   proinflammatory neurotransmitters, 26
   pulmonary, 26
   skin, human, 30, 31
   upper airway, human, 30
   vasodilation, 20, 27
Ipatropium bromide (*see* Pharmaceuticals)
Isoproterenol (*see* Pharmaceuticals)

L

Lansoprazole (*see* Pharmaceuticals)
Laryngopharyngeal reflux, 69–88, 228, 248
   arytenoid fixation, 70, 76
   carcinoma, 70, 75, 76, 78, 83
   degeneration, polypoid, 70, 75–77
   dysplasia, 76
   edema, laryngeal, 70, 71
   esophagitis, differences, 69
   globus, 56, 70, 72, 74–76, 79, 84, 98, 239, 242
   hematoma, 76
   injury, endotracheal tube, 70
   laryngomalacia, 70, 239, 240, 271, 275
   laryngospasm, paroxysmal, 70, 75–77, 240, 241, 273
   leukoplakia, 70, 76, 78
   nodules, vocal, 70, 75, 76
   pachydermia, laryngitis, 70, 76
   pediatric, 80, 237–243
   Reinke's edema, 75–77
   stenosis, posterior glottic, 70, 239, 243
   stenosis, subglottic, 70, 71, 75, 76, 78, 83, 239, 242, 243
   ulcers and granulomas, contact, 70, 76, 77, 117, 239
   voice disorders (*see* Voice disorders)
Larynx, 2, 7, 315
   aryepiglottic folds, 7

[Larynx]
  arytenoid, 7–8
  cricoid, 8
  infantile, 271
  laryngotracheal bud, 8
  ventricles, 7
Lidocaine, viscous (*see* Pharmaceuticals)
Lifestyle,
  alcohol, 78, 183
  chocolate, 183
  drugs, 183
  food,
    fatty, 183
    infantile, 271
    volume, 238, 271
  infantile, 271–272, 277, 278
  modifications, 71, 81, 83, 103, 116, 171, 181–184, 200–201, 210, 214, 238, 254, 255, 314
  obesity, 183, 238
  sleep time, 238
  tobacco, 78, 89
Lignocaine (*see* Pharmaceuticals)
Lung,
  abscess, 244, 245
  alveolar pneumocyte, 10
  amphibian, 4
  avian, 4
  bronchi, 8
  development, 9–10
  granulomatous pneumonia, recurrent, 244, 245
  lobes, 5
    tracheal (*see* Congenital anomalies)
  mammalian, 4
  parenchyma, 4
  pleura, 9
  pulmonary artery, 12
  pulmonary fibrosis, 215, 234, 244, 246, 305, 313
  reptile, 4
  segments, 4
  surfactant, 10
Lymphocytes,
  CD, 4, 21

[Lymphocytes]
  murine Th, 21, 23
  Th 1, 21
  Th 2, 21
  T helper, 21

M

Mediators of inflammation,
  autocoids, 20–24, 33
  bradykinin, 22, 26–28, 33, 36, 37
  cysteinyl-leukotrienes, 22, 24
  cytokines, 21, 24, 33, 38
  endothelins, 22, 33, 36, 37
  histamine, 22, 24, 26
  IL-1, 22
  IL-2, 21
  IL-4, 21, 23, 24
  IL-5, 23
  IL-8, 23–25, 33, 36, 37
  IL-13, 21, 24
  interferon-gamma, 21
  major basic protein, 22
  MIP-1 alpha, 24
  neurokinin A, 26, 27, 30
  neuropeptides, 26
  RANTES, 23
  substance P, 26, 27, 30, 34, 37
  tachykinins, 22, 26, 30, 31, 36, 37, 39
  TNF-alpha, 24
Meperidine (*see* Pharmaceuticals)
Methylanthines (*see* Pharmaceuticals)
Metoclopramide (*see* Pharmaceuticals)
Morphine (*see* Pharmaceuticals)

N

Neurotransmitters, 32
  acetylcholine, 35, 36, 37, 39
  autonomic, 38
  calcitonin gene-related peptide (CGRP), 37

[Neurotransmitters]
  cytokines (*see* Mediators of inflammation)
  galanin, 37
  neuropeptide Y, 37
  NO, 36, 37
  noradrenaline, 35
  relaxant type, 36
  substance P (*see* Mediators of inflammation)
  tachykinins (*see* Mediators of inflammation)
  VIP, 36, 37, 38
Nizatidine (*see* Pharmaceuticals)

O

Office approach, 317, 318
Omeprazole (*see* Pharmaceuticals)
Oral manifestations of GERD, 285–302
  dental erosions (*see* Dental erosions)
  eating disorders, 285 (*see also* Anorexia nervosa; Bulimia)
  mucosal lesions, 286
  periodontal, 286
  salivary gland, 286, 287 (*see also* Saliva)
Otitis media, 237, 239, 241, 242

P

Pantoprazole (*see* Pharmaceuticals)
Peripheral nervous system, 22
  airway adrenergic, 25, 26
  airway afferents, 31–33
  airway ganglia, 35
  autonomic, 25, 38
  capsaicin, desensitization, 26, 36, 37
  cholinergic, 34–38, 161
  dysfunction, 161
  esophageal myenteric plexus, 34, 35
  ganglion neurons, 31
  myelinated fibers, 307

[Peripheral nervous system]
  nociceptive afferent, 27
  NANC, 13, 36, 37, 38 (nonadrenergic noncholinergic)
  parasympathetic, 13, 161
  parasympathetic, adrenergic, 34, 35
  parasympathetic cholinergic, 34, 35, 37–39
  parasympathetic ganglion, 28, 34, 36, 37, 39
  parasympathetic postganglionic, 38
  peripheral efferent, 36
  phrenic nerve, 10–12, 34
  recurrent laryngeal nerve, 12
  retrograde tracing studies, 34
  sympathetic, 12, 34, 35, 38
  tachykinin-containing fibers, 39
  vagus nerve, 2, 4, 8, 12–15, 36, 38, 140
    efferent, 36
    inferior laryngeal, 8
    superior laryngeal, 12, 77, 306, 307
  visceral afferent, 27
Pharmaceuticals,
  albuterol, 168
  alginic acid, 181–184, 256, 278, 314
  alpha-adrenergic agonists, 183
  aminophylline, 165
  angiotensin-converting enzyme inhibitors, 90
  anticholinergic agents, 169
  atropine, 143, 147, 148, 151, 152, 158
  attapulgite, 299
  benzocaine, 299
  benzodiazepams, 185
  beta-adrenergic agonists, 19, 161, 183, 184, 187, 247
  bethanecol, 187, 257
  bronchodilators, 131–134, 306 (*see also* beta-adrenergic agonists, aminophylline, methylxanthines, theophylline)
  calcium channel blockers, 183
  capsaicin, 26, 29, 30, 33, 95
  cimetidine, 170, 182, 185–189, 197,

[Pharmaceuticals]
　256 (*see also* H$_2$-receptor antogonists)
　cisapride, 104, 105, 187–190, 257, 278, 312–314, 318 (*see also* prokinetic agents)
　corticosteroids, 19–21, 168, 169, 180, 192, 193, 196, 317
　cost (*see* Therapeutic trial)
　cytochrome p450, 312
　diazepam, 183
　diphenhydramine, 299
　domperidone, 182, 187, 257
　dopamine, 183
　dyclonine, 299
　epinepherine, 167
　famotidine, 182, 185, 256, 278, 313 (*see also* H$_2$-receptor antagonists)
　femoterol, 168 (*see also* beta-adrenergic agonists, bronchodilators)
　ganglionic blocker, 38
　hexamethonium, 38
　H$_2$-receptor antagonists, 58, 61, 74, 80, 81, 83, 103–105, 181, 182, 185–189, 202, 256, 313
　ipatropium bromide, 33, 94, 192
　isoproterenol, 167
　lansoprazole, 66, 81, 182, 190, 192, 256, 257, 313, 314
　lidocaine, viscous, 299
　lignocaine, 94
　meperidine, 183
　methylxanthines, 247
　metoclopramide, 104, 187, 257, 278, 312
　morphine, 183
　nizatidine, 182, 185, 313
　omeprazole, 66, 81, 83, 84, 104, 105, 170–172, 256, 257, 278, 298, 312–314
　orabase, 299
　pantoprazole, 182
　phytoin, 185
　pilocarpine, 298
　prednisone, 168

[Pharmaceuticals]
　progesterone, 183
　prokinetic agents, 58, 61, 103–105, 181, 257, 277, 318
　prostaglandins, 183
　proton pump inhibitors, 58–61, 66, 74, 77, 78, 80–85, 104, 105, 190–197, 210, 214, 215, 256, 312, 317, 318
　ranitidine, 105, 171–182, 185–189, 192, 200, 256, 278, 313, 314
　sucralfate, 258, 278, 313, 314
　theophylline, 161, 165–169, 183, 196, 247, 305
　warfarin, 185
　zilactingel, 299
Pregnancy, 184, 185, 187, 314
Prevalence, 56–57, 69
　cough, 98, 316
　gastroesophageal reflux, 56, 316, 317
　in asthma, 115–138, 180, 237, 316, 317
　incidence, 121–122
　laryngopharyngeal (LPR), 69, 84, 316, 317
　pulmonary disease, 316–317
　tooth erosions, 289
Progesterone (*see* Pharmaceuticals)
Progressive systemic sclerosis, 93
Prokinetic agents (*see* Pharmaceuticals)
Prostaglandins (*see* Pharmaccuticals)
Proton pump inhibitors (*see* Pharmaceuticals)
Pulmonary function tests,
　airway resistance, 95, 142, 145–147, 153, 154, 158, 249
　capsaicin inhalation challenge, 95
　closing volume, 143
　compliance, dynamic, 153
　cough threshold, 95
　flow volume loop, 317
　FEV, 95, 181, 186–189, 193, 200
　FVC, 95, 143, 186
　histamine challenge (*see* Asthma, airway hyperresponsiveness)
　hyperventilation, isocapnic, 150

[Pulmonary function tests]
  impedance, 144
  inductance, 249
  methacholine challenge, 94, 95, 120, 150, 151, 158, 161, 162, 188
  oxygen saturation, 143
  peak expiratory flow, 144–147, 158, 181, 187–189, 195, 200, 202, 249
  pressure pleural, 153, 162, 169, 243, 247
  restrictive changes, 305
  slope of alveolar plateau, 143
  spirometry, 144–147

R

Ranitidine (*see* Pharmaceuticals)
Receptors,
  acid sensitive, 170
  afferent esophageal, 92
  cholinergic, prejunctional, 36
  cough, 92
    rapidly adapting irritant, 92
  muscarinic,
    M2, 36, 37, 39
    M3, 30
    receptor antagonist, 33
  NK1, 39
  NK1 antagonist, 30
  NK 3, 39
  tachykinin, 30, 31
    preprotachykinin gene, 33
    receptor antagonist, 33, 34
Reflex,
  autonomic, 32
  axon, 26–28, 31
    esophagus and trachea, 28
  bronchoconstriction, 20
  central, 27
  defensive, 26
  esophagobronchial cardiac, 143, 246
  esophagoglottal closure, 93, 307, 309

[Reflex]
  geriatric changes, 307, 308
  inappropriate, 32
  inflammation, 26
  involuntary cough, 92
  peripheral, 34
  parasympathetic, cholinergic, 33, 34, 143
  pharyngoglottal, 93, 310
  respiratory, 10
  tracheobronchial cough, 92
  tracheobronchial–esophageal, 92, 94, 95
  vagal, 84, 85, 92, 97, 139–141, 147, 152, 170, 173, 241, 246, 273
    centrally mediated, 34
Rhinitis,
  allergic seasonal, 33
  chronic, 239, 241
  postnasal drip, 90–92
  rhinopharyngitis, 241

S

Saliva,
  artificial, 298
  buffering capacity, 291, 298
  flow, 291, 292, 298
  gum, sugar free, 298
  mucin levels, 292
  salivary glands (*see* Oral manifestations)
  sicca syndrome, 312
  xerostomia, 79
Sandifer's syndrome, 251
Sinusitis, 239, 305
Sjogren's syndrome, 79
Sleep,
  apnea, 162
  nasal CPAP, 162
  peristalsis, esophageal, 183
  saliva, decrease, 183
  upper esophageal sphincter (UES)

Stimulus for asthma,
  acid exposure time, 28, 211 (*see also* Acid)
  allergen, 28
  bradykinin (*see* Mediators)
  heartburn, 28 (*see also* Gastroesophageal reflux disease)
  hyperpnea, 28
  meals, 305
  ozone, 39
  positional changes, 305
  saline, hypertoic, 28
  smoke, cigarette, 28
  viral infection, 39
Stomach (gastric), 15
  emptying, 187, 210
    delayed, 161, 197
  distention gastric, 161, 210
    compliance, 270
  pain, 305
  parietal cell, 190, 191
  receptors, 190, 191
  volume ratio, to esophagus, 270
Sucralfate (*see* Pharmaceuticals)
Sudden infant death syndrome, 77
Surgery, 27, 60, 65, 67, 78, 80, 103, 105, 106, 117, 182, 196–201, 209–236, 278, 279, 313
  algorithm, 217, 219, 221, 231
  angelchik prosthesis, 259
  Belsey fundoplication, 105, 220, 222, 224, 229–232, 259
  Borema anterior gastropexy, 259
  compared to medical therapy, 197–200, 223
  Collis gastroplasty, 224–226, 231, 232
  complications, 225–228, 258, 259
    chest pain, 226
    dysphagia, 225–227
    gas bloat syndrome, 226, 228
    gastroparesis, 226
    herniation of repair, 226
    recurrent reflux, 226–228, 259
    vagal nerve injury, 226
  crural closure, 228

[Surgery]
  esophageal lengthening precedure, 220, 222, 225
  fundoplication, 78, 80, 82, 83, 90, 171, 197–200, 223, 224, 233, 278, 279
    redo, 226
  gastric antrostomy, 259
  gastrojejunostomy, 278, 279
  Hill posterior gastropexy, 105, 170, 197–199, 225, 259
  indications, 217
    intractable symptoms, 259
  laparoscopic, 222–229, 258, 259, 279, 313, 318
  laryngeal, 84
  Nissen fundoplication, 65, 105, 106, 171, 198–200, 220, 222, 229–231, 258–260
  proper procedure, 219
  pyloroplasty, 259
  results, 232, 233
  risks, 197
  short esophagus (*see* Esophagus)
  Thal procedure, 259
  Toupet procedure, 65, 222, 224, 226
  tracheotomy, 82
  transthoracic, 220, 222, 231
  vagotomy, 27, 95, 140, 142, 153, 154, 158, 160
Swallowing, 308–310
  laryngopharyngeal sensory test, 308
  primary, 309
  reflex changes, 307, 308
  videoendoscopy, 308
  videofluoroscopy, 308, 310

T

Theophylline (*see* Pharmaceuticals)
Theraputic trial, 58, 59, 64, 66, 98, 102, 180, 275
  cost, 180, 254, 312, 313, 317
  maintenance, 180
Tongue (*see* Geriatric)

V

Vocal cord dysfunction syndrome, 317
Vocal cords, 4, 7
  false, 5, 7
Voice disorders, 69–104, 305, 310
  breaks, 70
  dysphonia, 70, 75, 76, 84
  fatigue, voice, 70

[Voice disorders]
  singer, 76
  speaker, 76
  symptoms (*see* Symptoms)

Z

Zilactingel (*see* Pharmaceuticals)

HC
815.7
.G384

RC   Gastroesophageal
815.7   reflux disease and
.G384   airway disease.
1999

$179.95   45351

_____
  __   DATE   _ _   _____

SOUTH UNIVERSITY
709 MALL BLVD.
SAVANNAH, GA 31406